PHYSIOLOGICAL AND PHARMACOLOGICAL ASPECTS OF THE RETICULO-RUMEN

CURRENT TOPICS IN VETERINARY MEDICINE AND ANIMAL SCIENCE

PHYSIOLOGICAL AND PHARMACOLOGICAL ASPECTS OF THE RETICULO-RUMEN

Edited by

L.A.A. Ooms and A.D. Degryse
*Department of Veterinary Pharmacology, Janssen Pharmaceutica,
Beerse, Belgium*

A.S.J.P.A.M. van Miert
*Department of Veterinary Pharmacology, Pharmacy and Toxicology,
Faculty of Veterinary Medicine, Utrecht University,
Utrecht, The Netherlands*

1987 **MARTINUS NIJHOFF PUBLISHERS**
a member of the KLUWER ACADEMIC PUBLISHERS GROUP
DORDRECHT / BOSTON / LANCASTER
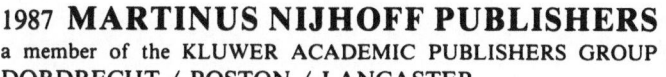

Distributors

for the United States and Canada: Kluwer Academic Publishers, P.O. Box 358, Accord Station, Hingham, MA 02018-0358, USA
for the UK and Ireland: Kluwer Academic Publishers, MTP Press Limited, Falcon House, Queen Square, Lancaster LA1 1RN, UK
for all other countries: Kluwer Academic Publishers Group, Distribution Center, P.O. Box 322, 3300 AH Dordrecht, The Netherlands

Library of Congress Cataloging in Publication Data

ISBN-13:978-94-010-7990-7   e-ISBN-13: 978-94-009-3319-4
DOI: 10.1007/978-94-009-3319-4

Copyright

PREFACE

The success of a scientific workshop depends on a delicate blend of many types of ingredients. Most important is to select a provocative topic which is at the forefront of a current investigative study. Coupled together with a relatively small but distinguished group of active research scientists known for their continued record of contributing significant findings, one has the firm foundation for an exciting and rewarding investment of time and effort. This was the setting for the first workshop organized by the European Association for Veterinary Pharmacology and Toxicology.

Ruminants have been domesticated for many centuries and have served mankind as a source of dairy products, meat, wool and power.

The ruminant stomach has long been - and still is - a major concern for physiologists, pathologists, clinicians and pharmacologists. This workshop was organized and convened in an attempt to strengthen the basic science of the ruminant stomach, as it applies to an economically important group of mammals. To achieve this, various topics were covered by specialists which ensured presentation of new data, followed by discussions.

In this book, reviews are presented on the different topics : motility (control and regulation, neurotransmitters and endogenous substances involved); flow of digesta (comparative aspects, role of content and metabolites); food intake; rumen metabolism (chemical manipulation, metabolism of xenobiotics and drugs); pharmacology of forestomach motility and, the reticulo-rumen as a pharmacokinetic compartment.

This book is dedicated to Dr. Paul Janssen, President and Director of Research of Janssen Pharmaceutica, on the occasion of his 60th birthday.

The editors would like to thank Dr. Robert Marsboom, Vice President and Head of the Veterinary Department of Janssen Pharmaceutica, for the facilities to organize the workshop.

The co-editors (L.O. and A.-D.D.) also wish to thank Mrs. C.W.P. Stigter-van Vliet from the Department of Veterinary Physiology (Utrecht) and Mr. J.M. Eijndhoven from the Department of Veterinary Pharmacology, Pharmacy and Toxicology (Utrecht) for technical assistance in preparing the manuscripts as well as Prof. Dr. A.S.J.P.A.M. van Miert for his encouragement and preparation of the book.

CONTENTS

LIST OF CONTRIBUTORS

J.A. BOGAN
Department of Veterinary
Pharmacology
University of Glasgow
Veterinary School
Bearsden Road, Bearsden
Glasgow GGI IQH
Scotland

S. BOUISSET
Docteur Vétérinaire
5 Route de Challans
85190 Aizenay
France

A.D. DEGRYSE
Department of Veterinary
Pharmacology
Janssen Pharmaceutica
B-2340 Beerse
Belgium

A. DE JONG
Institute for Chemotherapy
Bayer A.G.
P.O. Box 101709
5600 Wuppertal 1
Federal Republic of Germany

D.I. DEMEYER
Institute of Biotechnology
Free University of Brussels
Paardenstraat 65
B-1640 St.-Genesius Rode
Belgium

A.G. DESWYSEN
Nutritional Biochemistry Lab.
Department of Applied Animal Biology
Catholic University of Louvain-la-Neuve
Sciences 15-D2-tour Kellner
Place Croix du Sud, 3
B-1348 Louvain-la-Neuve
Belgium

R.N.B. KAY
Rowett Research Institute
Greenburn Road, Bucksburn
Aberdeen AB2 9SB
Scotland

P. KREDIET
Department of Veterinary Anatomy
and Embryology
Faculty of Sciences
University of Antwerp
Slachthuislaan 68
B-2000 Antwerp
Belgium

B.F. LEEK
Department of Veterinary Physiology
and Biochemistry
University College Dublin
Veterinary College, Ballsbridge
Dublin 4
Ireland

S.E. MARRINER
Department of Veterinary Pharma-
cology
University of Glasgow
Veterinary School
Bearsden Road, Bearsden
Glasgow GGI IQH
Scotland

L.A.A. OOMS
Department of Veterinary Pharma-
cology
Janssen Pharmaceutica
B-2340 Beerse
Belgium

TH. PEETERS
Gut Hormones Laboratory
Catholic University of Louvain
Louvain
Belgium

R.A. PRINS
Research Institute of Nature Management
P.O. Box 46
3956 ZR Leersum
The Netherlands

Y. RUCKEBUSCH
Department of Physiology and Pharmacology
National Veterinary School
23, Chemin des Capelles
31076 Toulouse Cédex
France

A.S.J.P.A.M. van MIERT
Department of Veterinary Pharmacology,
Pharmacy and Toxicology
Faculty of Veterinary Medicine
University of Utrecht
P.O. Box 80 176
3508 TD Utrecht
The Netherlands

L. van NASSAUW
Department of Veterinary Anatomy and
Embryology
Faculty of Sciences
University of Antwerp
Slachthuislaan 68
B-2000 Antwerp
Belgium

C.J. van NEVEL
Research Centre for Food, Animal Nutrition
and Meat Technology
Faculty of Sciences
University of Ghent
Proefhoevestraat 10
B-9230 Melle
Belgium

A. VERHOFSTAD
Department of Anatomy and Embryology
Catholic University of Nijmegen
Nijmegen
The Netherlands

A. WEYNS
Department of Veterinary Anatomy
and Embryology
Faculty of Science
University of Antwerp
Slachthuislaan 68
B-2000 Antwerp
Belgium

1. THE CONTROL OF THE MOTILITY OF THE RETICULO-RUMEN

B.F. LEEK

I. INTRODUCTION

In the absence of vagal and splanchnic nerves, the smooth muscle of the reticulo-ruminal walls undergoes low amplitude contractions ("intrinsic contractions"). The coordinated sequences of powerful contractions ("extrinsic contractions") constituting the 'primary' and 'secondary' cycle motility are dependent on bursts of efferent (motor) nerve impulses travelling in the vagal nerves. These bursts originate from the gastric centres located in the medulla oblongata of the hind-brain. The gastric centres do not appear to have a spontaneous rhythmicity but require an overall excitatory drive to be provided by inputs coming from other (mainly higher) parts of the central nervous system and from the periphery (mainly from the alimentary tract itself).

Situations which have general effects on the central nervous system or

which alter conditions within the gut, particularly within the reticulo-
-rumen, will therefore affect motility.

II. THE INTRINSIC CONTRACTIONS OF THE RETICULO-RUMEN

In the gut generally, two separate mechanisms exist for the production
of intrinsic contractions. First, there are "intrinsic myogenic
contractions" attributable to the rhythmic contractility of the muscle
cells themselves and, secondly, there are "intrinsic neurogenic
contractions" which require the involvement of the neurones of the
myenteric plexus. Evidence exists for both kinds of intrinsic contractions
in the reticulo-rumen.

Leek (1,2) recorded reticulo-ruminal tension receptor activity by a
'single afferent vagel fibre' technique in halothane-anaesthetised sheep.
In most cases, during the interval between extrinsic contractions, the
tension receptors exhibited phasic discharges of spikes (action
potentials) at a rate of about 10 cycles/min for the reticulum and 12
cycles/min for the cranial sac of the rumen. These rates were considered
to be indicative of the respective rhythmicities of the intrinsic
movements of these structures. Neither the phasic discharges of the
tension receptors nor the frequency of efferent vagal discharges responsible for extrinsic contractions were affected by the administration of
anti-cholinesterases (neostigmine), ganglionic blockers (tetraethyl-
ammonium chloride) or muscarinic blockers (probanthine hydrochloride),
even though, in contrast, the amplitudes of the extrinsic contractions
were enhanced with neostigmine and were reduced or abolished by tetraethylammonium chloride and probanthine. Therefore it was concluded that
these intrinsic contractions were probably myogenic in nature, because
they were not dependent on any tonically active neuronal mechanism with a
cholinergic synapse either at a ganglionic or at a post-ganglionic site.

When the reticulo-rumen was empty or when a reticular balloon was left
deflated, the resting discharges of tension receptors were either
non-existent or took the form of occasional spikes sometimes aggregated
into small bursts of activity. When the reticular balloon was lightly
inflated the discharges increased and generally appeared as phasic bursts
of activity with a few spikes in the interval between the bursts. Further
inflation caused the number of spikes to increase and the interval between

bursts to decrease. Even further inflation led to a continuous discharge with phasic peaks of activity at still shorter intervals. Thus passively distending the walls of the reticulum and of (the cranial sac of) the rumen caused an increased frequency and amplitude of the intrinsic myogenic contractions. Presumably this was a direct response of smooth muscle cells to being stretched: a general property of such cells in many other sites in the body.

An additional feature of the intrinsic myogenic contractions was that they tended to increase in circumstances where the extrinsic contractions were abolished, e.g. during the later stages of pyrogen-induced inhibition. When there had been recovery from the peripheral effects of pyrogen whilst the central nervous depression was still present, the intrinsic contractions became exaggerated until the extrinsic contractions returned (Leek & Van Miert (3) and unpublished observations). The possible effects on the intrinsic myogenic contractions of acids or other chemicals placed in the reticulo-ruminal lumen were not examined.

The existence and properties of the intrinsic myogenic contractions inferred from the characteristics of the resting discharges of reticular and ruminal tension receptors in halothane-anaesthetised sheep appear to have their counterparts in conscious sheep in the form of the slow-wave activity recorded by Ruckebusch (4) from EMG electrodes placed in the muscle layers of the reticulo-rumen.

Gregory (5) has studied the intrinsic movements in chronic vagally--denervated sheep kept alive with a special feeding technique to by-pass the forestomach. In these animals, in addition to slow-wave activity similar to that observed by Ruckebusch (4), there were large spike group discharges associated with almost simultaneous low-amplitude contractions of the reticulum and of the dorsal and ventral ruminal sacs. Gregory (6) showed that these group discharges which occurred at intervals of about 1 min were much enhanced by an anticholinesterase (eserine) and, conversely, were abolished by cholinergic blockers (hexamethonium, atropine). It was therefore concluded that the group discharges represented "intrinsic neurogenic contractions" involving cholinergic pathways and the myenteric plexus. These intrinsic contractions were accelerated by increasing ruminal volume and they were inhibited by acidifying the ruminal contents. The extent to which intrinsic neurogenic contractions may play a role in the normal conscious animal remains in doubt. Certainly the lack of a significant effect of anticholinesterases on the rate of extrinsic contractions suggests that cholinergic mechanisms such as the intrinsic neurogenic contractions are unlikely to be tonically active during the quiescent period between the primary cycle contractions. Furthermore, it is conceivable that the excitatory effect of increasing wall tension on intrinsic neurogenic contractions may be secondary to the more direct effect of tension on intrinsic myogenic contractions.

In addition to excitation by cholinergic mechanisms, the smooth muscle of the reticulo-rumen responds to other kinds of drugs. Adrenaline given with alpha- or beta-blockers or injection of specific alpha- or beta-adrenergic agonists demonstrate an alpha-adrenergic excitation and a beta-adrenergic inhibition of intrinsic contractions (7, unpublished observations by Leek and Van Miert). Other excitatory substances include pentagastrin (8 and unpublished observations), substance P, prostaglandin E_2 and bradykinin (7,9).

When a branch of a thoracic vagal nerve was electrically stimulated briefly at a site peripheral to an applied "cold block", the reticulo--ruminal smooth muscle was "toned up" and led to an enhancement of the next 3 or 4 extrinsic contractions (1). Thus, the tone of the smooth muscle during the period between contractions affects the ensuing extrinsic contractions. This involves a reflex mechanism for which some of the evidence is given later.

Because the magnitude of the intrinsic contractions reflexly influences the rate and amplitude of the extrinsic contractions, any factors which affect intrinsic contractions   will have consequential effects on extrinsic contraction. This may have considerable functional significance as a means of reflexly adjusting extrinsic contractions to the local needs of reticulo-ruminal function. Thus the extrinsic contractions may be reflexly modulated through the effects on the intrinsic contractions (a) of the physical and chemical state of the forestomach contents and (b) of peripheral humoral factors, such as digestive products (volatile fatty acids), hormones (adrenaline, gastro-intestinal hormones) and drugs. Circumstances which lead to a moderate increase in intrinsic contractions have a reflexly excitatory effect on extrinsic contractions but those which lead to a large increase in intrinsic contractions (as when drugs produce sustained contractures) have a reflexly depressing effect on extrinsic contractions.

III. THE EXTRINSIC CONTRACTIONS OF THE RETICULO-RUMEN

The gross movements of the ruminant forestomach are variously termed
"primary and secondary cycle movements", "A and B sequences" and "mixing
and eructation contractions". Detailed descriptions of this motility
were given first by Schalk & Amadon (10) in 1928 for cattle and by
Phillipson (11) in 1939 for sheep and a more recent comprehensive
exposition for sheep was provided by Wyburn (12). In essence, primary
cycles recur at intervals of approximately one minute and consist of
sequential contractions of the reticulum, then of the dorsal ruminal sac
and finally of the ventral ruminal sac. Secondary cycles occur, on average,
after every second primary cycle and consist of sequential contractions of
the dorsal ruminal sac and then of the ventral ruminal sac. The movements
are necessary for mixing and propelling the forestomach contents and,
particularly in the case of the secondary cycles, for the eructation of
the ruminal fermentation gases. The primary and secondary cycle movements
have an absolute dependence on efferent (motor) nervous activity carried
by vagal nerve fibres. For this reason they will be referred to as
"extrinsic contractions".

III.1. Efferent vagal nervous activity

Anatomical studies by Habel (13) have shown that each left and right
vagus divides in the thorax into a dorsal and ventral branch. The two
dorsal branches unite to form a dorsal vagal trunk (with a predominance
of right vagal fibres) and likewise the two ventral branches from a ventral
vagal trunk (with a predominance of left vagal fibres). The dorsal trunk
innervates all regions of the reticulo-rumen, whereas the ventral trunk
supplies the reticulum but little of the rumen. The vagi provide pathways
for afferent and efferent fibres in the ratio of 9:1 respectively. Duncan
(14) demonstrated in chronically denervated sheep, that extrinsic
contractions of normal amplitude and frequency required the presence of
not less than half of the total vagal supply and little difference was
observed between the apparent contributions of the different vagal
components.

In acute experiments on halothane-anaesthetised sheep, Leek (1)
produced temporary, reversible blockade of nervous conduction in the
various vagal branches by using a cooling thermode. Electrical stimulation

and single fibre recording were made simultaneously. Using rigorous criteria, it was concluded that, with regard just to efferent fibres, the right cervical vagus and dorsal thoracic vagal trunk made a greater motor contribution to contractions of the reticulum than did the left cervical vagus and the ventral thoracic vagal trunk. This last trunk provided no detectable supply to the rumen. These physiological results accord with the anatomical studies of Habel (13). Electrical stimulation of a vagal branch peripheral to a cold block or to a nerve section led to a reticular contraction and, in the case of the dorsal thoracic trunk or its contributors, also to a ruminal contraction. The durations, the forms and the amplitudes (subject to a maximum and to a degree of adaptation) of the evoked contractions were proportional to the durations, the patterns and the intensities of the stimulations. The ruminal contractions developed and decayed slightly later than the reticular contractions, presumably due to the length and polysynaptic nature of the efferent pathways postulated by the histological studies of Morrison & Habel (15). The correlation between the stimulus parameters and the ensuing contractions indicated that the efferent vagal nerve discharges did not act as triggers merely evoking peripherally-determined reticulo-ruminal sequences but acted as transmitters of a coordinated sequence of motor instructions, with each efferent fibre responsible for a discrete zone of activation. These conclusions were confirmed by the efferent unitary studies described below.

Using an electrophysiological ('single fibre') technique in halothane-anaesthetised sheep in which primary cycle movements were present (albeit subnormal in relation to the ruminal contractions), Iggo & Leek (16) were able to record the various patterns of nervous charges in individual efferent vagal fibres innervating different parts of the reticulo-rumen. In all cases there was no resting discharge, each cyclical burst of nervous activity had a fixed temporal relationship with the peak of the reticular contraction (which was used as the reference point) and the patterns of the discharges showed changes corresponding to reflexly evoked alterations in the duration, form and amplitude of reticulo-ruminal contractions. Similar unitary discharges in conscious sheep had been obtained earlier by Dussardier (17). He recorded unitary activity electromyographically from diaphragmatic muscle re-innervated by efferent vagal fibres which had grown from the central end of a cut vagus nerve into the cross-sutured peripheral stump of a cut phrenic nerve.

The efferent vagal pathways responsible for the extrinsic contractions involved cholinergic ganglionic and post-ganglionic transmission (1). Efferent gastric vagal discharges recordable in the pre-ganglionic axons in the cervical region failed to evoke extrinsic contractions after the administration of tetraethylammonium chloride (a nicotinic/ganglion blocker) or after giving atropine or probanthine hydrochloride (a muscarinic/post-ganglionic blocker). Conversely, the administration of neostigmine (an anticholinesterase) led to an enhancement of the amplitude and duration of the extrinsic contractions. Neither the cholinergic blockers nor the anticholinesterase changed the resting interval between the cyclical bursts of efferent discharges. It was therefore concluded that no cholinergic mechanism (such as intrinsic neurogenic motility) was tonically active during the resting interval, as this would have had a reflex excitatory effect on the rate of extrinsic contractions through the tension receptor mechanism described later.

For any given reticulo-ruminal efferent unit, its discharge could be altered reflexly (18). Acidification of the abomasum reduced the interval between the cyclical discharges or increased the number of action potentials and firing rate within each discharge. In turn this led to extrinsic contractions in the reticulo-rumen which had a higher rate, a greater amplitude and a longer duration. The converse effects were observed when the abomasum was distended. The reflex effects of distending the reticulum were more complicated. At low levels of distension there were increases in the cyclical rate of the discharges, in the number and firing rate of the action potentials (spikes) comprising each discharge and in the duration of the discharge. Moderate distension elicited even greater increases except that the peak firing rate associated with the second phase of the reticular contraction was less than expected. Extreme distension led to a reduction in the discharge and ultimately to a reduction in the rate of extrinsic contractions. The conclusions drawn from these experiments were that low and moderate tensions present in the wall of the reticulum during the resting period between contractions had a reflexly excitatory effect on the rate of contractions and on the spike composition of each efferent discharge. In contrast, extreme tensions present either passively at high levels of reticular inflation or actively during the reticular contraction had reflexly inhibitory effects which were persistent in the former case and transient in the latter. By using a variety of experimental manoeuvres, such as sudden reticular inflation or deflation at different points in the primary cycle and changing the contraction conditions from isometric to isotonic, it was possible to show that the tension developed during the early phases of the extrinsic contraction reflexly affected the efferent discharge and contraction characteristics of the later parts of the cycle. Minimum total reflex time of 1.3 s for reticulo-reticular and 2.1 s for reticulo-ruminal reflexes were measured, of which the central nervous integration was calculated to take at least 370 ms.

For the reasons given later, it is now possible to attribute the reflex excitatory effects to stimulation of reticulo-ruminal tension receptors and the reflex inhibitory effects to stimulation of reticulo-ruminal epithelial receptors.

III.2. Efferent splanchnic nervous activity

If the splanchnic nerves are stimulated electrically the overall effect is an inhibition of the extrinsic contractions (1). The administration of noradrenaline or alpha-adrenergic agonists leads directly to a contracture lasting several minutes and this can also been seen *in vitro*. As the contracture decays there may be very small extrinsic contractions super-imposed upon it. The associated efferent vagal activity for each contraction is very subnormal but the bursts recur after shorter than normal resting intervals. The reflex effect seems to be comparable with the situation of extreme reticular distension described earlier. Beta-adrenergic agonists or adrenaline given with an alpha-adrenergic blocker produce no contracture (7). They antagonise efferent vagal discharges peripherally.

Neither chronic splanchnic denervation in conscious sheep (14) nor acute splanchnic denervation in the halothane anaesthetised sheep (1,3) had any detectable effect on extrinsic contractions. Moreover, splanchnic denervation did not appear to affect the intrinsic neurogenic movements seen in the chronically vagotomised sheep of Gregory (5). The administration of alpha- and beta-adrenergic blockers did not affect the extrinsic contractions (3).

The conclusions from all of these studies are that the majority of the efferent splanchnic nerve fibres to the reticulo-rumen are potentially inhibitory. However these fibres are normally not tonically active and

make no detectable contribution to the occurrence of extrinsic contractions
or intrinsic myogenic contractions.

III.3. The gastric centres

The term 'gastric centres' is used to denote the bilateral areas of the
brain-stem responsible for producing the extrinsic movements of the
forestomach via discharges in the gastric vagal efferent nerve fibres. By
transecting the brainstem rostral and caudal to the medulla oblongata,
Iggo (19,20) demonstrated that the gastric centres were located in this
region. Subsequently, electrical stimulation of parts of the dorsal vagal
nuclei was shown by Bell & Lawn (21) to elict reticulo-ruminal movements
and records of neuronal activity in the dorsal vagal nuclei having a
fixed time relationship with the extrinsic motility of the forestomach were
obtained first by Beghelli, Borgatti & Parmeggiani (22) and later by
Harding & Leek (23,24,25).

Using the action potential collision technique, Harding and Leek (23)
distinguished between gastric centre activity present in motoneurons
and that in interneurons. The motoneuronal activity could be divided into
'early' and 'late' types on the basis of whether the peak of the
discharges occurred before or after the peak of the reticular contraction.
The early discharges were considered to be associated with the contraction
of the reticulum and related structures which contract early in the
primary cycle. The late discharges were attributed to the rumen and
related structures which contract after the reticulum. In a few
instances where secondary cycle contractions were present, the late
motoneurones(but not the early motoneurones) discharges both during the
primary and during the secondary cycles. These late motoneurones therefore
provided a 'common final pathway' for the quite different discharge
patterns for the activation of the ruminal muscle occurring in the primary
and in the secondary cycle sequence.

Three distinguishable types of interneurones were observed. One type
(Type A) had early and late discharge patterns which resembled those of
the early and late types of motoneurones and of the efferent gastric vagal
fibres described earlier. Presumably these were the interneurones which
drove the motoneurones. Another type of interneurone (Type C) had a
discharge pattern which started with a silent period during and shortly
after the primary cycle contractions and then slowly increased the rate of

its discharge in proportion to the level of primary cycle contraction. The behaviour of the interneurones suggested that their role was one of integrating and accumulating the tonic excitatory and inhibitory inputs arriving at the gastric centres from various reflexogenic sites during the quiescent period between contractions. The accumulation continued until the increasing level of activity in these interneurones reached a "firing level" which triggered the next primary cycle sequence. Consequently these interneurones came to be regarded as the major determinants of the rate of primary cycles and hence as the basis of the postulated 'rate circuits' of the gastric centres. A third type of interneurone (Type B) gave a steady discharge at all times except for a silent period. The discharge rate was not noticeably affected by different levels of excitatory input and it was postulated that these interneurones could have some kind of 'gating' function, being tonically inhibitory except during the silent period immediately before the start of the primary cycle sequences.

The ways in which the different gastric centre neurones react to different perturbations have thrown light on their probably mode of action. In halothane-anaesthetised sheep, when the spinal cord was sectioned just below the brainstem, there was usually little or not effect on extrinsic contractions. Thus splanchnic nerve afferents, which are generally considered to be mainly inhibitory, and afferents ascending the spinal cord from elsewhere in the periphery did not appear to be tonically active. In contrast, if, in addition to cord section, a brainstem section was made just caudal to the gastric centres, there was usually an immediate and sustained increase in the rate of primary cycle contractions. Thus the caudal regions of the medulla oblongata exerted a tonic inhibitory effect on the gastric centres.

If a second brainstem section was made rostral to the gastric centres, the primary cycle sequences were present but depressed. Thus rostral brainstem regions appeared to exert a tonic facilitatory influence on the gastric centres. If a median brainstem section either of full depth or restricted to the dorsal half was made between the left and right gastric centres, their activities were no longer synchronized. Primary cycle sequences attributable to the neuronal activity in the gastric centre on one side occurred and later there was a sequence attributable to the other side. Therefore commissural links were synchronizing the activities of the two centres. If, at this point, the vagal nerves were cut, no gastric centre interneuronal activity was observed. Therefore, the gastric centre neurones did not appear to possess an inherent rhythmicity but required to be driven by inputs from elsewhere.

If the vagal nerves were cut in a sheep in which the brainstem had not been transected rostral to the gastric centres, the interneuronal activity was still present, though less than before the vagal section, but there was no activity in the early and late vagal motoneurones. Thus it appeared that the gastric centre interneurones were capable of being driven by excitatory inputs coming *either* from the vagus nerves *or* from higher regions of the brain. However, at least in these anaesthetised sheep, vagal inputs were necessary to facilitate the synaptic transmission of Type A interneuronal activity across to the associated vagal motoneurones.

If the excitatory afferent vagal input to the gastric centres was varied, for instance by changing the volume of reticular distension, there was a short-term residual effect of the situation prior to the change on the Type C interneurones and this was reflected in the interval between the previous and the next primary cycle sequence, i.e. there was a residual effect on rate. In contrast, the discharges of Type A inter-neurones and the motoneurones were affected only by the changes in vagal input that occurred at the time of the discharges themselves. Indeed, as Iggo & Leek (18) observed even with efferent gastric vagal discharges at the cervical level, the tension conditions developed in the reticulo-rumen by the early part of the efferent discharge exerted a reflex effect, by way of tension receptors and vagal afferent pathways, on the later parts of the same efferent discharge.

Taking all of these results together, the general conclusion allows one to hypothesise on the mechanisms by which the gastric centres operate. Functionally, each centre behaves as if it contains two integrating circuits separated by a gate. A 'rate' circuit based on Type C inter-neurones accumulates over a short term the inputs from peripheral nerves and from higher and lower regions of the brain stem. When these inter-neurones reach a firing level they cause the opening of a gate, based on the Type B interneurones. For the few moments that the gate is open (i.e. whilst the Type B interneurones are silent), the various instantaneous inputs are integrated by the Type A interneurones which are the basis of a 'form and amplitude' circuit. This integrated input determines the pattern and the duration of the discharge in each Type A interneurone and

the lag between the various "early" and "late" interneurones. These
discharge patterns are in turn passed to the different reticular and
ruminal vagal motoneurones which result in the form and amplitude of the
contractions of the various regions of the forestomach during a primary
cycle contraction sequence.

Clearly the gastric centres are dependent on the overall excitatory
drive arising as a combination of inputs from other (probably mainly
higher) central nervous regions and from the periphery. Natural and
experimental situations which affect the general level of central nervous
activity are likely to have consequential effects on gastric centre
excitability and hence on reticulo-ruminal motility. Thus motility is
affected by excitement and drowsiness, environmental temperature and by
drugs. General anaesthetics depress central nervous activity and reduce or
abolish motility. Under halothane anaesthesia, it is possible to counter-
act the central nervous depression by increasing the level of an
excitatory input from the periphery, e.g. by inflating a balloon in the
reticulum. For this reason, the results of experiments obtained from
anaesthetised sheep require careful interpretation. In many conscious
animals reticulo-ruminal motility still occurs even after the reticulo-
ruminal contents have been removed, so that peripheral drives from the
reticulo-rumen itself would be minimal. Moreover, Falempin & Rousseau (26)
found that after selective chronic vagal de-afferentation, reticulo-
ruminal contractions in conscious sheep occurred more frequently and had
a longer duration. One interpretation of these results would be, that in
the conscious animal the peripheral inputs via the vagal nerves had a net
inhibitory effect on the gastric centres, rather than the net excitatory
effect deliberately created by reticular balloon distension in the
halothane-anaesthetised experiments described earlier.

III.4. Visceral sensory mechanisms
III.4.1. The effective stimuli

Classical reflex studies have shown that the mouth, the oesophagus,
the forestomach, the abomasum and the duodenum are important reflexogenic
areas for effects on reticulo-ruminal motility and often also on
salivation. Most attention has been given to various forms of mechanical
stimuli but chemical stimuli have been effective at some sites.

Borgatti (27) showed that mechanical stimulation of the oral mucous

membranes excited reticulo-ruminal motility. Receptors with afferent
pathways mainly in the second and third branches of the trigeminal nerves
were considered by Borgatti and Matscher (28) to be tonically active, as
primary cycle motility was reduced by trigeminal nerve section. During
mastication of food or of the cud, augmentation of this tonic activity
was considered to be responsible for the reflexly enhanced forestomach
motility. Chemical stimulation through the taste mechanism did not appear
to be involved. These conclusions are consistent with the results of sham
feeding and with the unilateral stimulation of parotid gland secretion
during mastication.

Balloon distension of the terminal oesophagus, cardia, reticulo-omasal
orifice, reticulum and the reticulo-ruminal orifice reflexly enhanced
primary cycle motility. Gaseous distension of the dorsal ruminal sac
enhanced secondary cycle motility. Balloon and manual distension of the
reticulum (29,19) and distension particularly of the reticulo-ruminal
orifice (30) were powerful means of promoting primary cycle contractions,
except when the stimulus became excessive and reflex inhibition of
motility ensued. Manual stretching the cardia, reticular groove, reticulo-
omasal orifice, reticulo-ruminal fold and cranial ruminal pillar was a
potent stimulus to parotid salivation in conscious sheep (29) and in
anaesthetised sheep (31).

Coarse fibre in the forestomach favours rumination. Conversely,
rumination was virtually eliminated by finely grinding the food (10,32).
Squeezing the reticulo-ruminal fold (33) and scratching the ruminal mucosa
(10,29) readily induced rumination.

Acidification of the reticulo-ruminal contents reflexly inhibited
forestomach motility (34,35). The potency of a particular acid was not
dependent on its pH *per se* but was more closely related to its titratable
acidity or to its concentration of undissociated weak acids (36). Acidification of the abomasum was a potent stimulus for primary cycle motility
(24,37) through a vago-vagal reflex (18). In contrast, balloon distension
of the abomasum and of the duodenum inhibited primary cycle motility
(37,18).

III.4.2. Visceral sensory receptors and their afferent pathways

At least three distinct types of visceral sensory receptors, classified
according to their sites (38), have been demonstrated electrophysiologi-

cally: (a) near to the basement membrane of the lining epithelium are located epithelial (mucosal) receptors, (b) in the muscle layers are tension receptors and (c) in the serosa and adjacent mesenteries are serosal receptors. In addition there is evidence of visceral thermo-receptors and the mesenteries contain many classical Pacinian corpuscles. The epithelial and tension receptors project via the vagi. The serosal receptors and perhaps a few tension receptors project via the splanchnic nerves.

III.4.2.1. Epithelial receptors

The epithelial receptors in sheep were first described by Harding and Leek (39,38) for the abomasum and the duodenum and later for the reticulo-rumen (40). They were rapidly-adapting mechanoreceptors which were also excitable with certain chemicals. As mechanoreceptors they gave a typical rapidly-adapting "on-off" response to a maintained moderate mechanical stimulus but an extreme stimulus could produce a persistent discharge.

Constant light brushing of the epithelium gave a repetitive discharge. The receptors have a superficial location and removal of the receptive field epithelium gave a loss of responsiveness. In the reticulum, the receptors were found particularly in the conical papillae surmounting the hexagonal ridges of the luminal epithelium and they were innervated by unmyelinated nerve fibres (41,42). Although the epithelial histology of the reticulo-rumen, of the abomasum and of the duodenum is very different, the epithelial receptors showed similar responses to a variety of chemicals, irrespective of their location. Most receptors were excited by mineral and organic acids, alkali, hyper-osmotic and hypo-osmotic sodium chloride or sucrose solutions and water. On the basis of their long response latencies and the published diffusion coefficients for the acids tested, it was calculated that the receptors were located about 150 um below the epithelial surface. This approximated to the position of the basement membrane where, histologically, the fine nerve fibres of the conical papillae appeared to terminate.

The acid-sensitivity of the reticulo-ruminal receptors appeared to depend on molecular 'size' (with the exception of butyric acid) and the degree of undissociation (association). In general, the higher the molecular weight of the acid then the longer was the latency of response and the higher was the threshold concentration (42). Presumably this was because the higher molecular weight acids had taken longer to diffuse across the epithelium and had consequently been neutralised to a greater extent *en route*. Butyric acid was specially potent on the epithelial receptors (43), as it had also been on the acid-induced inhibition of reticulo-ruminal motility in conscious sheep (34,44). This may have been due to special permeability or transport properties of the reticulo-ruminal epithelium for butyric acid absorption. Ruminal fluid samples taken from sheep at the point when reticulo-ruminal contractions had just been abolished by intra-ruminal infusion either of acetic or of butyric acid was capable of exciting epithelial receptors in another sheep (36). Furthermore the potency of this fluid was enhanced by lowering the pH, so that more of the acid was undissociated, and, conversely, the potency was reduced by raising the pH. The epithelial receptors are *not* pH or hydrogen ion receptors. In the case of weak organic acids, the effect of pH acted *indirectly* by causing a greater proportion of the total acid to be present in the undissociated form: a condition which is considered to favour epithelial permeability.

The physiological properties of the 'epithelial' or 'mucosal' receptors in the abomasum and proximal duodenum were similar to those of the reticulo-rumen (39,38) except that the estimated diffusion distance for test acids would place the receptors of the abomasum near to the opening of the gastric glands at the bottom of the gastric pits. More recent work by Cottrell & Iggo (46) has suggested that the duodenal mucosal receptors consist of one sub-group similar to that described above and another sub-group which is sensitive to KCl. In the small intestine of non-ruminants there is evidence of specific glucose sensitive receptors (47) and of amino-acid sensitive receptors (48) but no similar investigations have been carried out on the ruminant.

The epithelial receptors serve predominantly as mechanoreceptors. They are excited by even the lightest tactile stimulus. The repeated movement of fibrous digesta across the luminal epithelium and extreme distension situations could be expected to excite them.

Excitation of epithelial receptors in the reticulo-rumen acts as an inhibitory input to the gastric centres and reflexly reduces primary cycle motility (24). It is possible that they maintain a tonic inhibitory effect on the gastric centres, as selective vagal de-afferentation in conscious sheep has been shown to result in an increased rate of primary

cycle contractions, together with a lengthening of the contraction phase
of each compartment (26). They appear to have no reflex effect on salivation (31). Preliminary results by Leek and Stafford (49 and
unpublished observations) suggest that excitation of the epithelial
receptors in the reticulo-rumen serves as the peripheral trigger for
evoking rumination when the central nervous mechanisms are in a suitably
facilitatory state. The mechano-sensitive role of mucosal receptors in the
abomasum and in the duodenum is not known.

A physiological role for the epithelial receptors on the basis of their
chemo-sensitive properties is dubious but *pathological* and *experimental*
roles do exist. The inhibition of reticulo-ruminal motility evoked
experimentally by the intraruminal infusion of acids or arising
pathologically during the ruminal acidosis ('grain engorgement') syndrome
is undoubtedly attributable to reticulo-ruminal epithelial receptor
activation (36,50). It is conceivable that the abomasal epithelial
receptors may have a physiological role as monitors of abomasal acid
secretion and, experimentally, their activation would account for the
reflex enhancement of primary cycle motility arising from abomasal
acidification (37,18). Experimentally, the regulation of gastric emptying
based on the results of infusing acids and alkalis into the calf's
duodenum (51) is consistent with duodenal epithelial receptor activation.

III.4.2.2. Tension receptors

Tension receptors are slowly-adapting mechanoreceptors situated in the
muscle layers of all parts of the alimentary tract "in series" with the
smooth muscle cells (2). In the reticulo-rumen the tension receptors are
innervated by finely myelinated nerve fibres with conduction velocities
more than ten times faster than the unmyelinated nerve fibres which
innervated either tension receptors elsewhere or epithelial receptors.
The receptive fields of single afferent fibres innervating tension
receptors had diameters of 5-20 mm. When such a field is subjected to a
maintained mechanical stimulus (e.g. pressed with a probe) there is a
sustained receptor discharge which adapts only very slowly. If an
intrinsic or extrinsic contraction occurs there will be a large discharge
and this behaviour, which resembles that of the Golgi tendon organs in
skeletal muscle, is the basis of the "in series" concept. The discharge
rate of a tension receptor is therefore a composite feature reflecting the

passive tensions due to distension and the active tensions developed by intrinsic and extrinsic contractions. Any natural or experimental situations which affect these contractions will affect tension receptor activity accordingly.

In the reticulo-rumen, tension receptors are particularly densely located around the cardia, the reticulo-omasal orifice, the outer margins of the reticular groove, the reticulum (particularly its medial wall), the reticulo-ruminal fold and the cranial pillar and the longitudinal pillars (2). Few tension receptor fields have been located elsewhere in the rumen but they can be found in the floor of the omasal canal and they are plentiful in the terminal regions of the oesophagus. In the abomasum they are particularly abundant in the pyloric region. Recently Cottrell & Iggo (52) described the behaviour of tension receptors in the circular muscle of the sheep's duodenum.

The role of tension receptors are numerous. In the oesophagus they appear to elicit secondary contractions in the event of swallowed bolus falling behind the primary contractions. In the forestomach, tension receptors of the reticulum, of the reticulo-ruminal fold and probably of the reticular groove provide an excitatory input to the gastric centres leading to an increase in the rate, the duration and the amplitude of the primary cycle contractions. Tensions developed during the early phases of the contraction provide a reflex feed-back to influence the vagally-evoked later phases of contraction (18,24). It is perhaps for this reason that the reticulo-ruminal tension receptors are innervated by faster conducting fibres than are tension receptors elsewhere. Circumstances, such as feeding, which passively distend the reticulo-rumen with ingesta and gases enhance motility presumably by tension receptor activation, although some degree of reflex inhibition arising from epithelial receptors may also occur which would moderate the expected enhancement. Other circumstances, such as pyrogen production during febrile disease, may inhibit the intrinsic contractions and hence reduce the excitatory input from tension receptors to the gastric centres.

Tension receptors around the reticular groove, reticulo-ruminal fold and cranial pillar excite parotid salivary gland secretion (31). Tension receptors, perhaps in the cranial sac, facilitate secondary cycle contractions which in concert with the activation of other receptors (probably tension receptors) around the reticular groove lead to eructation. Tension receptors in the reticulo-rumen probably signal "rumen fill" to the appetite control centres. They do not provide the peripheral trigger for evoking rumination.

Tension receptors in the abomasum with afferent vagal pathways reflexly inhibit reticulo-ruminal motility (18) and this may provide a mechanism for regulating abomasal filling. Similarly tension receptors in the duodenum are presumably responsible for the inhibition of reticulo-ruminal motility which occurs during duodenal distension.

III.4.2.3. Serosal receptors

Serosal receptors have been studied in the sheep by Floy & Morrison (53). The receptors are located in the serosa near to the junction with the mesentery or in the mesenteries themselves. They are slowly-adapting receptors and they are affected not only by tension of the mesenteries but also by contractions of the neighbouring viscus. They are innervated by afferent fibres in the splanchnic nerves and therefore, as the splanchnic nerves do not appear to exert a tonically active or essential effect on forestomach motility, the serosal receptor input may be of limited significance. In nociceptive (pain-producing) situation, the serosal receptors may evoke reflexly inhibitory effects and they may have a minor part in the reflex inhibition of reticulo-ruminal motility elicited by abomasal distension.

IV CONCLUSION

The extrinsic contractions of the forestomach are essential for mixing and aboral propulsion of the contents, for eructation and for rumination. Their rate, form and amplitude are the consequence of central nervous activity, reflexly modified by sensory inputs largely from the alimentary tract itself. Any husbandry practices, clinical conditions or drug programmes which affect either the general level of central nervous activity or the volume, texture and composition of the gut contents will modify extrinsic contractions and may lead to digestive dysfunctions. As extrinsic contractions are readily examined clinically, abnormal motility should be an important early sign of many diseases (54,55).

REFERENCES

1. Leek, B.F.: Ph.D. Thesis (Edinburgh) (1967)
2. Leek, B.F.: J. Physiol. (London) 202, 585-609 (1969)
3. Leek, B.F. and Van Miert, A.S.J.P.A.M.: J. Physiol. (London) 215, 28-29P (1971)
4. Ruckebusch, Y.: J. Physiol. (London) 210, 857-882 (1970)
5. Gregory, P.C.: J. Physiol. (London) 328, 97-98P (1982)
6. Gregory, P.C.: J. Physiol. (London) 346, 379-393 (1984)
7. Van Miert, A.S.J.P.A.M.: In: Physiological and Pharmacological Aspects of the Reticulo-Rumen. Ooms, L.A.A., Degryse, A.D. and Van Miert, A.S.J.P.A.M. (eds), Martinus Nijhoff Publ., Dordrecht-Boston, 113 - 132 (1987)
8. Grovum, W.L. and Leek, B.F.: Ir. J. Med. Sci. 151, 86 (1982)
9. Maas, C.L. and Leek, B.F.: Vet. Res. Commun. 9, 89-113 (1985)
10. Schalk, A.F. and Amadon, R.S.: North Dakota Agricultural College Experimental Station Bulletin 216, 1-6 (1928)
11. Phillipson, A.T.: Quart. J. Exp. Physiol. 29, 395-415 (1939)
12. Wyburn, R.S.: In: Digestive Physiology and Metabolism in Ruminants. Ruckebusch, Y. and Thivend, P. (eds), MTP Press, Lancaster, pp. 35-51 (1980)
13. Habel, R.E.: Cornell Vet. 46, 555-628 (1956)
14. Duncan, D.L.: J. Physiol. (London) 119, 157-169 (1953)
15. Morrison, A.R. and Habel, R.E.: J. Comp. Neurol. 122, 297-308 (1964)
16. Iggo, A. and Leek, B.F.: J. Physiol. (London) 191, 177-204 (1967)
17. Dussardier, M.: D.Sc. Thesis (Paris) (1960)
18. Iggo, A. and Leek, B.F.: J. Physiol. (London) 193, 95-119 (1967)
19. Iggo, A.: J. Physiol. (London) 115, 28-29P (1951)
20. Iggo, A.: J. Physiol. (London) 131, 248-256 (1956)
21. Bell, F.R. and Lawn, A.M.: J. Physiol. (London) 128, 577-592 (1955)
22. Beghelli, V., Borgatti, G. and Parmeggiani, P.L.: Archs. Ital. Biol. 101, 365-384 (1963)
23. Harding, R. and Leek, B.F.: J. Physiol. (London) 219, 587-610 (1971)
24. Harding, R. and Leek, B.F.: J. Physiol. (London) 225, 309-338 (1972)
25. Harding, R. and Leek. B.F.: J. Physiol. (London) 228, 73-90 (1973)
26. Falempin, M. and Rousseau, J.P.: Ann. Rech. Vét. 10, 186-188 (1979)
27. Borgatti, G.: Nuova Veterin. 23, 187 (1947)

28. Borgatti, G. and Matscher, R.: Archs. Ital. Biol. 96, 38 (1958)
29. Ash, R.W. and Kay, R.N.B.: J. Physiol. (London) 149, 43-57 (1959)
30. Titchen, D.A.: J. Physiol. (London) 151, 139-153 (1960)
31. Grovum, W.L. and Leek, B.F.: J. Physiol. (London) 364, 35P (1985)
32. Freer, M., Campling, R.C. and Balch, C.C.: Br. J. Nutr. 16, 279-295 (1962)
33. Downie, H.G.: Am. J. Vet. Res. 15, 217-223 (1954)
34. Ash, R.W.: J. Physiol. (London) 147, 58-73 (1959)
35. Leek, B.F., Ryan, J.P. and Upton, P.K.: J. Physiol. (London) 263, 233-234 (1976)
36. Crichlow, E.C. and Leek, B.F.: J. Physiol. (London) 310, 60-61P (1981)
37. Titchen, D.A.: J. Physiol. (London) 142, 1-21 (1958)
38. Leek, B.F.: Br. Med. Bull. 33, 163-168 (1977)
39. Harding, R. and Leek, B.F.: J. Physiol. (London) 222, 139-140P (1972)
40. Harding, R. and Leek, B.F.: J. Physiol. (London) 223, 32-33P (1972)
41. Leek, B.F.: J. Physiol. (London) 227, 22-23P (1972)
42. Leek, B.F. and Harding, R.: In: Digestion and Metabolism in the Ruminant. McDonald, I.W. and Warner, A.C.I. (eds), University of New England, Armidale N.S.W., pp. 60-76 (1975)
43. Crichlow, E.C., Leek, B.F., Upton, P.K. and Ryan, J.P.: Fed. Proc. 39, 890 (1980)
44. Upton, P.K., Ryan, J.P. and Leek, B.F.: Proc. Nutr. Soc. 36, 9A (1977)
45. Crichlow, E.C. and Leek, B.F.: Am. J. Vet. Res. 47 (in press) (1986)
46. Cottrell, D.F. and Iggo, A.: J. Physiol. (London) 354, 497-522 (1984)
47. Mei, N.: J. Physiol. (London) 282, 485-506 (1978)
48. Jeanningros, R.: Physiol. & Behav. 28, 9-21 (1982)
49. Leek, B.F. and Stafford, K.J.: Ir. J. Med. Sci. in press (1986)
50. Crichlow, E.C. and Chaplin, R.K.: Can. J. Anim. Sci. 64, 5-7 (1984)
51. Bell, F.R. and Mostaghni, K.: J. Physiol. (London) 245, 387 (1975)
52. Cottrell, D.F. and Iggo, A.: J. Physiol. (London) 354, 457-475 (1984)
53. Floyd, K. and Morrison, J.F.B.: J. Physiol. (London) 237, 23P (1974)
54. Leek, B.F.: Vet. Rec. 113, 10-14 (1983)
55. Van Miert, A.S.J.P.A.M.: The Vet. Quarterly 7, 200-216 (1985)

2. RETICULO-RUMEN AND GASTRODUODENAL JUNCTION MOTILITY

Y.RUCKEBUSCH

I. INTRODUCTION

The ability of the reticulo-rumen to contract rhytmically is a result of a vagovagal reflex mediated by the gastric centre located in the medulla within the dorsal motor nucleus (8,37). The role of the central nervous system (CNS) is to achieve the integration of the activity of separate regions of the forestomach. Afferent impulses regulate their sequential contractile activity and control the frequency and amplitude of contractions, with feeding via tactile stimulation of the buccal cavity (26). This cyclical motor activity of the reticulo-ruminal and omasal muscular layer is impaired after bilateral vagotomy or anaesthesia. Within 1-2 weeks after vagotomy, the spike bursts reappear as stationary groups, and the resultant contractions occur over the whole reticulo-rumen. This is in contrast to the intact animal where the electrical activity and contractions are progagated from one location to another. These myoelectric activities are evidently organized by the ganglionic cells of neural plexuses, the enteric nervous system (ENS).

This intrinsic activity that develops in chronically vagotomized sheep persists after bilateral section of the splanchnic nerves and is stimulated by distension of reticulo-rumen (9), suggesting a major role for the ENS in the basal smooth muscle tone, although direct effects of Ca^{++} ions after tetrodotoxin suggest a myogenic control (5).

The true secretory stomach of the ruminant, the abomasum, is comparable to the simple stomach of other mammals. The continuous flow of ingesta from the reticulo-rumen through the reticulo-omasal orifice is the stimulus on the continuous abomasal secretion and emptying of acidic chyme through the antroduodenal junction (12,27). The emptying of liquid digesta (dry matter: less than 4%), at the rate of 6.1-6.8 litres per 24 h, from the ovine abomasum requires the duodenal bulb to propel it against gravity by means of propagated contractions which cease periodically at the end of a phase of intense activity. This cyclic activity of the junction is due to the migrating myoelectric complex (MMC) with a phase of irregular (ISA) and regular spiking activity (RSA) followed by quiescence at intervals of 90-120m min (31). Unlike the rhythmic reticulo-rumen movements, the cyclic motor events of the junction persist after vagotomy in the adult ruminants and are not modified by feeding. However, the duodenal area not only controls the transpyloric flow of digesta via neural and endocrine mechanisms, but also modifies the forestomach activity by acting as a brake by influencing abomasal emptying and gastric (abomasal) loading from the reticulo-rumen reservoir (33).

The rumen bypass in the milk-fed ruminant, and the ingestive behaviour and rumination in response to the coarse food, are also centrally-mediated and are associated with changes in the reticulo-rumen (RR) and gastro-duodenal junction (GDJ) activity. Emphasis in this study will be on the regulatory factors involved in the cyclic activity of the forestomach and those timing the gastric emptying. A detailed study of "the control of motility of the rumino-reticulum" has been recently published by Grovum in the Proceedings of the sixth International Symposium on Ruminant Physiology (Prentice-Hall, Englewood Cliffs, New Jersey, 1986, p. 18-40).

II. CHRONOTROPIC VERSUS INOTROPIC REGULATION OF RETICULO-RUMEN MOVEMENTS

The parasympathetic innervation is derived from the dorsal and ventral vagal trunks branched after a variable number of anastomoses from the two cervical vagus nerves. The dorsal vagal trunk supplies the prevertebral coeliaco-mesenteric plexus, the rumen, reticulum and omasum, and the visceral abomasal surface. The ventral vagal trunk also contributes to the coeliaco-mesenteric plexus and to the rumen, reticulum and omasum, as well as innervating the parietal abomasal surface (Fig. 1).

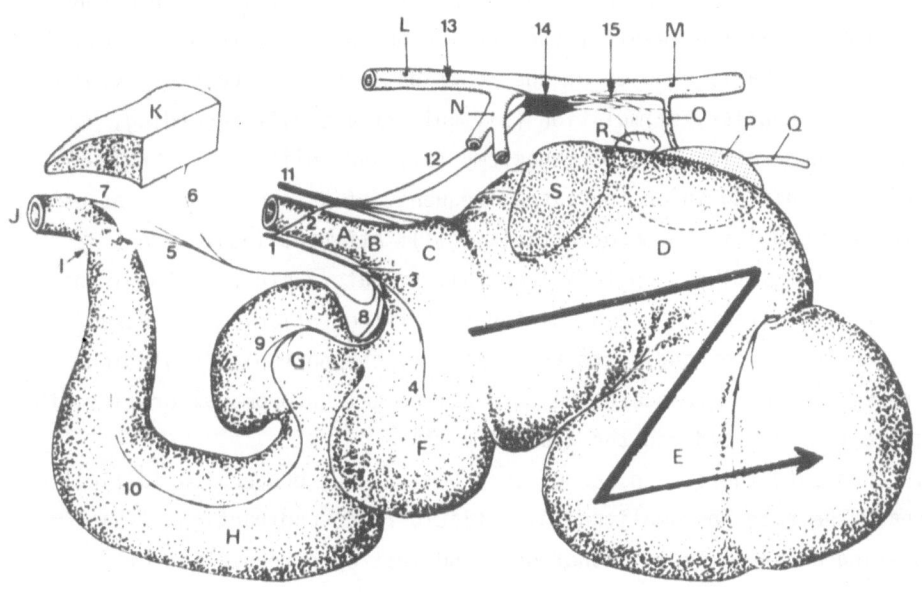

FIGURE 1. Extrinsic innervation of the ovine ruminant stomach and termination of ventral vagal trunk. A. oesophagus, B. cardia, C. atrium, D. dorsal sac of the rumen, E. ventral sac of the rumen, F. reticulum, G. omasum, H. abomasum, I. pylorus, J. duodenum, K. liver, L. thoracic aorta, M. abdominal aorta, N. coeliacomesenteric trunk, O. left renal artery, P. left kidney, Q. left ureter, R. left adrenal gland, S. spleen. 1. ventral vagal trunk, 2. communicating branch, 3. branches for the atrium and the reticulum (4), 5. long pyloric nerve, 6. hepatic branches, 7. duodenal branches, 8. branches of the reticular groove, the omasum (9) and abomasum (10), 11. dorsal vagal trunk, 12. coeliac branches, 13. splanchnic nerves, 14. coeliacomesenteric ganglia, 15. periaortic plexus.
The arrows correspond to the propagation of the primary ruminal contractions.

The long pyloric nerve, which gives off branches to the hepatic plexus and parallels the right gastric artery, innervates the duodenum and the antral region of the abomasum. The efferent vagal fibres are preganglionic and cholinergic (6). The splanchnic nerves which leave the plexus are

postganglionic adrenergic fibres mainly joining the arteries. Both
parasympathetic and sympathetic fibres are supposed to terminate in or
near the ganglions of the intramural plexuses of the ruminant stomach wall.
Since the sympathetic fibres do not directly innervate the gastrointestinal musculature, the effect of their stimulation may be the result
of an inhibition of parasympathetic activity and/or a decreased blood flow.

The vagovagal reflexes involved in the frequency of RR contractions
are integrated at the level of the medulla oblongata, outside the blood-
brain barrier. Early studies of the location of gastric centres involved
direct intramedullary stimulation (1), unitary activity recording,
cellular degeneration after rumenectomy (37) and spliting the brain
medially, resulting in an increased frequency of RR contractions as each
centre produced its own motor activity (11). Afferent inputs are
integrated cumulatively up to a 'central excitatory state' determining
the rate of contractions, e.g. distension of the reticulum increases
its frequency corresponding to an excitatory chronotropic regulation.
Other reflexogenic areas are the cardia, the reticulo-omasal orifice, the
reticulo-ruminal fold and the cranial pillar.

In contrast, the distension of the abomasum and duodenal acidification
decrease the rate and amplitude of reticulo-rumen contractions (15),
suggesting an inhibitory chronotropic and inotropic regulation of
motility. Efferent activity is the stimulus for the periodic and
sequential RR contractions or their inhibition, when the reticular
(oesophageal) groove is stimulated (Fig. 2).

An example of this regulation is given by the inhibition of reticulo-
rumen contractions associated with sucking in adult ruminant. The
closure of the reticular groove involves this cephalic phase characterized
by diminished intensity of reticulum contractions (Fig. 3). When the
abomasum is already filled, a new closure of the reticular groove with
further ingestion of milk reduces the frequency of contractions (rate),
proportional to the degree of distension of the abomasum. The inhibition
of this abomasal phase is, thus, mainly chronotropic (13).

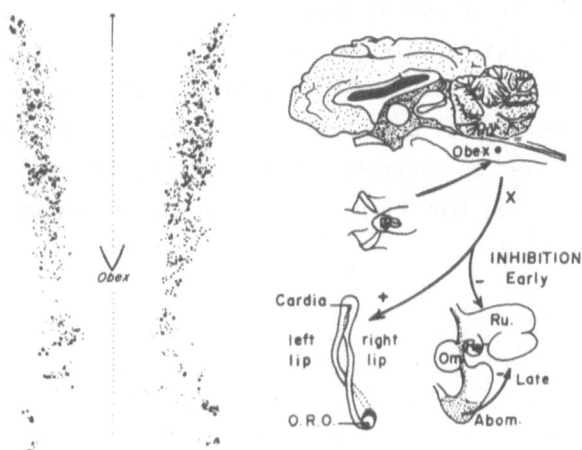

FIGURE 2. Gastric centres in the medulla are indicated by a dot located
near the obex under the cerebellum. Left: Retrograde cellular degeneration (black dots) 16 days after rumenectomy in a milk-fed lamb suggests
that the centres relative to the obex extent laterally and less caudally
than rostrally (from Szabo and Dussardier; 37). Right: Diagram showing
the opposite effects of vagal stimulation during sucking: stimulation
of the reticular groove and inhibition of reticulo-rumen activity.

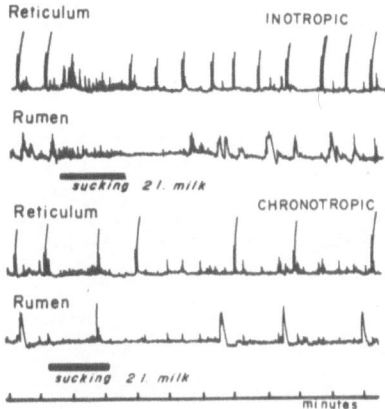

FIGURE 3. Inhibition of the reticulo-rumen response to sucking 2 l of warm
milk in an adult bull at 45-min intervals is indicated by the bars. The
cephalic phase (top) is inotropic since it is related to the amplitude.
The abomasal phase, when abomasum is already full (bottom), is related to
the frequency and therefore chronotropic. Small pressure fluctuations seen
during sucking are associated with swallowing. Time in minutes. (from
Kay & Ruckebusch, 13).

III. STIMULATION OF THE RETICULAR GROOVE REFLEX

A reason for stimulating this reflex in ruminants is its activation in calves thus avoiding the escape of milk into the rumen, e.g. when pharyngitis or oropharyngeal abcesses prevent the afferent arc of the reflex to be operative. In contrast, it might be of interest to avoid activation of the reflex from oropharyngeal origin in mature ruminants during oral dosing (17).

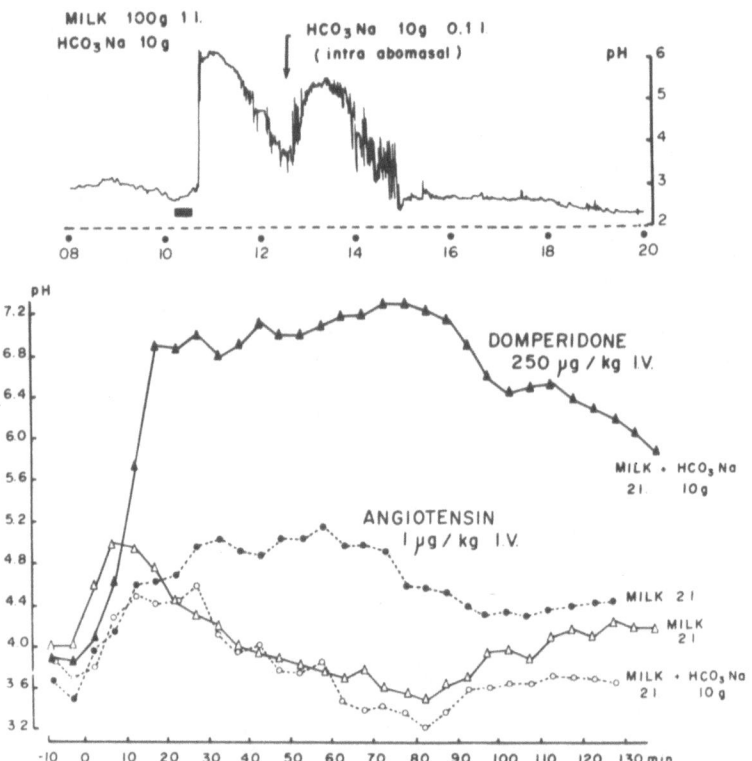

FIGURE 4. Top. Direct reading of pH distal to the pylorus in a calf during weaning, receiving milk and 10 g of sodium bicarbonate from a nipple with full closure of the reticular groove and high rate of salivation. The rise in pH is mimicked by bicarbonate administered directly into the stomach 2 h later.
Below. pH values of the chyme leaving the abomasum of a young steer drinking 2 l of milk after angiotensin or 2 l of milk plus sodium bicarbonate before and after prokinetic (domperidone) pretreatment.

The xylose absorption test has been applied to evaluate the degree of groove closure in sheep after cupric ions administration (10 ml of 10% $CuSO_4$). A detectable rise in xylosemia occurs when D-xylose (0.5 g/kg BW) is administered orally but not via a rumen cannula (19). In calves, at the time of weaning, no rise in xylosemia is detectable when bucked fed, even after a 24-h fast (food and water) whereas nipple feeding always results in a marked increase of xylosemia within 60 min. Direct reading of pH of the chyme in the proximal duodenum of calves shows a marked increase by 2 to 3 units due to saliva swallowed during nipple feeding, suggesting a full closure of the oesophageal groove, while there was only a tendency of increase in pH after bucket feeding (Fig. 4). A complete closure must occur for nipple feeding since duodenal pH values were similar to those seen after a direct abomasal administration (Fig. 4).

In adult sheep, to ascertain that a drug is delivered into the reticulo-rumen for a local action, three possibilities are at hand to prevent the activation of the reflex: injection of atropine, application of local anaesthetics to the oral cavity, and placing the drug into the thoracic oesophagus via a gastric tube. The latter procedure is generally recommended for its simplicity and effectiveness.

A major component of the oesophageal groove reflex has been noted by Orskov et al. (22): closure of the groove site seeing a nipple-bottle. The increased excitability provoked by showing the nipple-bottle was sufficient, in a trained sheep, to double or triple the volume of liquid collected from an abomasal fistula, after administration of that liquid into the lower oesophagus.

A significant ruminal bypass of drinking water also occurred in lactating cows. When water was withheld for 4.5 or 9 h following feeding, 18% of drinking water was found to bypass the rumen in 8 rumen-fistulated Holstein cows (39).

The inhibition of rumino-reticular contractions during the closure of the groove as reported in a 12 month-old bull when sucking 2 l of milk from a watering can (13), was mimicked by L-DOPA (1 mg/kg) and suppressed by metoclopramide (0.2 mg/kg) pretreatment (23). In young steers (6 month-old) fitted with reentrant cannula distal to the pylorus, the pH values were measured about 3 weeks after weaning during oral administration by bottle of 2 l milk and 10 g $NaHCO_3$. A more complete rumen bypass following domperidone (0.5 mg/kg i.m. or 0.25 mg/kg i.v.) was found (Fig. 4). In such cases the pH values remain at a very high level for about 2 h. In

28

similar trials using angiotensin II in order to elicit drinking behaviour, a gradual rise in pH was also recorded. However, a decrease in gastric acid secretion rather than a reflex closure of the groove could be involved. Nevertheless, it is noteworthy that the responses varied from day to day and among individuals as recently described by Wise and Anderson (38).

IV. RESETTING OF CYCLICAL OMASAL ACTIVITY

The omasal pressure in sheep recorded, by a balloon in the interlamellar space close to the greater curvature, shows a prolonged increase of smooth muscle tone. The high pressure phase which exists during half of the time interval between two reticular contractions, suddenly droped at the onset of each reticular contraction, an indication of involvement of a pump mechanism in the flow of digesta (4). The corresponding electrical activity was characterized by a series of slow waves and spikes termed group discharge, lasting from 12 to 40 sec and always ceasing at the onset of the reticular contraction in sheep. This resetting effect of the reticulum on the omasal cyclic activity is emphasized during feeding since the duration of omasal contractions is reduced as are the intervals

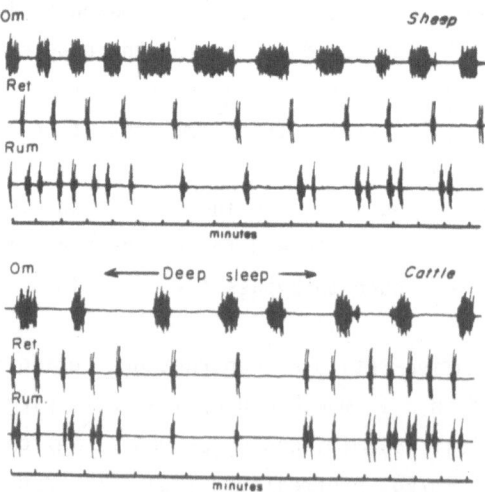

FIGURE 5. Electrical activity of the omasum (Om.) recorded as prolonged spike discharges occurring cyclically and which ceased at the onset of the reticulo-rumen (Ret-Rum) contractions. This was observed in sheep but not in cattle during the decreased reticulo-rumen contractions during deem sleep.

between reticular contractions. During sleep, the omasal activity is prolonged until the occurrence of a contraction of the reticulum. As shown in Fig. 5, this phenomenon did not occur for cattle in which the omasal body contracts less frequently than the reticulum.

The omasal activity which persists under general anaesthesia and during local anaesthesia of the cervical vagus nerves thus appears to be mostly influenced locally by the nature and volume of contents; e.g. pelleted food in contrast to hay causes a reduction of the motility index of the omasal body. The reticulo-omasal orifice opens to a diameter of 8-16 mm at the onset of a reticular contraction. This opening was followed by 4-5 alternating opening and closing which are progressively less pronounced (18). The rate of contractions of the omasal leaves which is increased by the presence of VFA (50 ml of 75 mM, pH 5.9) is different (2-4/min) from that of the omasal groove at 6-8 sec intervals. Of interest is the fact that in cattle, measurement of the digestive movements through the orifice showed the reflux of solid at irregular intervals (Dardillat, unpublished observations).

V. EXTRACONTRACTION OF THE RETICULUM

The sequence of reticulo-rumen contractions starts with a biphasic reticular contraction in sheep or goats, and two separated reticular contractions in cattle. When ruminating, a contraction of the reticulum alone precedes the normal reticular contraction.

Beside the communition of contents by masticatory movements, rumination has two effects on the passage of digesta: (i) an increased rate of digesta flow from the reticulo-rumen to the abomasum through the omasal canal in sheep, and (ii) the emptying of the material stored in the omasal body as a consequence of 2 or 3 long-lasting reticulo-rumen movements at the end of a period of rumination in sheep, hence a lower resetting effect on the omasal body contraction (14).

The role of central influences is demonstrated by the occurrence of an extracontraction of the reticulum preceding the normal biphasic reticular contractions as a conditioned reflex (7). The role of peripheral influences is demonstrated by the increase of up to 10 hr per day of the time spent ruminating in relation with the coarseness of food. The rumen is not actively involved in rumination so this terminology is somewhat a misnomer. The bolus rejected from the reticulum is actively carried past the zone where oesophageal distension evokes a secondary peristaltic wave.

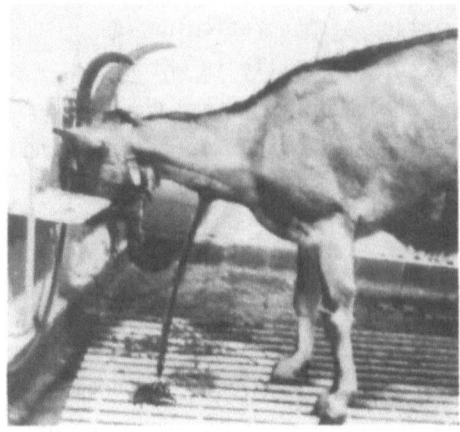
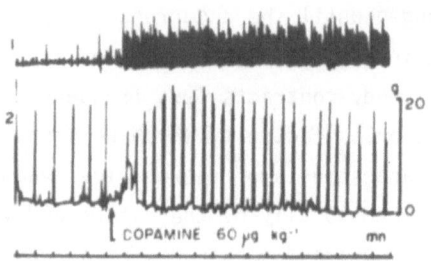
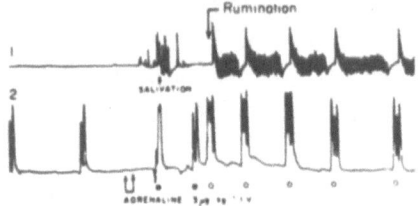

FIGURE 6. Left side: Regurgitation of reticulo-ruminal contents propelled at a velocity of 50 cm/sec from the cardia towards the oral cavity in the goat when an oesophageal cannula was opened as soon as the animal exhibited an inspiratory effort. The absence of chewing movements when the bolus was derived initiated a premature extra-reticular contraction. Right side, upper tracing: Recording of jaw movements (1) and reticular pressure by means of a strain gauge (2) in sheep showing a period of rumination following the intravenous administration of dopamine (60 μg/kg). Lower tracing: Recordings at a high speed of the increased salivary secretion and regurgitation efforts following the intravenous administration of adrenaline (3 μg/kg)

Velocity (50 cm/sec) and force (40 mm Hg) of the oesophageal contraction during regurgitation are sufficient to propel the bolus into the pharynx, without further active contraction in the proximal oesophagus (Fig. 6). The oesophageal reflux is facilitated by relaxation of the lower oesophageal sphincter (LOS). Manipulation of the LOS or reticulo-ruminal folds induces salivation and attempts to regurgitate within a few minutes, and when successful a series of rumination cycles. Other reflexogenic areas able to induce rumination in sheep are the contraction of the reticulum induced by dopamine or adrenaline (Fig. 6), omasal contractions elicited by pentagastrin or xylazine and also stimulation of the antroduodenal area evoked by several substances like naloxone, 5-HT, tolazoline (28).

Into explaining the mechanisms involved in the time spent ruminating in

relation with the amount of food and its texture, a major role is
attributed to the cranial pillars as peripheral sensors, as emphasized
by the observations of pseudorumination. Such a behaviour is observed
as brief periods of chewing movements following extracontractions of
the reticulum when regurgitation is impaired, e.g. in animals on a
liquid diet. When plastic fibres are introduced to an empty and isolated
rumen in calves fed via abomasal infusion, the time spent in pseudo-
rumination may reach 36% of the recording time versus less than 4-5%
when the rumen is emptied.

VI. INTRINSIC MOTOR ACTIVITY

Local motor activity of the reticulo-rumen wall is recorded as
bursts of spike potentials occurring at a high frequency during the
intervals of the phasic contractions in the rumen (14-18/min).
In agreement with a more dense network of multipolar neurons in the
plexuses in the reticulum than in the rumen, the intervals between
the bursts of spike potentials averaged 1.5-2 sec for the reticulum and
4-10 sec for the rumen. After section of the right vagus nerve in the
neck, these bursts have a tendency to be clustered in group discharges
occurring every 6 sec on the rumen dorsal sac. After section of the
left vagus nerve, group discharges are seen on the whole reticulo-rumen.
In contrast to the minor effects of the right or the left cervical
vagotomy, section of the dorsal vagal trunk mainly involves the dorsal
and ventral sacs of the rumen and considerably impairs their motor
activity (Fig. 7, bottom). Within 15 days, the activity becomes
polyphasic with rumen stasis, a low level rumination and bloating
suggesting an increased sphincteric tone at the LOS. After section
of the two vagal trunks (Fig. 7, top), the activity of the whole
reticulo-rumen consists of group discharges occurring at the same
frequency intervals of 4-10 sec (15). This activity, after 13-15 d,
resembles that of long-lasting group discharges seen after cervical
bivagotomy (9).

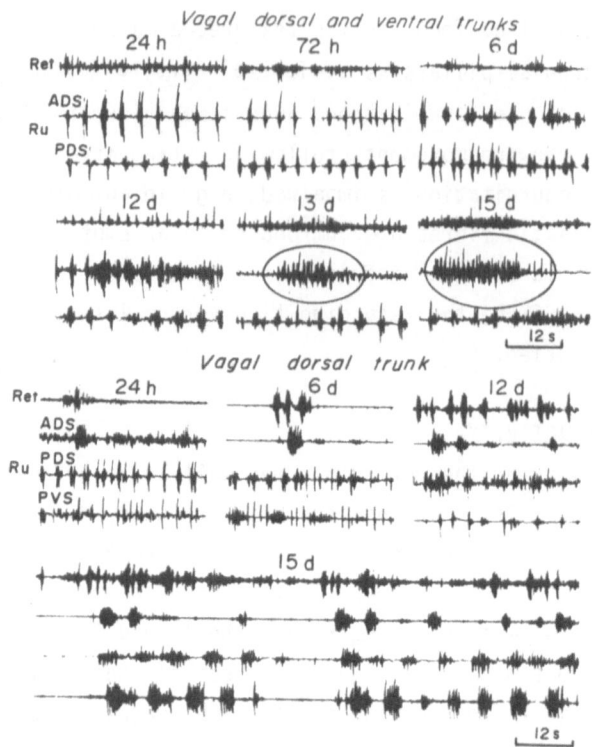

FIGURE 7. Intrinsic electrical activity of the reticulo-rumen after
section of either both vagal dorsal and ventral trunks (top) or vagal
dorsal trunk (bottom). Note that after bilateral vagotomy the local
discharges are grouped more rapidly on the anterior (ADS, 13 and 15
days after nerve section) than on the posterior dorsal sac (PDS) of
the rumen. After section of the vagal torsal trunk, the posterior
dorsal and ventral sacs of the rumen show isolated spike bursts (14/min
1 to 12 days after nerve section), and after 15 days group discharges
(6/min) are exhibited.

The patterns of intrinsic reticulo-ruminal motility in chronically-
vagotomized sheep depend upon the degree of distension, the post-
vagotomy time and the concentration of volatile fatty acids (VFA). The
consistent relationship which exists in vagotomized sheep between
the frequency of group discharges and the rumen volume suggests a
neurally-integrated activity at the myenteric plexus level. Atropine
(0.1 mg/kg) and hexamethonium (2 mg/kg), as well as cold water (30°C)
abolish this local activity with subsequent increase in ruminal volume
by 20% (9). Warmed 0.2 M acetic, propionic or butyric acids buffered to
pH 4.0 abolish the group discharges, the inhibition being more rapid

(3 min) for butyric and propionic than for acetic acid (7-17 min).
A major role for the enteric nervous system could therefore be the
maintenance of a basal smooth muscle tone in relation with the local
production of VFA. A myogenic origin however could not be excluded
(see chap. 4).

In vitro, the regular fluctuations of the resting membrane potential,
and hence of muscle excitability, are seen as minute rhythms with slow
waves when the longitudinal muscle layer is well-developed. The
spontaneous activity of isolated strips of the rumen is usually less
important for the ventral sax than for the dorsal sac to field
stimulation, suggesting a larger area of coordination by the enteric
neural network.

VII. SECONDARY CONTRACTIONS OF THE RUMEN

The ratio of primary to secondary ruminal contractions usually shifts
from 2:1 at rest to 1:1 after feeding as a consequence of ruminal
distension in sheep (35). An excess of VFA in the rumen (9) or fat in
the duodenum (20), decreases the rate of secondary ruminal contractions
enhanced by insufflatjon. In cattle, these secondary contractions may
persist during the inhibition of the primary ruminal contractions
induced by abomasal distension. The secondary ruminal contractions in
cattle thus appear to be "more intrinsic" than for small ruminants.

Accordingly, the secondary contractions of the rumen persist in
cattle but not in sheep after blockade of the reticulo-rumen movements
by xylazine which acts centrally at a presynaptic level; this effect is
relieved by tolazoline (25) or yohimbine suggesting that the presynaptic
receptors are α_2-receptors. In cattle too, after intramuscular injection
of an opiate agonist like fentanyl (30 µg/kg), the rate of reticulo-rumen
contractions was reduced by 50% during the phase of excitation and
bruxism. Such central effects of opiate agonists are potentiated by
pretreatment with H_1-receptor antagonist (promethazone, 0.3 mg/kg),
so that fentanyl becomes able to block the reticulo-rumen contractions.
However, the secondary ruminal contractions which are thus not drived
by reticulo-rumen contractions persist indicating an escape phenomenon
elicited at the enteric nervous system level. It is noteworthy that
sheep are not responsive to this opiate-antihistamine interaction.

VIII. BASIC REST-ACTIVITY CYCLE OF THE GASTRODUODENAL JUNCTION

The development of migrating myoelectric complexes (MMCs), initiated at the gastroduodenal junction (GDJ) at intervals of 90-120 min in sheep and of 40-60 min in cattle (30), corresponds to an antroduodenal interrelation in which antral activity ceases at the occurrence of a period of regular spiking activity (RSA phase or phase III of the MMC) in the duodenal bulb (34). This ultradian rhythm is generated locally by the enteric nervous system (36) and its frequency can be enhanced by the use of lysergic acid derivatives, e.g. methysergide (29).

Since the pancreatico-biliary duct opens into the duodenum far from the pylorus and that gastric emptying is almost continuous with a mean flow rate higher than 200 ml/hr in sheep, the ruminant duodenum, in contrast to many other monogastric species, is exposed to large amount of acidic digesta. The chyme is not neutralized by the duodenal secretions

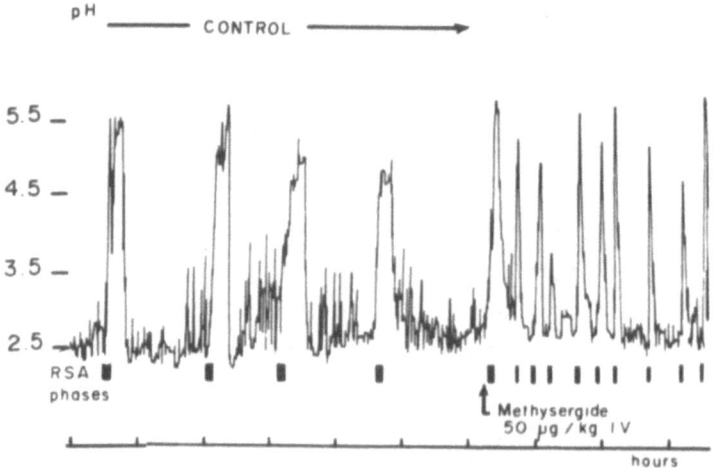

FIGURE 8. MMC-related changes in intraduodenal pH before and after 50 µg/kg methysergide IV in sheep (arrow). Solid bars indicate periods of RSA. Note the rise in pH at the end of RSA to 4.5-6.5 during the phase of quiescence (29).

which are less than 10-15 ml/h. The periodic interruption of abomasal emptying which coincides with the RSA phase development of the duodenum, is at the origin of duodenal pH rises. MMC-related changes of pH of duodenal contents measured via a small pH electrode introduced into the duodenal lumen consisted of a mean pH value of 2,9 during the ISA phase and of about 4.8 during the RSA phase and quiescence. Accordingly, the increased MMC rhythmicity by methysergide treatment was accompanied by concomitant cyclical changes in pH (Fig. 8).

IX. LOCAL DETERMINANTS OF ABOMASAL OUTFLOW

The electrical activity of the pyloric antrum is characterized by slow waves at a frequency of 6.5/min in sheep or goats, with almost continuous bursts of spike potentials of 2-sec duration (27). Some of these bursts are coupled with spike potentials in the duodenum which does not show slow waves over the first 10 cm beyond the pylorus. In cattle, the frequency of antral slow waves is less regular and about 50% of them are superimposed by bursts of spike potentials and pass aborally into the duodenum (21). However, the rate of emptying of the abomasum cannot be assessed from either the electrical or mechanical activity because of changes in pyloric diameter. Ultrasound imaging of the pylorus in cattle shows that the pylorus behaves as a ring muscle which closes the gastric outlet (16).

The pyloric sphincter activity assessed in the conscious sheep by continuous measurement of changes in impedance consisted of transient contractions following the antral contractions that propagated through the gastroduodenal junction. A long-lasting pyloric closure also occurred during the period of antral quiescence following the development of an RSA phase. The consequence of this pyloric closure is the transient absence of propulsion of acidic chyme through the pylorus as well as the absence of reflux of digesta from the duodenal bulb reservoir into the antrum (Fig. 9). Another pattern of activity indicated by changes in diffused fiberoptic light was periodical contractions at the rate of 4 to 6/min during the intervals of antroduodenal contractions. This pattern, which persisted after cholinergic and ganglioplegic blockade, was enhanced by cholecystokinin, indicating an intrinsic activity hormonally mediated.

Electromagnetic measurements of duodenal digesta flow in cannulated sheep (24) show that the increases in the cumulative flow are associated with an increased volume rather than the number of gushes at the GDJ level. Unlike for more aboral parts of the small intestine, the net aboral flow was not increased just before the development of the RSA phase of the migrating complex (Fig. 9).

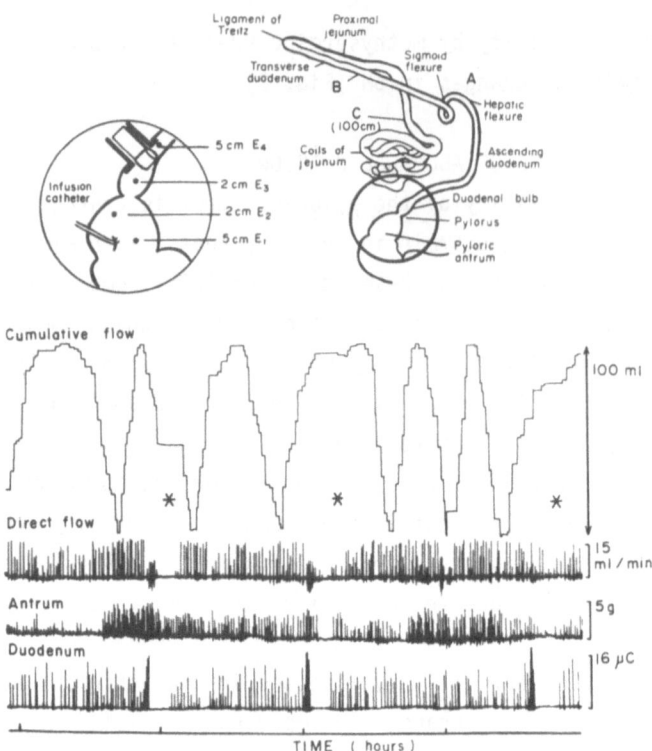

FIGURE 9. Composite line drawing illustrating radiographic anatomy of the ovine antroduodenal junction according to the studies performed at the Rowett Research Institute. Insert shows the position of the electro-magnetic flowmeter probe. Below, characteristics of the duodenal spiking activity associated to the abomasal outflow measured 5 cm distal to the pylorus. Note on the cumulative flow recording, the absence of passage of digesta (X) during antro-duodenal quiescence.

The relations between motility, abomasal outflow and digestive constituents were validated in sheep during continuous total enteral nutrition as described by Orskov et al. (23). In sheep receiving intra-abomasal infusion of casein solution at the rate of 166 ml/hr over period lasting 3 to 6 weeks, the outflow was linearly related to the stroke volume varying between 3.6 to 5.9 ml. In addition, diurnal variations were linked to a lower percentage of propagated contractions onward from the pyloric area. In this model, the outflow was decreased by 20-30% without major effects on motility for 1-2 h when the viscosity of the casein solution was increased by saline containing 100% guar gum. The infusion of saline instead of the casein solution had opposite effects

with again no changes in motor activity. In contrast with the results
recorded in neonate calves, acid solutions as well as hypertonic
solutions did not inhibit gastric emptying by a negative feedback
mechanism (2).

X. REGULATION OF MOTILITY PATTERNS

Depression of the gastric centres, lack of excitatory neural input,
increased inhibitory input from the omaso-abomasal compartment and
blockade of motor pathways are potential factors involved in the reduced
motor activity of the ruminant stomach.

X.1. Reticulo-rumen turnover rates of digesta

The characteristic patterns of reticulo-rumen motility are linked with
the intensity of masticatory movements during feeding. In addition, changes
in the ration of secondary to primary ruminal contractions from 0.5 to
0.67 indicate that the high rate of reticular motility reinforces the
mechanical performance of the rumen.

During rumination, the reticulo-rumen movements are more sustained and
prolonged in the ventral than the dorsal sacs of the rumen. The opening
of the reticulo-omasal orifice during the reticular extracontraction and
an increased rate of salivary secretion are additional factors which
facilitate the comminution and outflow of digesta. In sheep, the duration
of rumination increases from 5 to 6 h/kg intake of dry matter when eating lucerne with a reduction of 60-70% due to the size of particles.
Measurement of the reticulo-rumen motility and digesta turnover in the
forestomach of steers adapted to diets with varying proportions of hay
shows that the higher the frequency of reticulum contractions, the higher
turnover rate of liquid rumen digesta. Since the variations in such
processes were induced by changes in diet composition and not in the
rumen volume, a positive relationship between frequency of reticular
contractions and turnover rate of liquid rumen digesta is thus demonstrated.
Accordingly, the increase in reticulo-rumen turnover rate of digesta
during frequent versus infrequent feeding in cattle may be an effect of
the induced changes in the reticulo-rumen motor performance.

A positive relationship also existed between digestibility of a diet
and retention time of the food in the reticulum. The relation is
curvilinear for high fibre diet, because lignin sets an upper limit to the
digestibility of cellulose. For example, the lower digestibility of grass

pellets, observed in sheep during exposure to cold results from a reduced
retention time of the diet in the reticulo-rumen.

In recent studies performed in goats, distension of the cranial rumen
was associated with inhibition of growth hormone release and a fall in
plasma GH concentration, supporting the concept that inhibition of GH
release by the intake of roughage may be mediated by receptors which are
known to be concentrated in the cranial rumen and reticulum (15). Since
the major target sensory information is the nucleus of the solitary tract
which projects directly to hypothalamic nuclei, there is a well-defined
route for afferent neural input to reach the hypothalamus and influence
neuroendocrine mechanisms associated with gastric filling, concomitant
motility patterns and food intake (32).

X.2. Peripheral versus central control of rumination

The inherent drive for rumination occurs as early as 5 days after
birth in camels, and is present in preruminant lambs maintained on a milk
diet. Pseudorumination, which can reach very high levels, is an
alternative to rumination in milk-fed calves.

Central effects resembling those of GABA, a cerebral vasodilator which
facilitates drowsiness and rumination (unpubl. results), are also observed
with several substances which modify the metabolism of serotonin. However,
the site of action is presumably different from the area postrema (3).
It has been suggested that insulin hypoglycaemia may be a triggering
factor for the rumination centre, although the ruminant differs from
other mammals in that the most important source of glucose is the hepatic
gluconeogenesis from aminoacids and propionic acids.It is now well-
established that the role of insulin in the shortterm control of feeding
and/or rumination, if any, depends on the nutritional status. In
addition, factors involved in the decrease of immunoreactive serum insulin,
like clonidine in cattle, are able to depress central nervous system by
their alpha 2-adrenergic receptor agonistic properties, like xylazine (22)
and have no major effect on rumination.

In sheep fitted with a duodenal reentrant cannula, the physical
stimulation may be the cause of an excess of rumination. For example, in a
43-44 kg sheep, an increase by 30-40% of the time spent ruminating was
found related to the increased resistance of the flow of digesta. Factors
which induce satiety like gastrin-like peptides, when administered

centrally or peripherally (10) also enhance the occurrence of rumination. For example, the arrest of eating by cholecystokinin (CCK) which has been identified in sheep brain as a satiety factor, is then followed by rumination. The fact that several effects of CCK-like peptides are antagonized by enkephalins, is consistent with the involvement of a neuropeptidergic system in the initiation of feeding and with a role of an enkephalinergic pathway in the initiation of rumination.

X.3. Transpyloric flow of digesta

The regulating factors of the "steady" transpyloric flow involve the differential pressures between the fundus and antrum and between the pyloric antrum and duodenal bulb (34) and enterogastric reflexes originating in the duodenal bulb via tension and chemical receptors with vagal afferent fibres (6).

During duodenal acidification, the local release of somatostatin parallels that of 5-HT and it is possible that this peptide suggested in preruminant calves as a factor involved in the "duodenal brake" mechanism (2), may inhibit antral activity, and therefore the net effects would be a reduction in the flow of less acidic digesta.

According to Nicholson and Omer (20), the gradual inhibition of forestomach motility after the transpyloric passage of unsaturated long-chain fatty acids, suggests the involvement of an endocrine rather than a purely neural mechanism mediating the response. The release of CCK which reduces the frequency rather than the amplitude of forestomach motility could be this hormone.

The concept of a pyloric response mediated through a local neural path-way and involving an endogenous opioid peptide has been recently proposed in the cat. An opioid modulation of the passage of digesta through the pylorus could thus be the result of a local effect (36). Since the serotonin enhancement of the cyclical motor events at the GDJ also appears to be peripheral, an antagonism between these pathways should be noted. The enhancement of the cyclical activity of the junction by methysergide was prevented by methylnaloxone pretreatment (33).

XI CONCLUSIONS

In conclusion, the reticulo-rumen gastroduodenal junction interrelation-ship suggests that pharmacological advances should be based on agents able to reinforce the antropyloric pump activity or withdraw the duodenal braking mechanism. An innovative therapeutic approach to problems of gastric emptying, and a still more exciting possibility, concerns the restoration of the cyclical motor activity of the gastroduodenal junction when suppressed by metabolic, neural or hormonal derangements. Finally, the inhibition of growth hormone release by rumen distension in response to feeding suggests the possibility of increasing the amount of food intake by blocking or reducing the vagal information from the forestomach and antroduodenal area to the hypothalamus.

REFERENCES

1. Andersson, B., Kitchell, R.L. and Persson, N.: Acta Physiol. 46: 319-338 (1959).
2. Bell, F.R., Green, A.B., Wass, J.A.H., Webber, D.E.: J. Physiol. (Lond.) 321: 603-610 (1981).
3. Bost, J., McCarthy, L.E., Colby, E.D. & Borison, H.L.: Physiol. Behav. 3: 877-881 (1968).
4. Buéno, L. and Ruckebusch, Y.: J. Physiol. (Lond.) 238: 295-312 (1974).
5. Burgin, H.: J. Vet. Pharmacol. Therap. 2: 305-311 (1979).
6. Cottrell, D.F. and Iggo, A.: J. Physiol. (Lond.) 354: 477-495 (1984).
7. Dedashev, I.P.: Setchenov. J. Physiol (Paris) 45: 104-108 (1959).
8. Dussardier, M.: J. Physiol. (Paris) 40: 170-173 (1955).
9. Gregory, P.C.: J. Physiol. (Lond.) 346: 379-393 (1984).
10. Grovum, W.L. and Chapman, H.W.: Regul. Peptides 5: 35-42 (1982).
11. Harding, R. and Leek, B.F.: J. Physiol. (Lond.) 225: 309-338 (1972).
12. Hill, K.J.: Quart. J. Exp. Physiol. 40: 32-39 (1955).
13. Kay, R.N.B. and Ruckebusch, Y.: Br. J. Nutr. 26: 301-309 (1971).
14. Laplace, J.P.: Physiol. Behav. 5: 61-65 (1970).
15. Leek, B.F.: Vet. Rec. 97: 10-14 (1983).
16. Malbert, C.H. and Ruckebusch, Y.: Revue Méd. Vét. 136: 103-108 (1985).
17. Mathieu, C.M.: Ann. Biol. Anim. Bioch. Biophys. 8: 581-583 (1968).
18. Newhook, J.C. and Titchen, D.A.: J. Physiol. (Lond.) 237: 243-258 (1979).
19. Nicholson, T.: Can. J. Anim. Sci. 64: 187-188 (1984).
20. Nicholson, T. and Omer, S.A.: Br. J. Nutr. 50: 141-149 (1983).
21. Ooms, L. and Oyaert, W.: Zbl. Vet. Med. A25: 464-473 (1978).
22. Orskov, E.R., Benzie, D. and Kay, R.N.B.: Br. J. Nutr. 24: 785-795 (1970).

23. Orskov, E.R., MacLeod, N.A., Kay, R.N.B. and Gregory, P.L.: Can. J. Anim. Sci. 64: 138-139 (1984).

24. Poncet, C. and Ivan, M.: Reprod. Nutr. Dévelop. 24: 887-902 (1984).

25. Roming, L.G.P.: Dtsch. Tierärztl. Wschr. 91: 154-157 (1984).

26. Rousseau, J.P. and Falempin, M.: Reprod. Nutr. Dévelop. 25: 763-775 (1985).

27. Ruckebusch, Y.: J. Physiol. (Lond.) 254: 79-80 P (1976).

28. Ruckebusch, Y.: J. Vet. Pharmacol. Therap. 6: 245-272 (1983).

29. Ruckebusch, Y.: Gastroenterology 87: 1049-1055 (1984).

30. Ruckebusch, Y. and Bardon, T.: C.R. Acad. Sci. 296: 921-926 (1983).

31. Ruckebusch, Y. and Buéno, L.: Am. J. Physiol. 233: E484-E487 (1977).

32. Ruckebusch, Y. and Malbert, C.H.: Life Sci. 38: 929-934 (1986).

33. Ruckebusch, Y. and Merrit, A.M.: J. Vet. Pharmacol. Therap. 8: 339-351 (1985).

34. Ruckebusch, Y. and Pairet, M.: Zbl. Vet. Med. A31: 401-413 (1984).

35. Ruckebusch, Y. and Tomov, T.: J. Physiol. (Lond.) 235: 447-458 (1973).

36. Ruckebusch, Y., Bardon, T. and Pairet, M.: Life Sci. 35: 1731-1738 (1984).

37. Szabo, T. and Dussardier, M.: Z. Zellforsch. 63: 247-276 (1964).

38. Wise, G.H. and Anderson, G.W.: J. Dairy Sci. 67: 1983-1992 (1984).

39. Woodford, S.T., Murphy, M.R., Davis, C.L. and Homes, K.R.: J. Dairy Sci. 67: 2471-2474 (1984).

3. NEUROTRANSMITTERS / NEUROMODULATORS INVOLVED IN THE MOTOR AND SECRETORY FUNCTIONS OF THE RUMINANT STOMACH: A HISTOCHEMICAL, RADIOIMMUNOLOGICAL, IMMUNOCYTOCHEMICAL AND FUNCTIONAL APPROACH

A. WEYNS, L. OOMS, A. VERHOFSTAD, TH. PEETERS, A.D. DEGRYSE, L. van NASSAUW AND P. KREDIET

I. INTRODUCTION

The gastrointestinal tract of all mammals studied so far is richly
innervated by a remarkable complex and interconnected extrinsic and
intrinsic neuronal network which is heterogeneous in morphology,
histochemistry and function (1). The most important component in the neural
control of the gut is the enteric nervous system. This is an integrative
system that programs and coordinates the varied motility patterns of the
gut (2).

Morphologically and functionally there are two divisions of this system
the sympathetic and the parasympathetic, each made up of praeganglionic
and postganglionic neurons. The cell bodies of the praeganglionic neurons
lie in the brainstem or spinal cord and those of the postganglionic
neurons in the autonomic ganglia. The praeganglionic sympathetic neurons

are in the intermediomedial and intermediolateral cell columns of the
thoracic and upper lumbar cord. Some praeganglionic pathways remain
intraspinally for up to several segments before exiting through ventral
roots to reach the sympathetic trunk. Axons to thoracic ganglia arise
from ipsilateral sympathetic praeganglionic neurons but those reaching
lumbar ganglia are of bilateral origin. Therefore, crossed and uncrossed
intraspinal praeganglionic pathways exist. The praeganglionic fibers
synapse in the sympathetic chain or traverse several ganglia up or down
the chain before synapsing, or may pass through the ganglia to synapse in
ganglia near viscera (the coeliac-superior mesenteric complex and the
inferior mesenteric ganglion). These latter fibers form the splanchnic
nerves (3,4).

The praeganglionic neurons of the parasympathetic nervous system lie in
the visceral nuclei of the brainstem and in the intermediolateral column
of the sacral spinal cord. The major parasympathetic input of the gut
comes from the vagus. Its sensory fibers have their cell bodies in the
nodose ganglion and synapse in the dorsal nucleus of the vagus situated
in the medulla under the floor of the 4th ventricle. Axons from this
nucleus extend to the wall of the gut and make, via nicotinic cholinergic
receptors, synapses with the ganglionic cells within the myenteric and
submucosal ganglia (2). However catecholamine containing fibers originating
from some sympathetic ganglia i.e. the superior cervical and the stellate
ganglion were demonstrated in the vagal nerve too (5).

So the vagal nerves contain at least two distinct populations of
efferent axons: praeganglionic parasympathetic fibers and postganglionic
sympathetic axons. They make connection with intramural cholinergic
excitatory neurons and/or with intramural noncholinergic, nonadrenergic
inhibitory neurons. As a consequence the response to vagal stimulation
consists very often of a mixture of both excitation and inhibition (6).
The postganglionic parasympathetic fibers on the other hand originate
mainly in the gut wall receiving however a contribution from the dorsal
(vagal nerve) and the intermediolateral (sacral nerves) nucleus (4).

Intrinsic neurons have their cell bodies located in ganglionic
formations within the gut wall. The two ganglionated plexuses, Auerbach's
(myenteric) and Meissner's (submucous) plexus, are the principal sites of
these perikarya. Between the longitudinal and circular smooth muscle layer
of the intestine are prominent aggregates of ganglion cell bodies. They

are interconnected by a rich network of nerve fibers that is observed along the entire length of the gut.

Fibers run also across the circular muscle layer connecting the two main plexuses (7). Because of their position between the muscle layers the ganglia of the myenteric plexus must be greatly affected by the mechanical activity in the muscle. The myenteric ganglia reflect in their changeable shape the degree of contractions in the surrounding muscle layer. Indeed in the fully distended intestine the ganglia are spread out, the neurons are flattened and arranged in a thin cell monolayer. Conversely in the maximally contracted intestine the ganglia become thicker (2-3 times) and the neurons lie side by side and tend to form a palisade. It is not known whether this "message" affects the neuronal activity (8).

For a number of reasons (structural, chemical and functional) the enteric nervous system may be considered as an unique part of the autonomic nervous system. In structure the ENS differs from the peripheral autonomic nervous system. Indeed enteric neurons are histologically different from the neurons of other autonomic ganglia: there is a compact organization of neural and glial elements in the ganglia of the ENS resulting in little or no extracellular space; they lack collagen (endoneural supporting sheats); the supporting cells resemble the glia of the central nervous system rather than Schwann cells; axons of the ENS are not individually enveloped in mesaxons and finally specialized blood vessels just outside the myenteric plexus give rise to a blood-myenteric barrier analogous to the blood-brain barrier.

The most striking chemical feature of the ENS is the abundance of putative and established neurotransmitters. No other region of the autonomic nervous system has yet been found to have such an abundance of neuroactive substances that characterize the ENS. Moreover many of these substances exist in the cell bodies and neuritic processes of intrinsic enteric nerves.

Functionally the ENS is unique in that it is the only part of the peripheral nervous system that can manifest reflex activity in vitro (9). This intrinsic capacity to give rise to neurally mediated reflexes includes that the gut must contain primary afferent neurons, interneurons and motor neurons able to excite or relax smooth muscles (9). For that purpose the system receives sensory informations from different types of receptors (chemo-, mechano- and tensionreceptors located in the intestinal wall), processes this information and generates an output that is appropriate for the control of the effector system (motility, secretion/absorption process). These are properties that are normally associated only with the central nervous system (2). Furthermore there is a discrepancy between the number of efferent fibers and the number of intramural nerve cell bodies. So many enteric neurons do not receive any direct input from the CNS (10,11). In fact only a small proportion of the enteric ganglion cells make a direct contact with vagal nerve fibers, so there is only a small morphological basis for any direct vagal control. This arrangement emphases the physiologically independence of the enteric nervous system from the central nervous system control (11). However the degree of the CNS control varies from region to region: oesophagus, stomach and large intestine are more dependent on the CNS input for the normal function than the small intestine, which appears to function quite normally in the absence of the CNS input (2).

Thus it is suggested that the autonomic outflow from the CNS serves only to modulate the activity of the enteric system which not only sends excitatory and inhibitory messages to the muscles of the gut but likewise contains in the interneurons of the ganglia the "programs" for gut activity (2).

Classically the autonomic efferent nerves have been divided into adrenergic and cholinergic. However a number of observations indicate the existence of other types of nerves distinguisable on morphological ground (p-type nerves) and on electrophysiological and pharmacological ground (non-cholinergic, non-adrenergic nerves) from the classical adrenergic and cholinergic nerves (see 7,12).

The existence of a large and complex peptidergic system in the gut wall has recently be recognized. Peptide containing nerves form a complex mesh of nerve fibers and cell bodies with a well defined architecture forming newly described peptidergic pathways. VIP, sub. P and the enkephalins are the most abundant peptides of the gut wall. They all display a characteristic distribution pattern and architecture providing anatomical support for a separate and well defined set of actions (1). In addition it was found that some neuropeptides have a dual localization in the gut in that they occur in the endocrine cells as well.

Notwithstanding the enormous importance of the ruminant stomach pathology in veterinary medicine (and hence in economy) and the fact that

motility of the ruminant stomach wall depends upon the integrity of the
enteric nervous system (afferent/efferent nerves, intramural nervous
system), it is rather surprising to ascertain that little or no basic
morphological data concerning the intramural innervation of the ruminant
stomach are available from the literature.

However on morphological (complexity and volume) and functional (energy
production, gasproduction, secretion/absorption) grounds the ruminant
stomach may be considered as the most important and critical part of the
ruminant gastrointestinal tract. As a consequence this complex is
frequently involved in a broad spectrum of pathologies including
carbohydrate engorgement, acute and chronic ruminal tympany, vagus
indigestion, parakeratosis, villus atrophy, abomasal displacements,
primary acetonaemia etc., resulting every year in substantial economical
losses (low conversion of food, retardation of growth, premature
slaughtering, long lasting expensive medication).

The ruminant stomach is capable of a more complex pattern of activity
than simply the peristaltic reflex. Indeed not all motility is propulsive.
Several events are accomplished in complex but coordinated cycles of
forestomach motility: mixing and retaining of the ingesta for microbial
digestion, regurgitation, eructation of large quantities of gas and
finally controlled and ordely transport of the ingesta within the
forestomach complex (13). These different motility patterns have to be
appropriately controlled and coordinated with propulsive activity (14).
Certainly this is one of the main functions of the intramural enteric
nervous system.

Further one has to realise that the different parts of the stomach of
ruminants are closely associated anatomically and functionally. As a
consequence damage to one or other of these parts causes interference with
the normal stereotyped movements (mixing contractions, eructation
contractions etc.) resulting in the classical spectrum of the ruminant
stomach pathology (15).

Considering the vital importance of a perfectly functioning enteric
nervous system for the normal digestive functions and finally the health
of the ruminants and the fact that so little essential information
concerning the intramural enteric nervous system is available today, a
multidisciplinary study (morphological, radioimmunological and functional
approach) was undertaken.

Aims

The aims of this study are:

- to gain insight, primo in the basic morphological structure of the
  intramural nervous system of the ruminant stomach, secundo in the
  presence and typical distribution pattern of the different
  neurotransmitters/neuromodulators possibly involved in the functioning
  of the enteric nervous system.
- to provide basic morphologic and quantitative data for further
  physiological and functional research concerning the fundamental
  mechanisms controlling and coordinating the secretion/absorption
  process and the different motility patterns in the ruminant stomach.
- to increase our understanding of
  * the normal function of the ruminant stomach
  * the pathogenesis of the abnormalities in motility and in the
    secretion/absorption processes.
- to provide basic knowledge for appropriate therapy.

II MATERIAL AND METHODS

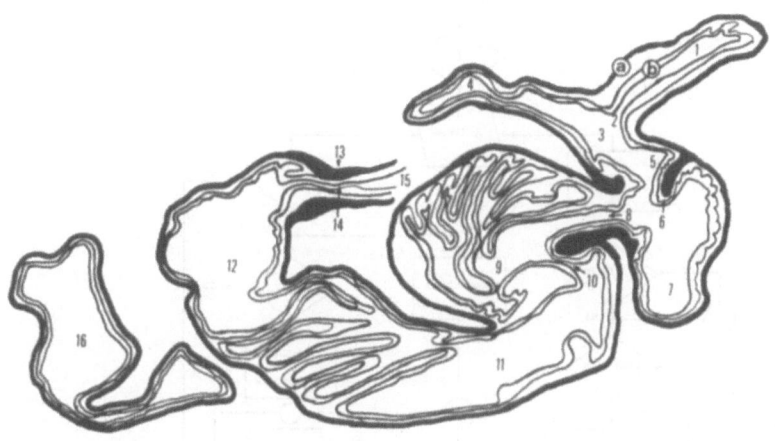

FIGURE 1. Reconstructive morphological picture of the ruminant stomach of
the sheep (foetus) illustrating the different segments investigated*.
a. tunica muscularis b. tunica mucosa
1. oesophagus 2. cardia 3. atrium ruminis 4. onset of the ruminal dorsal
sac (RDS)* 5. sulcus reticuli (oesophageal groove (OG))* 6. labium
dextrum 7. reticulum (Ret)* 8. ostium reticulo-omasicum 9. omasum
(OMA)* 10. ostium omasoabomasicum 11. abomasum (ABO)* 12. antrum
pyloricum (AP)* 13. sphincter pyloricus 14. canalis pyloricus (PYL)*
15. duodenum 16. onset of the ruminal ventral sac (RVS)*

Material

In this study six adult sheep (3 males and 3 females) and three foetuses (12, 20 and 37 cm) were investigated.

For each sheep specimens from the different stomach segments studied (see fig. 1), were taken for the morphological and radioimmunological study. For radioimmunoassay a part of all specimens was stripped (separation mucosa and submucosa from the muscularis).

The specimens from the foetuses were only histochemically (in toto preparations) and immunocytochemically studied.

Methods

It is beyond the scope of this contribution to describe in detail the different methods used in this study. Therefore they are only mentioned very briefly here and for more detailed information the reader is referred to the original articles (e.g. 16,17,18). An outline of our methodological approach is presented in fig. 2.

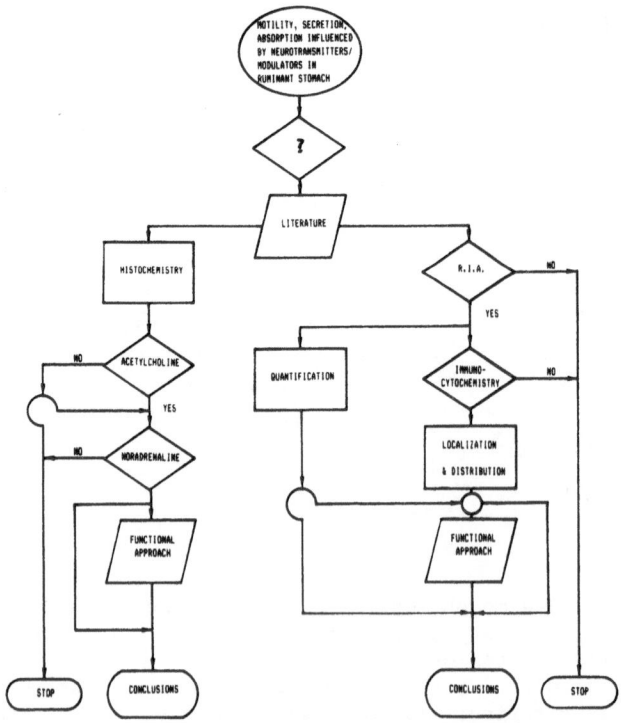

FIGURE 2. Outline of the methodological approach of the present study.

II.1. Histochemical study

- acetylcholinesterase (16)

  The different specimens were first fixed in a 6% buffered
  paraformaldehyde solution (pH: 7,4; $4^{o}C$; 48 h). After rinsing in buffer
  ($4^{o}C$; 48 h) they were incubated in toto with acetylthiocholine. After
  incubation they were washed, stored in 100% glycerin and micro-
  photographed.

- noradrenaline (17)

  Stripped pieces of the muscularis from the different segments were
  immersed in glycoxylic acid solution (1%). After the appropriated
  incubation time, the specimens were air dried, spread out, pinned up
  on a cork-plate and dried at $100^{o}C$.
  Small samples were then mounted in Entellan, serosal side up, and
  studied under the epifluorescence microscope (Leitz Orthoplan with
  Ploem Opak).

II.2. Immunocytochemical study (18)

After fixation in 10% buffered paraformaldehyde (pH 7,4; $4^{o}C$; 24h) the
specimens were embedded in Paraplast[R] following the classical histological
procedures. 5 micron thick serial sections were cut. Consecutive sections
were tested against serotonin (dilution 1/1000), vasoactive intestinal
polypeptide (dilution 1/1300) and substance P (dilution 1/1600) using
the unlabelled antibody peroxidase-antiperoxidase technique (P.A.P.) (19).

After the immunocytochemical procedure the sections were slightly
counterstained with cresylviolet 1% and evaluated under the light
microscope (Reichert Univar). Microphotographs were taken.

For the immunocytochemical part of this study the following specificity
tests were performed:

- absorption control. The specific primary antiserum was first incubated
  with the specific antigen followed by the immunocytochemical test.
- Omission of a stap in the immunocytochemical procedure i.e. incubation
  without primary antiserum. Thereafter the immunocytochemical reaction
  was performed.
- Incubation of some sections with a nonimmune or inappropriate
  antiserum.

II.3. Radioimmunoassay

Specimens for RIA were cut in two parts. One part was frozen immediately

in 2-methylbutane cooled with solid CO_2 (-70°C); the other part was first
stripped and than frozen. All the pieces were stored at -80°C.

VIP was measured using the procedure described by Long and Bryant (20).
Labeled VIP was from New England Nuclear (6072 Dreieck, D.B.R.), antibody
and porcine VIP standard were obtained from U.C.B. Bioproducts (B 1420
Braine - L'Alleud).

The assay system has a detection limit of 0,16 fmol/tube.

III HISTOCHEMICAL STUDY

III.1. Acetylcholine

It must be pointed out in advance that there are no good histochemical
methods for the detection of cholinergic nervous tissue. Although some
enteric neurons and nerve fibers contain AchE, this enzym can not be
relied upon a specific cholinergic marker. So it cannot be excluded that
other types of nerve fibers may stain for AchE without being cholinergic
(see 14,21,22).

It is argued that the myenteric plexus is primarily concerned with
motility, whereas the submucous plexus is thought to control absorptive
and secretory functions (12). As ruminal motility
can most readily be examined, it may be used as an index for the digestive
function in the ruminant (15). Therefore the presence and morphology
of Auerbach's plexus in the ruminal stomach wall was studied first.

The truncus vagalis dorsalis/ventralis were seen as very large AchE+
nerves. During their course over the ruminant stomach complex large AchE+
nerve fibers branch off. They terminate in part by branching into
mediumsized fibers either in the subserous or myenteric plexus. The latter
plexus is confined to the space between the circular and longitudinal
muscle layer where presumably certain mechanical conditions prevail (8).

The arrangement of the myenteric plexus in the different segments
examined, follows an essentially similar pattern throughout the ruminant
stomach complex. Passing from one ganglion mass to another are
interconnecting nerve strands forming a continuous open two dimensional
network, with the ganglia lying at irregular intervals in the nodes of
this meshwork.However differences in the prominence of the plexus, in the
size and shape of the ganglia, in the interganglionic nerve fibers and in
the density and distribution of nerve fibers between the muscle bundles
were observed. No discontinuity in the transition zones (oesophageal

53

groove, ostium reticulo-omasicum, pylorus) was observed.

In the ganglia of the myenteric plexus a range of intensity of AchE activity was regularly observed. Some cells show strong reactivity with other being moderately or very weakly stained. It has been suggested that sensory neurons may exhibited a low level of AchE activity. So no or lightly stained neurons possibly represent sensory neurons (see 23).

The mesoscopic picture of Auerbach's plexus, in the different segments investigated, will be discussed now briefly.

Ruminal dorsal sac (RDS) (see fig. 3).

Large polygonal ganglia alternate with more elongated ones. Large to mediumsized nerve bundles interconnect these ganglia forming an irregular nervous network. On the course of the interconnecting bundles small ganglia were regularly encountered. Small nerve bundles branch off from the interconnecting strands forming within the meshes of the network a clear interlacing plexus (secundary and tertiary plexus).

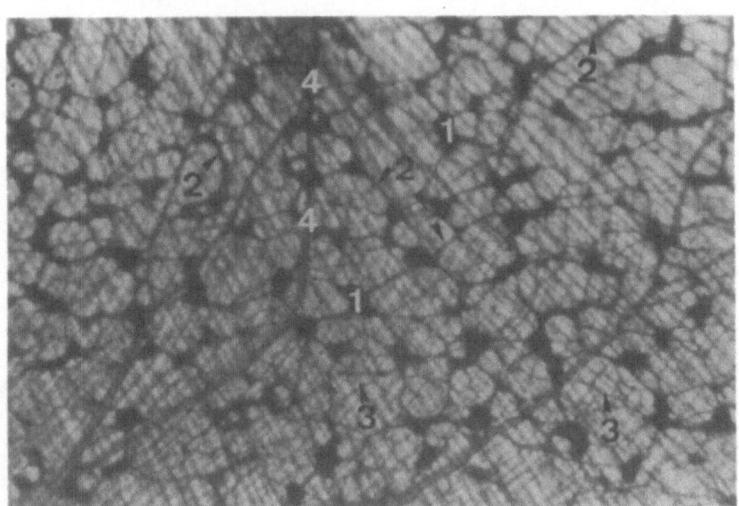

FIGURE 3. Ruminal Dorsal Sac (RDS; foetus sheep: 18 cm; 77x) Auerbach's plexus after in toto staining for AchE.
1. ganglion.   2. interganglionic nerve bundles (internodal strands).
3. interlaching AchE+ nervous network.   4. branch of the truncus vagalis dorsalis.

Ruminal ventral sac (RVS) (see fig. 4)

Taken as a whole the myenteric network of the RVS seems to be not so dense as in the RDS. Larger elongated and smaller more rounded ganglia together with thin and thick interganglionic nerve bundles constitute Auerbach's plexus. The meshes of this network are wider and more angular than in the RDS. The secundary and tertiary plexus is clearly established.

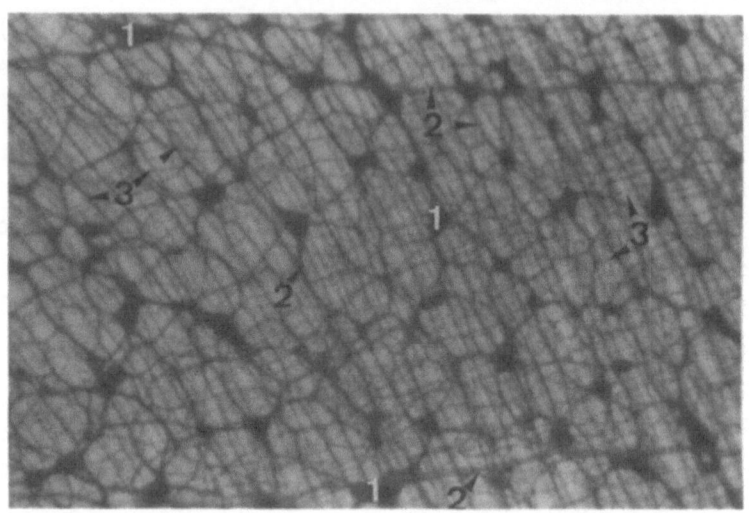

FIGURE 4. Ruminal Ventral Sac (RVS; foetus sheep: 18 cm; 113 x). Auerbach's plexus after in toto staining for AchE. Legend: see fig. 3.

Reticulum (RET) (see fig. 5).

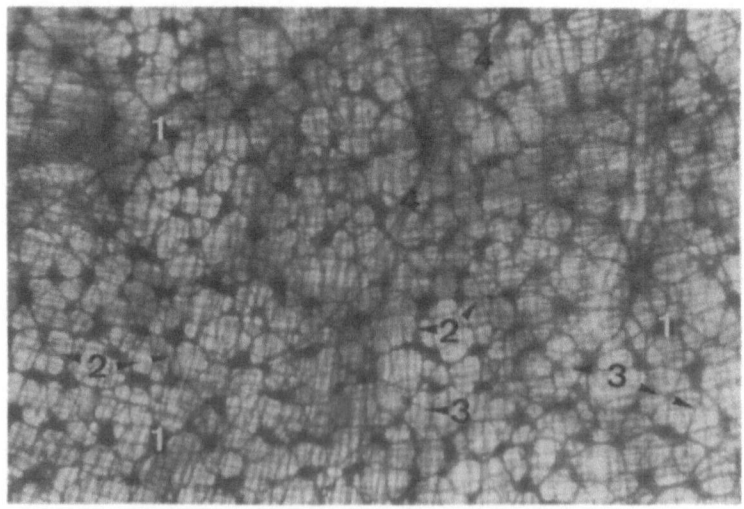

FIGURE 5. Reticulum (Ret; foetus sheep: 18 cm; 70 x). Auerbach's plexus after in toto staining for AchE. 1. ganglion 2. internodal strands. 3. interlaching AchE+ nervous network. 4. branch of the truncus vagalis ventralis.

A dense AchE+ nervous network is formed by large polygonal ganglia, thick interconnecting nerve strands and a distinct interlacing secondary and tertiary plexus. Comparing the rumen and the reticulum it is the impression that the weave pattern of the myenteric plexus in the reticulum is much denser than in the rumen.

Omasum (OMA) (see fig. 6)

Very large polygonal ganglia interconnected by thick bundles of nerve fibers were evidenced. They form a very dense AchE+ nervous network characterised by small, rounded meshes. The smaller nerve bundles, branching off from the large interganglionic bundles, form a distinguished interlacing plexus. It seems most probably that the densest AchE+ nervous network of the whole ruminant stomach complex is found in this segment.

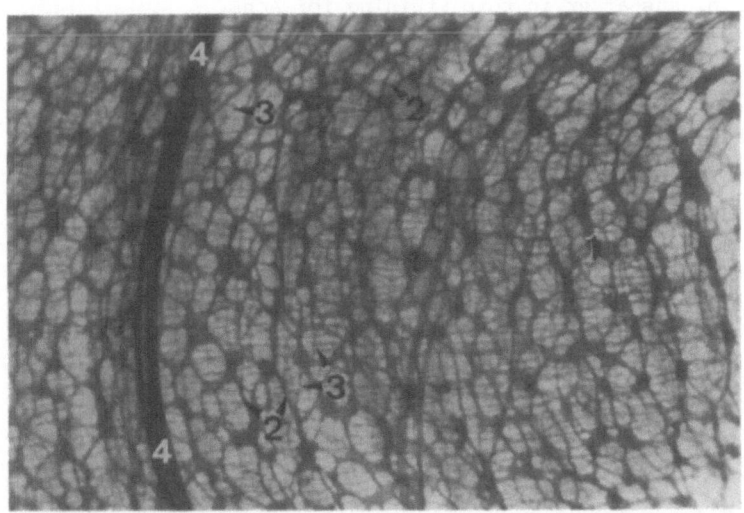

FIGURE 6. Omasum (OMA; foetus sheep: 18 cm; 70 x).
Auerbach's plexus after in toto staining for AchE. 4. truncus vagalis ventralis. Legend: see fig. 5.

Abomasum (ABO) (see fig. 7)

Large and small ganglia alternate and are connected by respectively thick and small nerve bundles. They constitute an uninterrupted nervous network characterised by more or less elliptical meshes of different dimensions. The secondary and tertiary plexus however seems not so distinctly developed as in the previous segments.

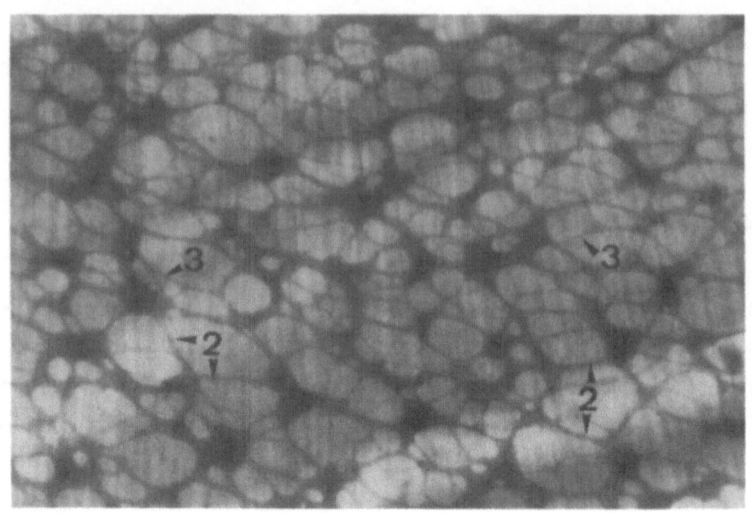

FIGURE 7. Abomasum (ABO; foetus sheep: 18 cm; 113 x).
Auerbach's plexus after in toto staining for AchE.
1. ganglion. 2. interganglionic nerve bundles. 3. interlaching AchE nervous
network.

Pylorus (PYL) (see fig. 8)

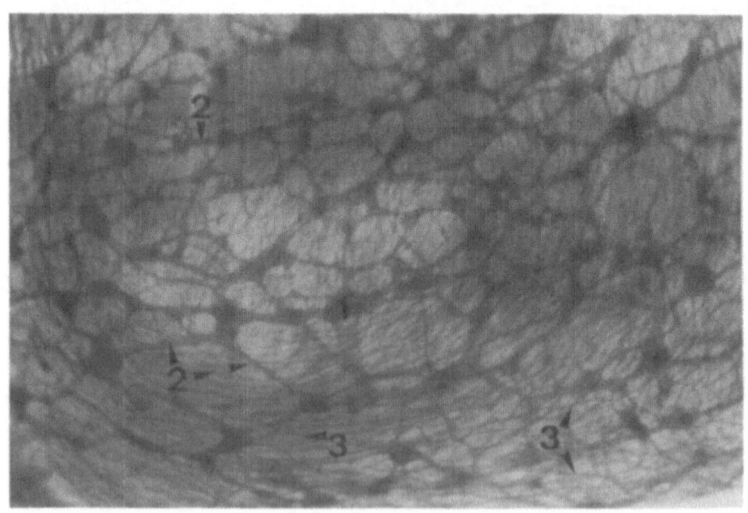

FIGURE 8. Pylorus (PYL; foetus sheep: 18 cm; 106 x).
Auerbach's plexus after in toto staining for AchE. Legend: see fig. 7.

In essence the same picture as described for the abomasum could be
evidenced. However a dense and well developed secundary and tertiary

plexus was always present and this may be the most striking feature of this segment. As already stated no discontinuity in the plexus between the pylorus and the duodenum could be demonstrated.

III.2. Noradrenaline

Most adrenergic nerves in wall of the ruminant stomach of the adult sheep terminate in the myenteric plexus, while the terminals in the smooth muscle of the gut are not well visualized. Thus the primary adrenergic innervation of the different segments seems to be contained within the myenteric plexus at all levels of the ruminant stomach.

In essence no basic difference in the adrenergic supply of the myenteric ganglia in the different segment of the ruminant stomach could be evidenced, although the size and shape of the ganglia do differ.

There is a dense supply of noradrenaline containing axons to the enteric ganglia and comparatively a sparse supply to the non sphincter smooth muscle (whereas cholinergic innervation is comparatively dense (vide supra)). So there is little morphological evidence for a direct innervation of the smooth muscle by these fibers. In small mammals there are practically no adrenergic fibers within the longitudinal muscle layer of small and large intestine except in some species (guinea pig, cat and dogs) and in these segments where the longitudinal muscle layer is gathered into taeniae (see 24). Although sparse there is some adrenergic innervation of the circular muscle layer of both small and large intestine (see 24).

Intensely green fluorescent varicose adrenergic terminals were abundant and form networks around the non fluorescent ganglion cells of the myenteric plexus. Most or all enteric ganglion cells of the myenteric plexus may have varicose noradrenergic axons close to them. Beaded fluorescent fibers are also observed in the internodal strands. Thus a close topographic relationship between the adrenergic varicose axons and the neurons in Auerbach's plexus was demonstrated (see fig. 9).

Intramural arteries and arterioles are also well supplied, while veins are more sparsely innervated with noradrenergic axons.

In conclusion the morphological picture of the noradrenergic innervation of the ruminant stomach resembles strongly the results described by other investigators for other species (25,24,26,21,27,28,29,30,31,32,33,34).

Consequently there is a solid morphological basis to speculate on the functions of noradrenaline in the ruminant stomach wall.

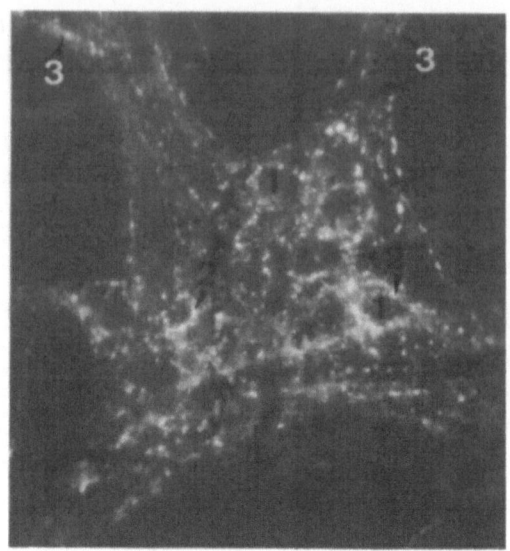

FIGURE 9. Omasum (OMA) of an adult sheep (688 x).
Auerbach's plexus after in toto staining for noradrenaline.
1. nonreactive nerve cell bodies. 2. pericellular noradrenergic network
surrounding 1. 3. varicous noradrenergic nerve fibers in the internodal
strands.

The presence of dense pericellular noradrenergic networks in the
myenteric plexus and the general sparseness of adrenergic nerves in the
ruminant stomach musculature may be in accordance with the view that the
adrenergic effects on the mammalian gastro-intestinal motility are mainly
indirect. In other words the adrenergic control would occur mainly at the
ganglionic level (35).

Fluorescence histochemistry of the adrenergic transmitters and
physiological experiments have convincingly demonstrated that adrenergic
sympathetic nerve fibers mediate inhibition of contraction and activate
relaxation of the smooth muscle layer (see 32).

Indeed noradrenaline is released at the periphery of the enteric
plexuses where it acts on receptors on cholinergic nerves to inhibit
praesynaptic release of acetylcholine (2).

So it is most probably that the adrenergic inhibitory mechanism takes
place primarily at the myenteric plexus by inhibiting the nerve impulse
transmission of the cholinergic ganglion cells (14,30). It was assumed that
catecholamines inhibited cholinergic nerve mediated motor activity via
praesynaptic alpha receptors and relaxed or inhibited spontaneous activity
via beta receptors. So the side of action of noradrenaline released from

sympathetic nerve terminals seems more likely to be on praeganglionic than on postganglionic cholinergic nerve endings (see 36). On the other hand, postsynaptic alpha receptors presumably mediated the contraction in response to catecholamines (see 36).

In addition some postganglionic sympathetic fibers enter the circular muscle coat. Noradrenaline released by these nerves also inhibits motility by producing hyperpolarisation of muscle cells through action on beta adrenoreceptors.

IV. IMMUNOCYTOCHEMICAL AND RADIOIMMUNOLOGICAL STUDY.

In this study we describe the literature from which we have destilled the general sentence, own research and results, preliminary conclusions and functional considerations concerning serotonin (5-HT), vasoactive intestinal polypeptide (VIP) and substance P (SP).

IV.1. Serotonin (5-HT)
IV.1.1. Review of the literature
IV.1.1.1. Presence of 5-HT in gut epithelium (enterochromaffin and enterochromaffin-like cells).

SEGMENT	SPECIES	REFERENCES
*oral cavity in association with gustatory epithelia	frog rabbit	see (37)
*oesophagus	bullfrog	(37)
*stomach small & large intestine	different species (chicken, mice, rat, guinea pig, rabbit, cat, pig, horse) including man	see (38) see (39) see (40),(41),(42),(43), (44),(45),(46),(47),(48), (49),(50),(51),(52),(53), (54),(55),(56)
*possible costorage with motilin or SP		(57)
SP enkephalin motilin	different species (rat, guinea pig, cat)	(58),(59),(60),(61),(62)
*gastrointestinal and peritoneal mast cells	rat & mice	see (39)

Presence of 5-HT in neural elements (neurons and nerve fibers).

SEGMENT	LOCALISATION	SPECIES	REFERENCES
*stomach small intestine large intestine gall bladder	intramural plexuses (mainly myenteric plexus) immunoreactive neurons and nerve fibers	#species in- cluding (mice, rat, guinea pig, rabbit)	(63) (64) (65),(66),,(38), (67),(68),(39)
*intestine (small & large)	enteric neurons high affinity uptake mecha- nism for L tryptophan	guinea pig	(69),(70)
	myenteric neurons synthesizes 5-HT from L tryptophan	guinea pig	(71)
	intramural plexuses high affinity uptake mechanism for ^{3}H-5 HT	guinea pig rabbit	(71),(72) (43)
	tryptophan hydroxylase present in muscle layer suggesting the presence of 5-HT neurons	rat	(41)
	in myenteric plexus 5-HT stored & released together with serotonin binding protein (SBP)	guinea pig	(66),(69)
*foetal intestine	immunoreactive neurons in Auerbach's plexus; some in Meissner's plexus, immunoreactive nerve fibers in ganglia & internodal strands, wall some small mesenteric blood vessels outside intestine	man	(73)
*vagal nerve	serotoninergic system in vagal afferents	cat	(74)
*(brain)	SBP in central 5-HT neurons	rat	(75),(76)

N.B. In some species 5-HT is localized in mast cells (52).

IV.1.1.2. Release of 5-HT.

From entero-endocrin cells (mucosal pool)	

Stimuli from mucosal side

Stimulus	References
*food intake	(77),(78),(79)
*change in intraluminal pH	(80),(81),(85),(82),(84),(45),(40)
*increase in intraluminal pressure	see (85),(86),(39),(87),(88),(89), (90),(91)
*peristalsis	(39),(92),(93),(87),(88)
*hypertonic glucose	see (80),(45),(94),(90),(89)
*mechanical stimulation	(95)
*absorbable fat	(39)
*application catecholamines acetylcholine	(85),(96),(88)
*cholera toxin	(97),(98)
*mechanical obstruction small bowel	see (39)
*autotransplantation small bowel	see (39)
*pyloroplasty with or without vagotomy	see (39)

N.B. small quantities 5-HT continuously released into lumen (91,99,100).

Stimuli from serosal side

Stimulus	References
*transmural electrical stimulation (blocked by tetrodotoxin)	(85)
*scratching serosal surface	(87)
*vagal nerve stimulation	(101),(102),(86),(103),(87),(88),(78), (14),(83),(104),(105),(106),(107),(39), (94)
*splanchnic nerve stimulation	(86),(87),(88),(105),(104),(108),(109), (107),(94)
*intraarterial infusion of drugs (nicotine, morphine, catecholamines, Ach)	(110),(92),(93),(87),(88),(111)
*vagotomy	see (94)

From intramural neural elements	
*electrical stimulation (vagal nerve, myenteric plexus) transmural electrical stimulation	see (72),(64),(66)

IV.1.1.3. Effects of 5-HT on motility

EFFECT	SEGMENT	SPECIES	REFERENCES
*contraction smooth muscle	oesophagus	guinea pig	(112),(113), see (39)
	stomach	rat	(114),(115)
	ileum	guinea pig	(99)
	jejunum	rabbit	(99)
	small intestine	man	(116)
	colon	man	(117)
by blocking c-AMP inhibition effects	small intestine	dog	(118)
direct and indirect ex-citatory effect	small intestine	dog	(110)
direct effect via D receptors	duodenum	mouse	(119)
via cholinergic pathway	ileum	guinea pig	(120),(39)
direct action on 2 separate receptors	intestine fundus & antrum	cat guinea pig	(121),(122)
via M receptors on nerve cells; D receptors on smooth muscle cells	stomach	rat	(119), see (123), see (124)
followed by relaxation ("fade")	ileum	guinea pig	(125)
tachyphylaxis of 5-HT on nerve and direct mediated effects	small intestine & colon	guinea pig	(126)
acts indirectly through inhibitory & excitatory neu-rons (M receptors)	duodenum	mouse	(119)

EFFECT	SEGMENT	SPECIES	REFERENCES
participate in response intestine to morphine & related agents	intestine	dog	(92)
*induction short contractions decreases primary & secondary contractions	forestomach	sheep	(127)
inhibition extrinsic reticulo-rumen contractions	forestomach	goat	(128)
increases eructation rate reflex inhibition normal cyclic contraction	forestomach	goat	(129)
*direct stimulatory action on smooth muscle fiber; participate in genesis spontaneous movements fetal rumen	rumen	bovine foetus	(130)
*relaxation receptive relaxation	fundus & antrum	guinea pig	(122)
longitudinal muscle layer	colon	man	(117)
after 5-HT IV infusion	colon	man	(116)
*changes in motility			
stimulation	stomach & intestine	#species including man	(116),(131),(132)
hypermotility in carcinoid syndrome	small intestine	man	(116),(38)
increase volume fluid transport	ileum jejunum	guinea pig rabbit	(99)
depression of motility in carcinoid syndrome hypomotility	colon	man	(116),(133)
decrease motility	stomach & colon	man	(116)

EFFECT	SEGMENT	SPECIES	REFERENCES
*modulation peristalsis, involved in descending suppression of vagal excitation	gut	mammals	(134)
by action on mucosal sensory receptors	jejunum ileum	rabbit guinea pig	(93) (99)
possible role in initiating peristaltic reflex	ileum	guinea pig	(87),(91)
involved in ascending excitatory neural pathway	distal colon & rectum	guinea pig	(135)
inhibition peristalsis due to praesynaptic blockade in the myenteric plexus	ileum	guinea pig	(136)
regulation peristalsis	ileum jejunum	guinea pig rabbit #species	see (131) see (131) (99), see (91), see (87), see (132)
neurotransmitter role between sensory & motor neurons in the peristaltic reflex	small intestine	mouse	(137)
decreases intraluminal pressure threshold for peristaltic reflex	intestine	man	(116)
*inhibits cholinergic excitatory neurons for smooth muscle	proximal colon	rabbit	(138)
*prevent presynaptic release Ach in myenteric ganglia	small intestine	guinea pig	(139)
*neurotransmitter in intrinsic inhibitory & excitatory enteric neurons	small intestine	mouse guinea pig	(119) see (72), see (66), (140)

EFFECT	SEGMENT	SPECIES	REFERENCES
*participate in vagal inhibitory pathway			see (66)
*production of slow EPSP in myenteric neurons	small intestine	guinea pig	(141),(142),(143)
*depolarizes neurons submucous plexus (5-HT neurotransmitter in plexus submucosus)	small intestine & colon	guinea pig	(126)
*stimulation mucosal afferent nerve endings; excitatory & inhibitory ganglion cells	review		see (39),(113)
*regulation cholinergic transmission in general	lumbar sympathetic ganglia; sciactic nerve	bullfrog frog	(144)
*activates afferent elements of mesenteric nerves in the submucosa	duodenum	rat	(145)
*neurotransmitter in enteric interneurons	ileum & colon	guinea pig	(126)
*excites intramural neuronal elements	small intestine	rat	(146)
*causes release ACH from myenteric ganglion cells	ileum	guinea pig	(120)
*transmitter in non adrenergic non cholinergic inhibitory nerves of the gut, acts on postganglionic cholinergic nerve fibers	review		see (39)
*activates specific receptors at intramural parasympathetic ganglion cells	ileum	guinea pig	(140)

EFFECT	SEGMENT	SPECIES	REFERENCES
*inhibition synaptic transmission in sympathetic ganglia by reducing evoked release Ach	superior cervical ganglion	rabbit	(147)
*increases release excitatory transmitter	nerve terminals	lobster	(148)
*decreases affinity Ach to nicotine receptor sites	sympathetic ganglia	bullfrog	(149)
*induces long term metabolic changes in nerve terminals	nerve terminals	lobster	(148)
*alter metabolism catecholamines		review	see (39)
*inhibtion AchE	striatum	rat	(150)

IV.1.1.4. Effects of 5-HT on secretion

EFFECT	SEGMENT	SPECIES	REFERENCES
*stimulation of secretion by intramural nervous reflex(es) in which VIP may be involved	small intestine	cat	(97)
*increases secretion	intestine	rat	see (151)
stimulates ileal secretion depresses mid-jejunal absorption H_2O & electrolytes	small intestine	rabbit	(133) see (151)
*high doses 5-HT cause ↓ gastric acid secretion	stomach	#species	see (39) see (43)

EFFECT	SEGMENT	SPECIES	REFERENCES
↓ basal gastric juice volume acid & pepsin output	stomach	rat	see (39)
↓ basal & induced gastric acid secretion	stomach	dog	see (39)
↑ mucus production, secretion and pepsin output		man	see (39)
biphasic effect on pepsin secretion	stomach	guinea pig	see (39)
*involved in diarrhoea induced by cholera toxin	small intestine	cat	(98)
*water resorption	gut	#species	see (131)
*stimulates secretion from salivary glands	salivary glands	#species	see (39)
*carcinoid syndrome 5-HT changes in intestinal water & electrolyte transport	small intestine	rabbit	see (38),(133)

IV.1.1.5. Miscellaneous effects

EFFECT	SEGMENT	SPECIES	REFERENCES
*constriction gastric and colonic vein & artery (artery less sensitive)	stomach & colon	man	(152)
*contraction saphenous vein	saphenous vein	dogs	(153)
*vasoconstriction	intestine	#species	see (131)
*reduces mucosal blood flow	gut	#species	see (39)
*decreases protein synthesis in intestine and brain	intestine	rat	(154)

EFFECT	SEGMENT	SPECIES	REFERENCES
*involved in vasomotor compo-nent of dumping syndrome (cfr basic defect in dumping is abnormality in distribution, bin-ding and release of 5-HT)	small intestine	dog	(89) see (39)
*modulate uptake, storage or release gastrointestinal polypeptide hormones	review		see (39) (155)
*proliferation of the gastrointestinal epithelium	review		(155)
*5-HT transmitter in some autonomic nerves of the gut	review		(156) see (157)

IV.1.1.6. General sentence of 5-HT.

In all species examined until now 5-HT is localized in EC cells. Number and distribution of EC cells varies in different gastrointestinal parts and also from one species to another, perhaps depending upon the development of the adrenergic innervation (158). Within mammals the gastrointestinal tract seems to be quantitatively the most important source of 5-HT. In the gut serotonin has a dual localisation: primarily in the enterochromaffin cells and in smaller quantities in the intramural nervous elements (immunoreactive neurons and nerve fibers). 65% of the total body 5-HT is stored in the 5-HT containing entero-endocrine cells. It is most interesting to mention that there is evidence for a costorage of 5-HT with some regulatory peptides i.e., enkephalin, motilin and SP within these cells. A variety of stimuli either acting from the mucosal side (food; fat; change in intralum. pH, somotic pressure, pressure; motility; mechanical stimulation; cholera toxin; mechanical obstruction) or from the serosal side (transmural electrical stimulation; vagal and splanchnic nerve stimulation, vagotomy; drugs) cause a release of 5-HT from its mucosal and/or intramural neural pool.

At the level of the gastrointestinal tract serotonin may influence motility and the secretion/absorption process as well:

by increasing the tonus of the smooth muscles; inducing contractions;

increasing the electrical activity (small intestine); inducing the release of acetylcholine from Auerbach's plexus; increasing the sensitivity of the smooth muscles for acetylcholine and finally by inhibiting acetylcholinesterase serotonin is able to control (modulate) the peristaltic reflex and the gastrointestinal motility. Also the secretion/absorption process may be controlled by serotonin. Due to an inhibition of the electrogenic Na^+-transport and a stimulation of the Ca^{2+}-influx into the epithelial cells, by inducing a local release of VIP from the submucosal pool and finally by causing a vasodilation of the mesenterial vessels and intramural arterioles on one hand and a vasoconstriction of venules on the other hand -consequently resulting in a congestion of the intestinal mucosa- 5-HT may stimulate the secretion and suppress the absorption.

IV.1.2. Own research and results

IV.1.2.1. Immunocytochemistry

The results of the immunocytochemical study concerning 5-HT are summarized in Table 1.

TABLE 1. 5-HT immunoreactive musocal cells in the ruminant stomach wall of the sheep (n=3)

	Adult	Foetus
OG	-	+
RET	-	+
RDS	-	+
RVS	-	+
OMA	-	+
ABO	+	+
AP	+	+
PYL	-	-

This study shows that in the adult sheep 5-HT can only be demonstrated in the glandular part of the ruminant stomach i.e. in the abomasum and the antrum pyloricum. Within these segments 5-HT seems to be pooled only in the lamina epithelialis. Here the 5-HT containing cells are principally encountered in the base of the gastric glands, less frequently in the surface epithelium (see fig. 10). The morphological appearance of the 5-HT immunoreactive epithelial cells in the sheep resembles the picture described in other species; i.e. triangle to flask shaped cells sometimes showing a long slender apical process directed towards the lumen and/or a short basal process probably making contact with adjacent structures.

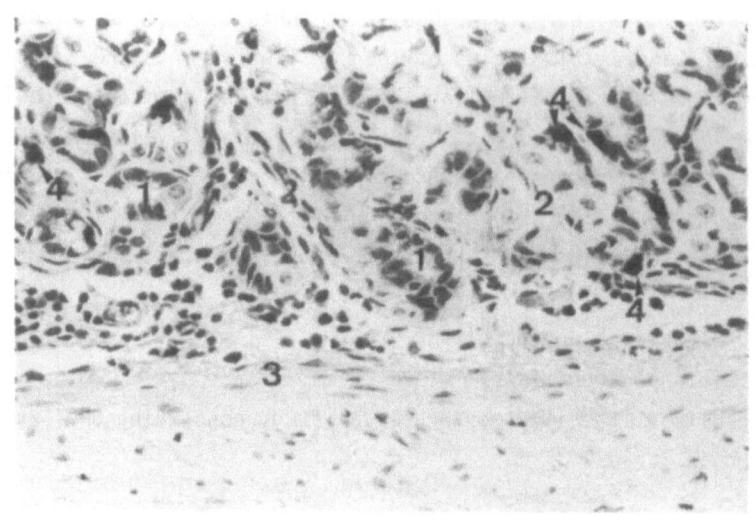

FIGURE 10. 5-HT immunoreactivity in the omasum (OMA) of an adult sheep (2000 x).
1. gastric glands   2. lamina propria.   3. lamina muscularis mucosae.
4. 5-HT containing epithelial cells.

Contrary to these findings in the adult sheep, the distribution of the 5-HT pattern in the stomach of the foetus seems to be totally different. Indeed 5-HT immunoreactive epithelial cells could, with exception of the pylorus, be demonstrated in every segment investigated.

IV.2. Vasoactive intestinal polypeptide (VIP)
IV.2.1. Review of the literature
IV.2.1.1. Presence of VIP in the gastrointestinal tract (immunocyto-
          chemistry)

SEGMENT	LOCALIZATION	SPECIES	REFERENCES
*oesophagus	circular & longitudinal muscle layer	rat, cat, pig, man, other mammals	(159),(160),(161), (162),(163),(164), (165),(166), see (1)
	immunoreactive epithelial cells	cat, man (foetus)	(167)

SEGMENT	LOCALIZATION	SPECIES	REFERENCES
*L.E.S.	circular muscle layer, plexus myentericus	rat, guinea pig, cat, rat, pig man	(159),(168),(160), (161), see (12), (169) (162)
*stomach	both muscle layers, both plexuses, lamina propria	chicken, cods mice, rat, guinea pig, cat, dog, man	(159), see (170), (171), (160),(161),(12),(172), (173),(174),(175), (176),(177), see (178), (7)
*pylorus	both muscle layers, plexus myentericus	cat, man	(171),(160),(161), see (12),(179)
*intestine (small & large)	both muscle layers, both plexuses, submucosa, lamina muscularis mucosae, lamina propria	mice, rat guinea pig, cat, dog, pig, man	(159), see (170),(180), (160),(161) (12),(172),(173),(181), (175),(176),(177),(1), see (178), see (7), (182),(183),(184), (167),(185),(186),(187), (171),(188)
	immunoreactive epithelial cells	quail, dog, pig, baboon	(189)
*blood vessels	immunoreactive fibers in wall intramural blood vessels	mammals	(7)
*peripheral nerves (vagal nerve, sciatic nerve)	immunoreactive fibers	man	(190),(191)

IV.2.1.2. Release of VIP from intramural nervous elements

Stimulation

STIMULUS	SPECIES	REFERENCES
*food and pentagastrin in stomach	cat	(192)
*acidification of the duodenal content	mammals	(193)
*fat, bill, HCl and high concentration ethanol in duodenum	dog	(194)

STIMULUS	SPECIES	REFERENCES
*acetylcholine IV	pig	see (195)
*cholinesterase inhibitors (neostigmine)	mammals	see (195)
*calcium IV	mammals dog	see (195) see (191)
*cholera toxin	cat	(170), see (196)
*intestinal ischemia	mammals	see (195)
*stimulation mechanoreceptors pharynx and oesophagus leading to gastric receptive relaxation	mammals	(163)
*electrical stimulation parasympathetic nerves (n. vagus, nn. pelvici)	guinea pig cat pig mammals	(163) (161), (197), see (195), (198),(199),(188),(200), see (7), see (195),(193)
	different species	see (1)
*electrical stimulation nonadrenergic noncholinergic inhibitory fibers	cat	(168)
*electrical field stimulation gut	rabbit	see (191)
*distention gastric fundus	dog	see (191)
*mechanical stimulation intestinal mucosa	cat	see (191)
*E coli endotoxin shock	pig	(201)

Inhibition

STIMULUS	SPECIES	REFERENCES
*electrical stimulation splanchnic nerves	pig	see (195)
*tetrodotoxin	cat mammals	(170) (168),(196)
*somatostatin	pig mammals	(199) (202),(163)
*H_1 & H_2 receptor antagonists	guinea pig	(203)
*atropine	rat dog guinea pig	(204) (166) (185)
*nicotine antagonists	mammals	(160),(163),(161)

IV.2.1.3. Effects of VIP on motility

EFFECT	SEGMENT	SPECIES	REFERENCES
*relaxation	oesophagus	mammals	(163),(165)
*relaxation	L.E.S.	cat	(168),(160),(161), see (195)
		opossum	(160),(161),(173), see (195)
		baboon	(160),(161),(173),(205)
		man	(160),(161),(173),(195)
		mammals	(193),(163)
*relaxation (gastric receptive relaxation)	stomach & pylorus	rat	(160),(161)
		guinea pig	(160),(161),(206),(207), see (195)
		cat	(193),(171),(160),(163), (161),(165), see (195)
		dog	(160),(161),(173)
		man	(160),(161)
		mammals	(193),(163),(165)
*dual effect of VIP on smooth muscle of the gut - relaxation of circular muscle layer (specially sphincters)		small & large rat	(261),(208)
		guinea pig	(161),(207),(209),(185), see (195)
- contraction of longitudinal muscle layer (high concentration of VIP)		rabbit	(161)
		opossum	(173)
		dog	(161)
		man	(210),(193)
		mammals	(193),(165),(1),(7), see (4), (12)
*potent vasodilation	blood vessels	#species	(191),(1),(7), see (1), (170),(12)

IV.2.1.4. Effects of VIP on secretion and absorption

EFFECT	SEGMENT	SPECIES	REFERENCES
*inhibition acid and pepsin secretion	stomach	cod	(211)
		rat	see (195)
		guinea pig & dog	(211),(212),(213), see (195),(214),(215),(173)
*stimulation mucus and peptic secretion		guinea pig	(192)
*stimulation secretion somatostatin		rat	(216)
*stimulation intestinal secretion, inhibition normal absorption	intestine (small & large)	shark	(217)
		goldfish	(186)
		Tilapia	(218)
		rat	(219),(220),(173),(169), (217),
		guinea pig	(180),(220)
		rabbit	(221),(219),(181),(222), (220),(173),(169)
		dog	(223),(187),(219),(181), see (195)
		man	(224),(219),(225),(226), (220),(173),(227),(181), (228), see (195)
		mammals	(202),(183),(193),(196), see (191),(1),(7), see (1),(170),(12)
*stimulation bicarbonate secretion from Brunner glands		rat	(229),(204)
*stimulation secretion pancreatic juice and bicarbonate	pancreas	birds, chicken & turkey	see (195),(177)
		rat	(160),(169),(230)
		cat	(160),(231),(169), see (195)
		dog	see (195)
		pig	(164),(160),(200), (169), see (195)

EFFECT	SEGMENT	SPECIES	REFERENCES
		man	see (195)
		mammals	(193),(163),(165), see (195),(188)
stimulation secretion insulin and somatostatin		dog	(232),(173)
stimulation secretion amylase, lipase and trypsin		rat, guinea pig, dog	(173)

NOTE: VIP acts on the adenylate-cyclase system: Ca^{2+} mobilisation and increase in cAMP concentration followed by membrane fosforylation

		SPECIES	REFERENCES
		shark	(161)
		mammals	(220),(173),(233), (217),(170),(230)

IV.2.1.5. General sentence of VIP

The gut contains large quantities of VIP throughout its entire length and as a consequence VIP containing structures are always found in the gastrointestinal wall.

Most, if not all, VIP in the gastrointestinal tract is contained within the nervous tissue. A substantial fraction of these VIPergic nerves is probably intrinsic to the gut wall. So VIP fibers apparently constitute a quantitatively (most) important nerve population in the gut. However VIP immunoreactive epithelial cells are found in the oesophagus of the cat and human foetus, while in the small and large intestine of the quail, dog, pig and baboon these cells have also been demonstrated (vide supra).

Varicose VIP fibers are seen to ramify extensively around non-immunoreactive nerve cell bodies in Auerbach's and Meissner's plexus.

Numerous VIP positive perikarya seems to be present in the gastrointestinal wall, where they are found in both plexuses but in the submucosus plexus in particular. These neurons innervate all cell types of the gut.

VIP immunoreactive nerve fibers are numerous in the muscular coat and especially in regions having a sphincter function. However there seems to be a difference in the density of the VIP-ergic innervation of both muscle layers being very rich in the circular muscle layer and sparse (or absent in some species) in the longitudinal layer.

In the mucosal layer VIP nerves form a network around the gastric and intestinal glands. In the small intestine they extend up in the core of the villi. Small terminals are demonstrated just beneath the epithelium giving the impression that they are able to control secretory and/or absorptive functions. Finally a rich perivascular VIP-ergic innervation was also found in the wall of intramural blood vessels.

Under a variety of experimental conditions a release of VIP from its principal source -the gut- has been demonstrated. They include: electrical stimulation of the vagal and pelvic nerves; transmural electrical stimulation; intraluminal perfusion of the intestine with various chemicals; gastric distention and mechanical stimulation of the intestinal mucosa; intestinal ischemia; acetylcholine IV and cholinesterase inhibitors.

The biological actions of VIP include a potent relaxant effect (being slow both in onset and recovery) on the gut muscle especially sphincters; a potent vasodilation promoting the bloodflow to splanchnic and other organs: a suppression of the gastric acid secretion and an augmentation of the intestinal secretory activity (water & ions). This is most probably mediated by an increase in the intracellular cyclic AMP.

The fact that VIP immunoreactive fibers are numerous beneath the intestinal epithelium, around perikarya in both plexuses and in autonomic ganglia outside the gut suggests additional roles for VIP including a neuromodulatory one and may be the coordination of functions of both plexuses (10,234).

IV. 2.2. Own research and results
IV.2.2.1. Radioimmunoassay

The results of the radioimmunological study are illustrated in table 2.

TABLE 2. Concentration of VIP (picogram/mg tissue) in stripped specimens of the ruminant stomach wall (n = 6).

	OG	RET	RDS	RVS	OMA	ABO	AP	PYL
Mucosa & Submucosa	228	44	23	11	180	224	237	279
Muscularis	353	371	330	304	500	387	356	323

One may conclude that:
- VIP is present in all the segments of the ruminant stomach studied so far
- the VIP concentration is always higher in the muscular coat as compared to the mucosa, suggesting that in the ruminant stomach wall most of the VIP is pooled in the tunica muscularis.
- with exception of the OMA, comparable VIP concentrations seem to be present in the tunica muscularis over the whole ruminant stomach.'
- there is no evidence for a higher VIP concentration in the tunica muscularis of sphincters (PYL) or sphincter-like regions (OG).
- the mucosa contains only small quantities of VIP.

However in the glandular part of the stomach the mucosal VIP concentration tend to be higher than in the aglandular part. This may, at least in part, be explained based upon the following morphological data. In the glandular stomach the tunica musoca is very thick with a well established lamina propria and lamina muscularis mucosae. Furthermore one has to realize that "the mucosa" in our stripped specimens holds also the tunica submucosa. This layer is provided with a considerable number of blood vessels and a well established neural network (Meissner's plexus). All these forementioned structures (lamina propria, lamina muscularis mucosae, submucosal blood vessels, Meissner's plexus) show in our immunocytochemical study a clear VIP immunoreactivity.

The higher VIP concentration in the pyloric mucosa, as compared to the rest of the gastric mucosa, may partly explained by the fact that in this region the submucosa is very well established and contains a relative large number of smooth muscle fibers most probably deriving from the internal circular muscle layer.

Nevertheless in the mucosa of some segments (the oesophageal groove and the omasum) of the aglandular stomach high VIP concentrations are also found. These findings too may have a morphological background.

In the oesophageal groove the lamina muscularis mucosae is continuous with the same layer of the oesophagus and is especially prominent along the margins of the sulcus.

For the omasum the mucosa is characterized by numerous foliated primary folds (laminae = leaves) and smaller papillae as well. The thick muscularis muscusal forms, following the contours, within the laminae a double layer of smooth muscle.

Also the innermost layer of the circular muscle layer is continued into the primary omasal folds. Consequently in a cross section a triple-layered smooth muscle layer can be seen in the center of the primary omasal folds.

So in both cases the mucosal specimens of the OG and the OMA may contain a considerable portion of smooth muscle. In the immunocytochemical part of this study a clear VIP immunoreactive innervation of the lamina muscularis mucosae and the inner circular muscle layer was demonstrated.

IV.2.2.2. Immunocytochemistry

Table 3 represents the immunocytochemical evaluation of the VIP immuno-reactivity in the different segments of the ruminant stomach wall.

TABLE 3. Distribution pattern of VIP immunoreactivity in the ruminant stomach wall (n = 6).

	OG	RET	RDS	RVS	OMA	ABO	AP	PYL
Mucosa & Submucosa	++	+	-	-	++	++	+	+
Muscularis	++	++	+	+	+++	++	++	+

In general the results of this study are in fairly good agreement with the quantitative results obtained in the RIA.

VIP immunoreactivity was always found in the wall of the ruminant stomach, where it was exclusively encountered within the nervous tissue.

VIP containing varicose nerve fibers are sparse, sometimes absent, in the longitudinal muscle layer. No specific distribution pattern along the ruminant stomach wall could be evidenced.

In contrast VIP immunoreactive nerve fibers are clearly seen in Auerbach's plexus, where they ramify around some non-immunoreactive perikarya. This picture was in particular evident in the OMA. Seldom and only in some segments (ABO, AP) immunoreactive nerve cell bodies could be seen.

By far the most dense network was always found in the inner circular muscle layer principally in the OMA, ABO, AP and OG. VIP immunoreactive fibers run parallel to the smooth muscle cells following the delicate connective tissue strands separating the muscular bundles (see fig. 11). Under our experimental conditions there was no evidence for a different

distribution pattern of VIP containing nerve fibers in the inner circular
layer of sphincter region.

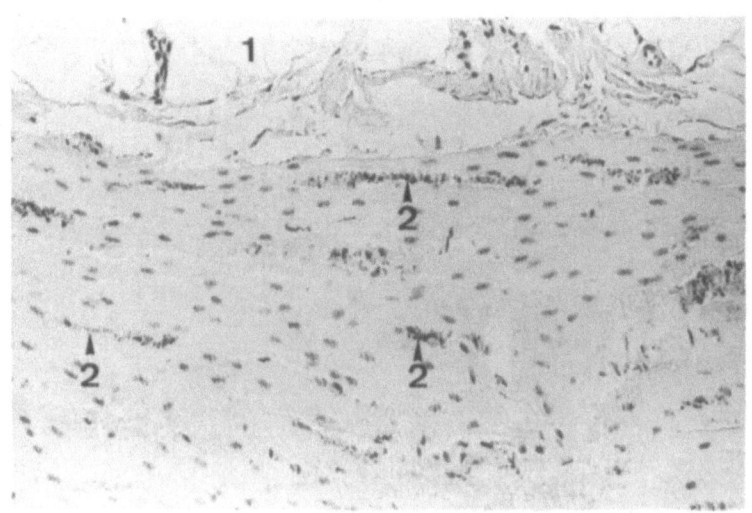

FIGURE 11. VIP immunoreactivity in the circular muscle layer of the omasum
(OMA) of an adult sheep (1250 x). 1. submucosa. 2. VIP immunoreactive
nerve fibers.

In the submucosa the picture is not uniform. A distinct reaction was
only demonstrated in the glandular part of the stomach especially in
Meissner's plexus where VIP containing nerve fibers, as in Auerbach's
plexus, ramify around non-immunoreactive nerve cell bodies (see fig. 12).
Immunoreactive perikarya were not seen. In the aglandular part of the
stomach immunoreactivity against VIP can hardly be ascertained.

In the mucosa VIP immunoreactivity was never found in the epithelium.
Delicate VIP containing fibers can be seen in the lamina propria of the
glandular part of the stomach.Noteworthy is the fact that in the ABO and
AP small ganglia (3 to 5 nerve cell bodies) were frequently found between
the base of the gastric glands and the lamina muscularis mucosae. Here
VIP containing fibers were also seen to surround some of the non-immunoreactive neurons.

A VIP-ergic innervation of the lamina muscularis mucosae was in
particular evident in those segments where this smooth muscle layer is well
established i.e. the OG, OMA and the glandular stomach as a whole. The
reaction is of course absent in these segments were the lamina muscularis

80

mucosae is lacking (RDS and RVS).

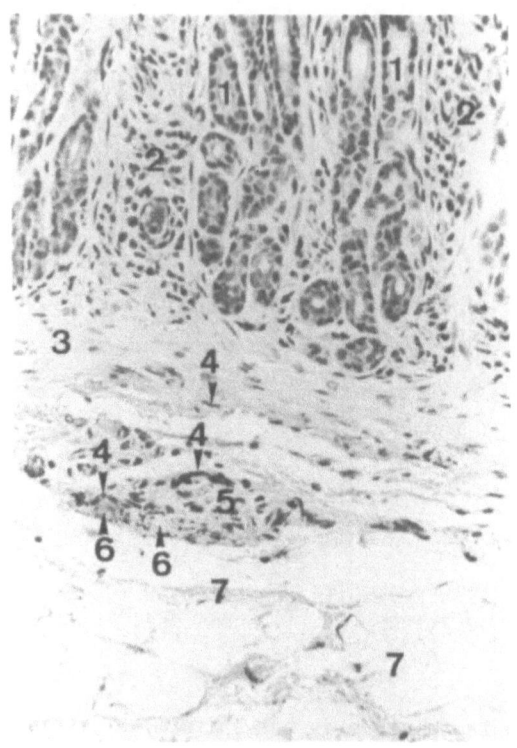

FIGURE 12. VIP reaction in the antrum pyloricum (AP) of an adult sheep
(880x).
1. pyloric glands. 2. lamina propria. 3. lamina muscularis mucosae.
4. VIP containing nerve fibers. 5. ganglion from Meissner's plexus with
VIP immunoreactive nerve fibers (4) surrounding non-immunoreactive nerve
cell bodies (6). 7. submucosa.

Finally VIP immunoreactive fibers are regular found in the wall of
larger intramural blood vessels.

IV.2.2.3. Preliminary conclusions and functional considerations.
The overall picture of the intramural VIP-ergic innervation of the
ruminant stomach in this immunocytochemical study resembles strongly the
picture as described by other investigators for different animals
including man (vide supra). Although basic information concerning the
functional consequences of VIP on some ruminant stomach functions is still

very scanty or lacking, it is -based upon the above-mentioned morphological
similarities-, tempting to speculate on a similarity in functions too.

The ruminant stomach is anatomically a complex and highly compart-
mentalized intestinal segment in which specific functions may be correlated
to (a) specific compartment(s). So it may be possible that in the ruminant
stomach VIP is at least partly involved in the control and coordination of
motility, the critical control of the secretion/absorption process and
intramural bloodflow. Consequently VIP may be an essential link in the
normal functioning of this by far most important part of the ruminant
gastrointestinal tract.

IV.3. Substance P (SP)
IV.3.1. Review of the literature
IV.3.1.1. Presence of SP in the gastrointestinal tract.

SEGMENT	LOCALISATION	SPECIES	REFERENCES
*intestine (small & large)	both muscle layers, both plexuses, submucosa, epithelial endocrine cells	chicken mouse rat & guinea pig	(235) (58) (236),(237)
		cat	(238),(239)
		dog	(240)
		horse	(241),(242)
		man	see (243)
		mammals	(183),(62), see (178), see (7),(1)
	costorage with somato-statin in nerve fibers	mouse	(58)
		rat	(224)
		mammals	(62)
*primary sensory neurons of visceral receptors		rat	(178)
		guinea pig	(178)
		cat	(178)
*blood vessels	mucosal layer	mammals	(245),(1)
*vagal nerve	small quantities	mammals	(183),(242),(246)

SEGMENT	LOCALISATION	SPECIES	REFERENCES
*inferior mesenteric ganglion	immunoreactive fibers around principal ganglion cells	rat	see (247),(248)
coelicac superior mesenteric ganglion complex		guinea pig	see (247),(248)
		cat	(247),(248)

Note: Species differences (colon)

plexus submucosus numerous, the plexus myentericus small number immunoreactive nerve cell bodies		horse, man	(183)
opposite in		guinea pig & cat	(183)
even distribution of immunoreactive nerve fibers in both muscle layers		cat, man	(183)
circular muscle layer highest density of immunoreactive nerve fibers		dog, horse	(183)
sparse immunoreactive nerve fibers in mucosa		cat	(183)
numerous immunoreactive nerve fibers in mucosa		dog, horse, man	(183)

IV.3.1.2. Release of SP

Stimulation

STIMULUS	SPECIES	REFERENCES
*acidification distal oesophagus	cat	(249)
*acidification duodenum	cat	(249)
*increase intraluminal pressure	guinea pig	(250)
*stimulation vagal nerve and splanchnic nerves	cat	(251),(239),(252)
*neurotoxins (capsaicin)	guinea pig	(250)
Inhibition		
*atropin	cat	(238),(239),(252)
*tetrodotoxin	guinea pig cat	(250) (249)

IV.3.1.3. Effects of SP on motility

EFFECT	SEGMENT	SPECIES	REFERENCES
*contraction muscularis mucosae (direct effect)	oesopha-gus	guinea pig	(237)
*contraction	L.E.S.	cat pig	(249) (253)
*contraction direct stimulation circular muscle layer indirect stimulation longitudinal muscle layer	stomach	cat dog	(251) (254) (255) (256) (257) (258) (259)
*inhibition contraction	stomach	rat	(260)
*increase pressure in gastric wall	stomach	cat	(261)
*contraction	pylorus	cat dog	(238),(239) (258)
*contraction both muscle layers	small & large intestine intestine	chicken guinea pig rat rabbit cat pig dog mammals	(235) (262),(263),(264),(265), (266),(267),(268), see (1) (264) (264) (264) (264) (269),(270) (183),(1), see (12)
direct effect	intestine	guinea pig mammals	(268), (12),(7),(4),(1),(271)
indirect effect -stimulation afferent nerve fibers in peri-staltic reflex arch	intestine	guinea pig mammals	(271) see (12)
-by modulating choli-nergic transmission in intramural neurons	intestine	mammals	(7),(271),(183)
-by modulating adre-nergic transmission	intestine	mammals	(183)

EFFECT	SEGMENT	SPECIES	REFERENCES
-by depolarising the myenteric neuron membrane primarily by an inactivation of resting potassium conductance	intestine	guinea pig	(272)
*contraction longitudinal muscle layer direct stimulation	intestine	chicken guinea pig guinea pig rabbit cat dog	(235) (273),(274) (262),(275),(264) (266),(267),(268) (264) (264) (269),(270)
indirect via Ach	intestine	rat cat dog pig	(264) (264) (276) (264)
*contraction muscularis mucosae (via release bombesin)	intestine	dog	(277)
*sensory neurotransmitter involved in peristalsis	intestine	mammals	(278)
*modulator muscular tone	intestine	mammals	(1)
*excitatory transmitter of interneurons with peripheral branches in mucosa & lamina propria	intestine	guinea pig & other species	(1) (279)
*excitatory transmitter motorneurons		mammals	(7)
vasodilation (splanchnic area)	blood vessels	mammals	(12),(246),(7)

IV.3.1.4. Effects of SP on secretion and absorption

EFFECT	SEGMENT	SPECIES	REFERENCES
*inhibition secretion induced by pentagastrin	stomach	dog	(281)
*stimulation secretion and reduction absorption	intestine	rat guinea pig rabbit	(282) (283) (284)
*stimulation secretion (direct effect)	pancreas	dog mammals	(281) (7),(12)
*stimulation secretion	exocrine glands	mammals	see (7), see (12)

IV.3.1.5. Miscellaneous effects

EFFECT	SEGMENT	SPECIES	REFERENCES
functional role in some type of visceral sensory function and in special types of reflex arches in primary sensory neurons	extramural ganglia	guinea pig rat cat	(247) (280)
facilitation neuro-muscular transmission	neuromuscular junction	frog	(260)

IV.3.1.6. General sentence of SP

SP resides in all layers of the gut. Here it has a dual localisation i.e. in some mucosal endocrine cells (principally in small & large intestine) and in SP immunoreactive nerve fibers and cell bodies along almost the entire length of the gut, being however least prominent in the upper portion of the gastrointestinal tract (oesophagus, stomach). SP containing nerve cell bodies are mainly localised in Auerbach's plexus. A very dense network of SP positive nerve terminals is found around perikarya of both intramural plexuses but in the myenteric plexus in particular. SP containing nerve fibers were also seen to extend from the plexus in between the bundles of smooth muscle cells. By so doing the circular muscle layer becomes richly, the longitudinal muscle layer on the contrary scarcely innervated by these nerves. Some SP containing nerve fibers are also demonstrated in the lamina propria.

Evidence has been provided that SP is present in the dorsal root of the spinal cord suggesting that it is involved in the transmission of sensory information. So it may be possible that SP nerves in the gut wall are processes from sensory neurons coming from visceral receptors. Also the morphological features of SP fibers in ganglia outside the gut wall may evoke the idea that these fibers may be involved in some type of visceral sensory function or special types of reflex arches.

The distribution of SP immunoreactive nerve fibers within the gut wall suggests that the smooth muscle cells and neurons are the main target organs. The contracting action of SP on the non-vascular smooth muscle might be twofold: a direct effect and an indirect one involving the stimulation of afferent nerve fibers in the peristaltic reflex arc or by its release from non-cholinergic interneurons in the myenteric plexus.

On the contrary SP is a potent vasodilator in different vascular beds among them the splanchnic area.

Finally it was also shown that SP increases the secretion and reduces the absorption.

IV.3.2. Own research and results

IV.3.2.1. Radioimmunoassay

TABLE 4. Concentration of SP (picogram/mg tissue) in stripped specimens of the ruminant stomach wall (n = 6)

	OG	RET	RDS	RVS	OMA	ABO	AP	PYL
Muscosa & Submucosa	66	55	34	31	53	77	90	76
Muscularis	75	78	55	65	59	69	67	78

From the results of the radioimmunological study, summarized in table 4, the following conclusions may be drawn:
- although in considerable lower concentrations than VIP, SP is demonstrated in both the mucosa, with adhering submucosa, and the muscular layer of all segments investigated.
- considering the aglandular part (OG, RET, RDS, RVS, OMA) first it seems that the mucosal-submucosal strips contain only small quantities of SP. Low SP concentrations are found in both (RDS and RVS) ruminal compartments, while higher values are demonstrated in those segments (OG, RET, OMA) where the mucosal strip holds also a more or less developed smooth muscle layer.
Compared to the mucosa, SP concentrations are normally higher in the muscular layer. This is clearly demonstrated in those segments (OG, RET) with a well developed muscular coat.
- in the glandular part of the stomach (ABO, AP, PYL) the reversed situation holds true. The SP content of the mucosa tend to be higher as compared to the muscularis and to the mucosa of the aglandular part. This finding may partly be explained by the presence of a well developed lamina muscularis mucosae and Meissner's plexus in which immunocytochemically SP like neurons and fibers are found. However in the pyloric sphincter a higher SP content was evidenced. In this respect the pylorus follows the trend seen in the aglandular part.

IV.3.2.2. Immunocytochemistry

Table 5 summarizes the results of the immunocytochemical study.

TABLE 5. Distribution pattern of SP immunoreactivity in the ruminant
stomach wall (n = 6)

	OG	RET	RDS	RVS	OMA	ABO	AP	PYL
Mucosa & Submucosa	+	+	-	-	++	+	+	+
Muscularis	++	++	+	+	++	++	++	++

Neither in the epithelial cells nor in the lamina propria of any
segment SP immunoreactivity was seen. Only in these segments where the
muscularis mucosae is well established (OG, RET, ABO) and in the OMA in
particular varicose SP containing nerve fibers were evidenced. With
exception of the ABO, where some SP containing neurons were seen and
where some SP immunoractive fibers surround non-immunoreactive neurons
in the plexus submucosus, SP immunoreactivity can hardly be detected in
the submucosa (see fig. 13).

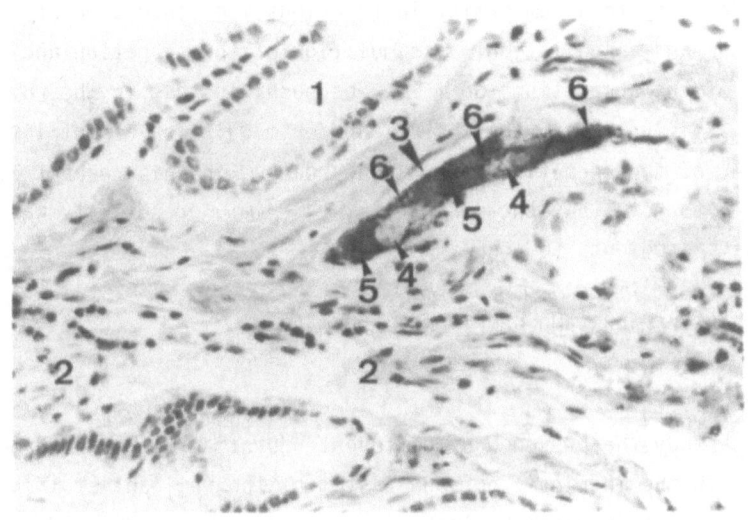

FIGURE 13. SP immunoreactivity located in the transitional zone between
pylorus and duodenum in a ganglion of Meissner's plexus. 1. onset Brunner
glands. 2. submucosa. 3. ganglion. 4. non-immunoreactive nerve cell
bodies. 5. SP containing nerve cell bodies. 6. SP containing nerve fibers.

The most clear and notable reaction is always found in the circular muscle layer. This is especially the case in the OG, RET, OMA and ABO. Although not evidenced in every segment investigated, SP containing nerve fibers were seen to encircle non-immunoreactive neurons in Auerbach's plexus. Immunoreactive neurons were not found. Finally the longitudinal muscle layer of the ruminant stomach seems to be only faintly innervated by SP nerves. In fact in most segments SP immunoreactivity was even not demonstrable in this muscle layer. Regularly very fine SP immunoreactive fibers are seen in the wall of some intramural blood vessels.

In conclusion SP immunoreactivity was found in the wall of every segment studied. However, after examinating consecutive sections of the same segment, the impression exists that the immunocytochemical reaction against SP was not as pronounced as for VIP.

IV.3.2.3. Preliminary conclusions and functional considerations

SP was demonstrated in the wall of every segment of the ruminant stomach studied so far. Broadly spoken the microscopial picture of the SP immunoreactivity in this study seems to be in agreement with this described in other species. This similarity in morphology may as a consequence refer to a comformity in functions i.e. induction of contractions and vasodilation, a stimulation of the secretion and a reduction of the absorption. So it may be possible that in the ruminant stomach SP is involved in the control and/or modulation of motility and the control of the secretion/absorption process. In this respect it is interesting to note that the most striking SP immunoreactivity was found in "decisive" segments (OG, RET, OMA, ABO).

V. CONCLUSIVE REMARKS AND FUNCTIONAL APPROACH

V.1. Conclusive remarks.

In this study the presence of different neurotransmitters/neuro-modulators in the intrinsic nervous system of the ruminant stomach was studied particularly using histochemistry, radioimmunoassay and immuno-cytochemistry.

Acetylcholinesterase, biogenic amines (noradrenaline, serotonin) and regulatory peptides (VIP, SP) -having a characteristic region specific distribution within the stomach wall- were demonstrated (see fig. 14).

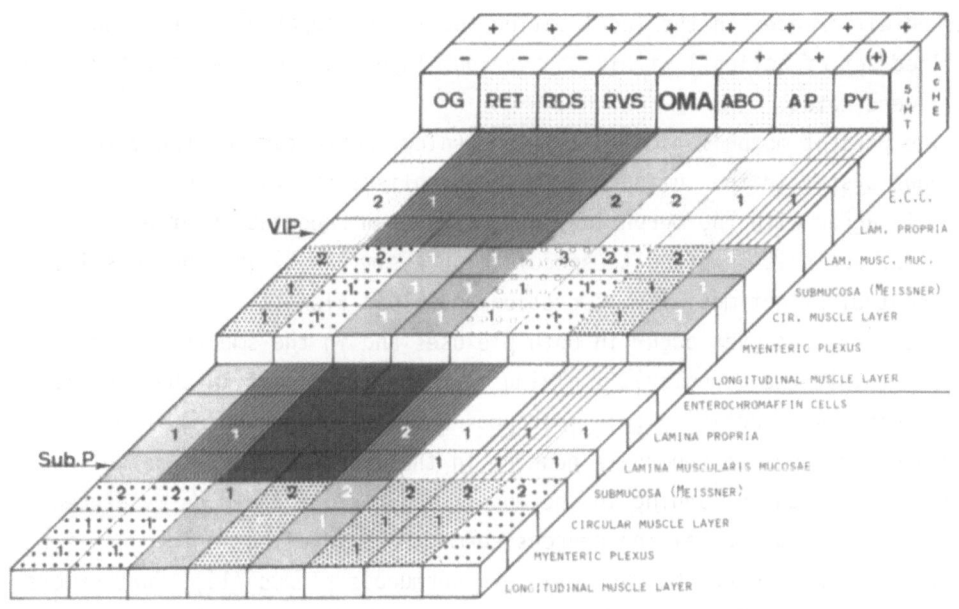

FIGURE 14. Diagram representing the results of a histochemical (5-HT, AchE), immunocytochemical (VIP, Sub. P) and radioimmunological (VIP, Sub. P) study on the ruminant stomach of the sheep.
For the peptides VIP and Sub. P the density of the lattice is inversely related to the content (RIA) of the regulatory peptide in the different layers and segments.
The results of the immunocytochemical evaluation are represented by the number 1 to 3.

+ = present, - = absent; 1 = low, 2 = moderate, 3 = high immunoreactivity; OG = oesophageal groove; RET = reticulum; RDS = ruminal dorsal sac; RVS = ruminal ventral sac; OMA = omasum; ABO = abomasum; AP = antrum pyloricum; PYL = pylorus; 5-HT = 5-hydroxytryptamin; AchE = acetylcholinesterase; VIP = vasoactive intestinal polypeptide; Sub. P = substance P.

Based upon these findings it is most likely that, beside the classical cholinergic and noradrenergic innervation, the ruminant stomach is also richly innervated by a complex peptidergic system. Although this system seems to be distributed throughout the length of the ruminant stomach, marked differences in the localization (possibly compatible with a well defined set of actions) within the various layers of the ruminant stomach wall were noted.

The present morphological data, concerning the texture of the enteric nervous system in the ruminant stomach established in this study, broadly agree with the morphology of this system reported in other species. So it is tempting to speculate on a similarity in functions i.e. the control of gut motility, secretion and blood flow (1).

Peptidergic nerves occur in both plexuses and in the smooth muscle layer (mainly the circular), implying that they take part in the regulation of smooth muscle activity (7). Thereupon a VIP pathway running from the submucous neurons to innervate neurons in the myenteric plexus as well as substance P pathway running in the opposite direction could be evidenced. Thus, the peptide containing neurons seems to be involved in the communication between the myenteric and submucous plexus (12). Furthermore VIP and substance P are found in the submucosal plexus and the mucosal layer in the glandular part of the ruminant stomach and thus may be involved in the regulation of epithelial functions (7). The system of peptide containing neurons may provide therefore the morphological basis for functional coordination and autonomy of the gut (see 12).

Beside the classical neurotransmitters (acetylcholine, noradrenaline) it is generally believed that 5-HT and the regulatory peptides (peptidergic neuronal system) function within the context of the autonomic nervous system (7). Most likely the intramural neurons of the gut modulate the response(s) to the extrinsic nerve impulses. Conceivably the intramural peptidergic neurons can mediate and modulate the response(s) to an extrinsic nerve impulse flow according to local needs (7). Due to the relative independence of the enteric nervous system from the central nervous system control the different type of neurons in the enteric plexuses are most likely involved in local reflex mechanisms either as sensory neurons, interneurons or efferent neurons (7). When the proposed actions of the various peptides are viewed with the distribution pattern of the peptide containing nerve fibers in mind, it is tempting to speculate that they serve a neurotransmitter role. This view is, at least in other species, further favored by morphological and physiological data (see 12).

In conclusion, the intramural innervation of the ruminant stomach seems to be far more complex than originally stated and our classical morphological and functional picture of a bipartite innervation of the ruminant stomach has to be reconsidered.

Although morphological studies may contribute significantly to our current understanding of the neuronal topography in the ruminant stomach wall, the functions of most of these substances remain to be adequately defined. However their localization in the intramural nerves elements and endocrine cells has given rise to reasonable speculations about the role they may play (e.g. neurotransmitter, neuromodulatory, endocrine and paracrine).

Nevertheless if we will have any chance of understanding and treating the abnormalities in the mechanisms that occur in various diseases of the ruminant stomach (chronic ruminal tympany, displacement of abomasum etc.), it is imperative to increase further our understanding of the basic morphologic, functional and neurological mechanisms proceeding in the intramural nervous system in the ruminant stomach wall and of the different links in the delicate equilibrium between the different elements of this ruminant stomach "brain".

V.2. Functional approach

In the ruminants, a considerable bacteral- and protozoal metabolism is observed in the rumen. The rumen is also important for its reservoir function and for the absorption of the endproducts of fermentation. The reticulum functions as a cyclic pump controlling the flow of contents between the oesophagus, rumen and omasum in adult animals. The omasum is involved in the absorption of ions and fluid, while the abomasum has the classical functions of monogastric animals.

To fulfil all the functional requirements on motility, the smooth muscles of the different compartments have to be adapted to the specific function of the different compartments during the evolution. Contraction of smooth muscles can be initiated by changes in membrane permeability after either binding of agonists to the receptors or exposure to high K^+ concentrations (285). Two pathways of transmembrane flux of Ca^{2+} exist: a voltage-dependent (Ca^{2+} channel), activated by changes in membrane potential, and a receptor-linked Ca^{2+}-channel, activated by binding of agonists to their receptors. The electrical and chemical membrane signals indirectly activate contractile elements by releasing membrane-bound Ca^{2+}, or increasing Ca^{2+} influx, or both. Activation of the voltage-linked channel results in a phasic contraction while activation of the receptor--linked channel results in a tonic contraction. In some muscles, there is an overlapping of the sensitivity for activation between both types of channels. The phasic contractions are involved in the regulation of the transport and mixing of contents while the tonic contractions are involved in the regulation of the reservoir function and the function of sphincters.

A group of organic Ca^{2+} antagonists or Ca^{2+} channel blockers (including verapamil, methoxyverapamil, nifedipine, diltiazem and flunarizine) have been described as specific inhibitors of Ca^{2+} influx through voltage--dependent Ca^{2+} channels (286,287,288). These agents inhibit both the contraction and the increase in Ca^{2+} influx induced by high concentrations of K^+, whereas little effect was observed on both the contraction and Ca^{2+} movements elicited with norepinephrine or histamine in rabbit aorta smooth muscles. Sodium nitroprusside seems to be a selective inhibitor of the receptor-linked Ca^{2+} channel (289). The mucosa free strips of ruminal smooth muscles of sheep, exhibit no (or limited) spontaneous electrical and contractile activity but showed a spontaneous myogenic tone.

The tone was completely eliminated in Ca^{2+}-free solutions and also by sodium nitroprusside (290). Similar results were obtained with sodium nitroprusside on circular and longitudinal ruminal smooth muscle strips in cattle and calves. These muscles showed rather frequent spontaneous contractions. Sodium nitroprusside inhibited muscle tone but also the spontaneous contractions. Similar, but long-lasting inhibition of muscle tone and spontaneous contractions was observed with ritanserin (291).

Neurotransmitters and hormones present in the wall of the rumen, as shown in this study, are of importance in modifying and regulating the tonic type of activity and the phasic contractions. Both are of importance for the control of each compartment (e.g. adaptation of volume, sphincter activity, pump mechanism, absorption of fluid and metabolites) and the coordination between the different compartments (e.g. between reticulum and orificium reticulo-omasale).

One of the transmitters involved is serotonin. On circular smooth muscle of the different compartments, 5-HT (10^{-10} - 10^{-7} M) increased muscle tone of RDS, RVS and OMA (see fig. 15).

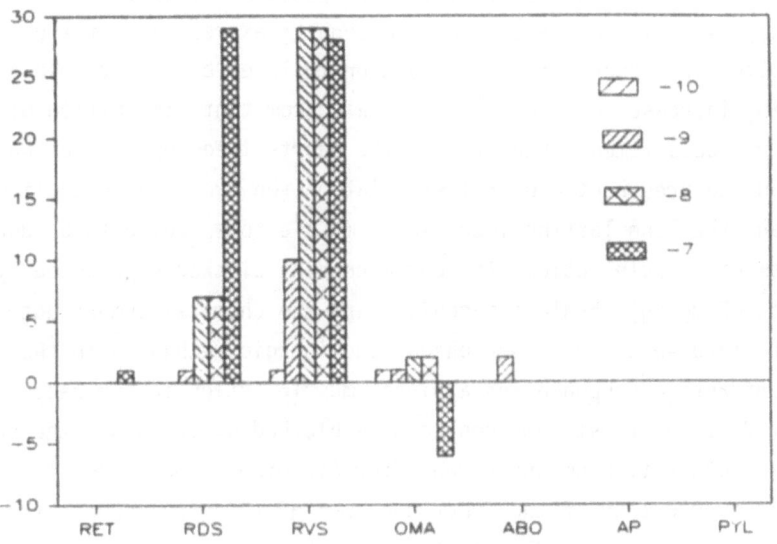

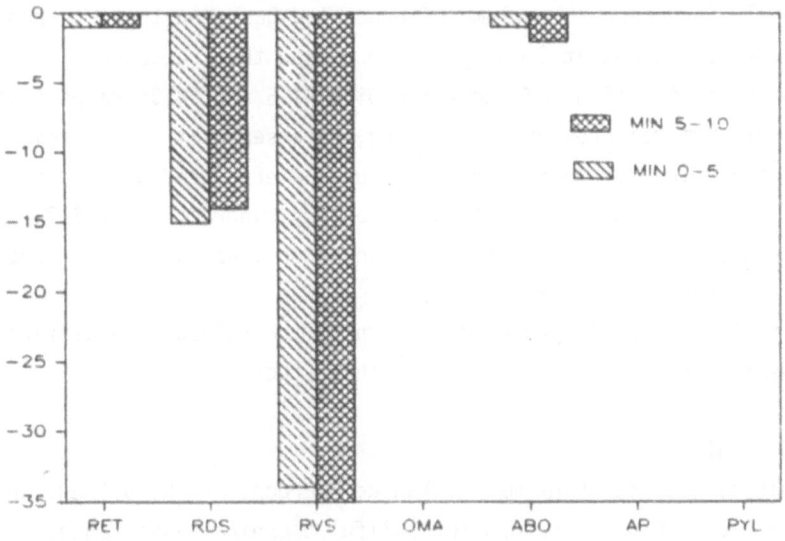

FIGURE 15 and 16. Effects of endogenous substances on circular smooth muscle tone. Upper part: serotonin (5-HT). Lower part: VIP (10^{-9} M). RET = reticulum, RDS = rumen dorsal sac, RVS = rumen ventral sac, OMA = omasum; ABO = abomasum, AP = antrum pyloricum and PYL = pylorus.

On the contrary, VIP (10^{-9} M) reduced muscle tone of RET, RES, RVS and ABO (fig. 16) both from 0-5 and 5-10 min. after addition of VIP.

I.V. administration of serotonin (6 microg/kg expressed as the base) in sheep resulted in a short-lived contraction followed by a sustained and long lasting increase in muscle tone and a concomitant inhibition of the extrinsic reticulo-rumen contractions. The short-lived contraction was probably due to presynaptic neural stimulation (on presynaptic cholinergic neurons) and the long lasting increase of muscle tone seemed to be due to a direct smooth muscle action. The corresponding blockades produced by atropine (0.05 mg/kg), $5-HT_2$ antagonists and the chemical sympathectomy suggest the involvement of a peripheral cholinergic mechanism in the initial contractile response and a direct muscle action in the second response (292). The first component can be blocked by morphine, the second persists in both reticulum and rumen after atropine or morphine. The increase in muscle tone of the rumen due to 5-HT (5 µg/kg) under atropine blockade is inhibited by $5-HT_2$ blockers. In sheep it was also shown that a specific serotonin 2 (S_2) antagonist at a dose level of 0.05 mg/kg significantly increased the volume of eructated gas when the intraruminal pressure was maintained at 2 mm Hg and increased the frequency of primary and secondary contractions of the rumen with 41.5 and 24.3% respectively.

At an intraruminal pressure of 4 mm Hg, ketanserin at a dose level of 0.1 mg/kg significantly increased the volume of eructated gas and also the frequency of both primary (23.6%) and secondary contractions (23.7%) (293).

Also spontaneous bloating can be prevented or treated with a serotonin 2 antagonist (ritanserin) (see 294).

Further studies are in progress concerning the role of the different neurotransmitters and hormones shown in this study.

ACKNOWLEDGEMENTS

The authors wish to thank Mr. A. Van de Mieroop, Mr. W. Willems and Mrs. N. Verhaert, Miss A. Dendas for skilful technical assistance. We are grateful to Mrs. D. Verhoeven and Miss K. Willems for typing the manuscript.

REFERENCES

References especially on introduction, methodology, acetylcholine and noradrenaline
1. Polak, J.M. and Bloom, S.R.: In: Cellular Basis of Chemical Messengers in the Digestive System. Grossman, M.I. et al. (eds), Acad. Press Inc., 267-282 (1981)
2. Hendrix, T.R. and Castell, D.O.: In: Alimentary Tract Motility. American Gastroenterological Association (eds), Milner-Fenwick, Inc., 1-15 (1982)
3. Appenzeller, O.: In: The Autonomic Nervous System, Chapter I. Anatomy and Histology. Appenzeller, O. (ed), Elsevier Biomed. Press, 1-29 (1982)
4. Polak, J.M. and Bloom, S.R.: In: Gut Peptides. Bloom, S.R. and Polak, J.M. (eds), 2nd ed., 487-494 (1981)
5. Slader, J.R. and McNeill, T.H.: Cell Tissue Res. 210, 181-189 (1980)
6. Roman, C. and Gonella, J.: In: Physiology of the Gastrointestinal Tract, Chapter IX. Extrinsic control of digestive tract motility. Johnson, L.R. (ed), Raven Press, N.Y., 289-334 (1981)
7. Sundler, F., Hakanson, R. and Leander, S.: Clin. Gastroenterol. 9, 517-543 (1980)
8. Gabella, G.: In: Basic Science in Gastroenterology. Structure of the gut. Polak, J.M. et al. (eds), Glaxo, 193-203 (1982)
9. Gershon, M.D., Payette, R.F. and Rothman, T.P.: Fed. Proc. 42, 1620-1625 (1983)
10. Jessen, K.R., Polak, J.M., Van Noorden, S., Bloom, S.R. and Burnstock, G.: Nature 283, 391-393 (1980)
11. Riemann, J.F.: In: Basic Science in Gastroenterology. Structure of the Gut. Polak, J.M. et al. (eds), Glaxo, 289-302 (1982)
12. Hakanson, R., Leander, S., Sundler, F. and Uddman, R.: In: Cell Basis of Chemical Messengers in the Digestive System. Grossman, M.I. et al. (eds), Acad. Press Inc., 169-199 (1981)
13. Argenzio, R.A.: In: Veterinary Gastroenterology, Chapter XII. Comparative physiology of the gastrointestinal system. N.V. Anderson, Lea & Febiger (eds), 172-198 (1980)
14. Gershon, M.D.: Ann. Rev. Neurosci. 4, 227-272 (1981)
15. Blood, D.C., Henderson, J.A. and Radostits, O.M.: In: Veterinary

Medicine. A textbook of the diseases of cattle, sheep, pigs and horses. London, B. Tindall (eds) 1135 (1981)

16. Baljet, B. and Drukker, J.: Stain Technology 50, 31-36 (1975)
17. Furness, J.B. and Costa, M.: Histochemistry 41, 335-352 (1975)
18. Forssmann, W.G., Pickel, V., Reinecke, M., Hock, D. and Metz, J.: In: Techniques in Neuroanatomical Research. Heym, Ch. and Forssmann, W.G. (eds), Springer Verlag,171-205 (1981)
19. Sternberger, L.A.: Mikroscopy 25, 346-361 (1969)
20. Long, R.G. and Bryant, M.G.: In: Radioimmunoassay of Gut Regulatory Peptides. Bloom, S.R. and Long, R.G. (eds), W.B. Saunders Company Ltd., London (1982)
21. Malfors, G., Leander, S., Brodin, E., Hakanson, R., Holmin, T. and Sundler, F.: Cell Tiss. Res. 214, 225-238 (1981)
22. Marani, E.: Thesis, Leiden (1982)
23. Silva, D.G., Farrell, K.E. and Smith, G.C.: Anat. Rec. 162, 157-175 (1968)
24. Furness, J.B. and Costa, M.: Ergebn. Physiol. 69, 1-51 (1974)
25. Jacobowitz, D.H.: Pharmacol. Exp. Therap. 149, 358-364 (1965)
26. Llewellyn-Smith, I.J., Furness, J.B., Wilson, A.J. and Costa, M.: In: Autonomic Ganglia. Lars Gösta Elfin (eds) 145-182 (1983)
27. Furness, J.B. and Costa, M.: Neuroscience 5, 1-20 (1980)
28. Costa, M. and Gabella, G.: Z. Zellforsch. 122, 357-377 (1971)
29. Wood, J.D.: In: Physiology of the Gastrointestinal Tract. Johnson, L.R. (ed), Raven Press, New York, Chapter I, Physiology of the enteric nervous system, 1-37 (1981)
30. Burnstock, G.: In: Integrative Functions of the Autonomic Nervous System. Brooks, C.McC., Koizumu, K. and Sato, O. (eds), University of Tokyo Press Elsevier/North-Holland Biomedical Press, 145-158 (1979)
31. Degabriele, R.: Scientific American , 94-99 (1980)
32. Baumgarten, H.G., Holstein, A.-F. and Owman, Ch.: Zeitschrift Zellforsch. 106, 376-397 (1970)
33. Scheuermann, D.W. and Stach, W.: Histochemistry 77, 303-311 (1983)
34. Stach, W.: Z. Mikrosk. Ant. Forsch. Leipzig 95, 161-182 (1981)
35. Read, J.B. and Burnstock, G.: Comp. Biochem. Physiol. 27, 505-517 (1968)
36. Seno, N., Nakazato, Y. and Ohga, A.: Eur. J. Pharmacol. 51, 229-237 (1978)

References especially on 5-HT

2. Hendrix, T.R. and Castell, D.O.: In: Alimentary Tract Motility. American Gastroenterological Association (eds), Milner-Fenwick, Inc., 1-15 (1982)

3. Appenzeller, O.: In: The Autonomic Nervous System, Chapter I. Anatomy and histology. Appenzeller, O. (ed), Elsevier Biomed. Press, 1-29 (1982)

5. Sladek, J.R. and McNeill, T.H.: Cell Tissue Res. 210, 181-189 (1980)

6. Roman, C. and Gonella, J.: In: Physiology of the Gastrointestinal Tract, Chapter IX. Extrinsic control of digestive tract motility. Johnson, L.R. (ed), Raven Press, N.Y., 289-334 (1981)

9. Gershon, M.D., Payette, R.F. and Rothman, T.P.: Fed. Proc. 42, 1620-1625 (1983)

11. Riemann, J.F.: In: Basic Science in Gastroenterology. Structure of the Gut. Polak, J.M. et al. (eds), Glaxo, 289-302 (1982)

13. Argenzio, R.A.: In: Veterinary Gastroenterology, Chapter XII. Comparative physiology of the gastrointestinal system. N.V. Anderson, Lea & Febiger (eds), 172-198 (1980)

37. Nada, O., Hiratsuka, T. and Komatsu, K.: Histochemistry 81, 115-118 (1984)

38. Donowitz, M., Charney, A.N. and Tai, J.H.: In: Mech. Intestinal Secret., Kroc Foundation Series, vol. 12. Binder, H.J. (ed), Alan R. Liss Inc., New York, 217-230 (1979)

39. Thompson, J.H.: Res. Commun. Path. Pharmacol. 2, 688-772 (1971)

40. Resnick, R.H. and Gray, S.J.: Gastroenterology 42, 48-55 (1962)

41. Legay, C., Faudon, M., Héry, F. and Ternaux, J.P.: Neurochem. Int. 5, 571-577 (1983)

42. Legay, C., Faudon, M., Héry, F. and Ternaux, J.P.: Neurochem. Int. 5, 721-727 (1983)

43. Ternaux, J.P., Gonella, J., Legay, C., Faudon, M., Barrit, M.C. and Héry, F.: J. Physiol. (Paris) 77, 319-326 (1981)

44. Rubin, W. and Schwartz, : Gastroenterology 84, 34-50 (1983)

45. Nemoto, N., Kawaoi, A. and Shikata, T.: Biomed. Res. 3, 181-187 (1982)

46. Weyns, A., Stoppie, P., Verhofstad, A.A.J., Degryse, A.-D. and Ooms, L.: Acta Morphol. Neerl. Scand. 23, 59 (1985)

47. Weyns, A., Stoppie, P., Ooms, L., Verhofstad, A.A.J., Van de Mieroop, F. and Krediet, P.: Proc. XXII World Vet. Congress Perth (1983)

48. Weyns, A., Apers, C., Ooms, L. and Krediet, P.: Proc. XV Congress Eur. Vet. Anatomists Utrecht (1984)

49. Butler, S.P. and Hinterberger, H.: Pathology 12, 219-222 (1980)

50. Grube, D. and Forssmann, W.G.: Z. Zellforsch. 140, 551-565 (1973)

51. Grube, D.: Progress in Histochem. & Cytochem. 8, 1-128. Grammann, W., Loyda, C., Pearse, H.G.E. and Schiebler, T.H. (eds), Gustave Fischer Verlag, Stuttgart (1976)

52. Pentilla, A.: Acta Physiol. Scand. 69,281, 1-69 (1966)

53. Pentilla, A.: Histochemie N., 185-194 (1967)

54. Pentilla, A.: Z. Zellforsch. 91, 380-390 (1968)

55. Pentilla, A. and Hirvonen, J.: Scand. J. Gastroenterol. 4, 489-496 (1969)

56. Pentilla, A. and Lemfinen, M.: Gastroenterology 54, 375-381 (1968)

57. Polak, J.M., De Mey, J. and Bloom, S.R.: In: 5-Hydroxytryptamine in Peripheral Reactions. De Clerck, F. and Vanhoutte, P.M. (eds), Raven Press, NY, 23-35 (1982)

58. Nilsson, G., Larsson, L.I., Hakanson, R., Brodin, E., Pernow, B. and Sundler, F.: Histochemistry 43, 87-99 (1975)

59. Pearse, A.G.E. and Polak, J.M.: Virchows Arch. B. Cell Pathol. 16, 111-120 (1974)

60. Alumets, J., Hakanson, R., Sundler, F. and Chang, K.J.: Histochemistry 56, 187-196 (1978)

61. Heitz, P.V., Kasper, M., Krey, G., Polak, J.M. and Pearse, A.G.E.: Gastroenterology 74, 713-717 (1978)

62. Pearse, A.G.E., Polak, J.M., Bloom, S.R., Adams, C., Dryburgh, J.R. and Brown, J.D.: Histochemistry 41, 373-375 (1975)

63. Furness, J.B. and Costa, M.: Neuroscience 7, 341-349 (1982)

64. Gershon, M.D. and Sherman, D.L.: J. Comp. Neurol. 204, 407-421 (1982)

65. Costa, M., Furness, J.B., Cuello, A.C., Verhofstad, A.A.J., Steinbusch, H.W.W. and Elde, R.P.: Neuroscience 7, 351-363 (1982)

66. Gershon, M.D.: In: Cell Basis Chemical Messengers in the Digestive System. Grossman, M.I. (ed), Acad. Press Inc., 285-298 (1981)

67. Gershon, M.D.: In: Nerves and the Gut. Brooks, F.J. and Evers, P.W. (eds), Slack Ch.B. U.S.A., 197-206 (1977)

68. Gershon, M.D., Robinson, R.G. and Ross, L.L.: J. Pharmacol. Exp. Therap. 198, 548-561 (1976)

69. Gershon, M.D.: J. Physiol. (Paris) 77, 257-265 (1981)

70. Gershon, M.D. and Dreyfus, C.F.: Brain Res. 184, 229-233 (1980)

71. Dreyfus, C.F., Bornstein, M.B. and Gershon, M.D.: Brain Res. 128, 125-139 (1977)

72. Dreyfus, C.F., Sherman, D.L. and Gershon, M.D.: Brain Res. 128, 109-123 (1977)

73. Griffith, S.G. and Burnstock, G.: Gastroenterology 85, 929-937 (1983)

74. Gaudin-Chazal, G., Seyfritz, N., Araneda, S., Vigier, D. and Puizillout, J.J.: Brain Res. Bull. 8, 503-509 (1982)

75. Tamir, H.: J. Histochem. Cytochem. 30, 837-840 (1982)

76. Tamir, H. and Gershon, M.D.: J. Physiol. (Paris) 77, 283-286 (1981)

77. Brown, J.E.: J. Nutrition 109, 300-303 (1979)

78. Ferrara, A., Jaffe, B.M., McFadden, D.W. and Zinner, M.J.: Surgical forum 35, 198-199 (1984)

79. Forsberg, E.J. and Miller, R.J.: Gastroenterology 82, 1254 (1982)

80. Forsberg, E.J. and Miller, R.J.: J. Pharmacol. Exp. Therap. 227, 755-766 (1983)

81. Kellum, J.M., Donowitz, M., Cerel, A. and Wu, J.: J. Surg. Res. 36, 172-176 (1984)

82. Kellum, J.M., Wu, J. and Donowitz, M.: Surgery 96, 139-145 (1984)

83. Kellum, J., McCabe, M., Schneier, J. and Donowitz, M.: Am. J. Physiol. 245, G824-G831 (1983)

84. Kellum, J.M., McCabe, M., Schneier, J. and Donowitz, M.: Gastroenterology 82, 1098 (1982)

85. Pettersson, G.B., Newson, B., Ahlman, H. and Dahlström, A.: J. Surg. Res. 29, 141-148 (1980)

86. Ahlman, H., Lundberg, J., Dahlström, A. and Kewenter, J. et al.: Acta Physiol. Scand. 98, 366-375 (1976)

87. Burks, T.F. and Long, J.P.: Am. J. Physiol. 211, 619-625 (1966)

88. Burks, T.F. and Long, J.P.: J. Pharm. Sci. 55, 1383-1386 (1966)

89. Drapanas, T., McDonald, J.C. and Stewart, J.D.: Ann. Surg. 156, 528-536 (1962)

90. Peskin, G.W. and Miller, L.D.: Arch. Surg. 85, 701-704 (1962)

91. Bülbring, E. and Crema, A.: J. Physiol. (London) 146, 18-28 (1959)

92. Burks, T.F. and Long, J.P.: J. Pharmacol. Exp. Therap. 156, 267-276 (1967)

93. Burks, T.F. and Long, J.P.: Br. J. Pharmacol. Chemother. 30, 229-239 (1967)

94. Tobe, T., Izumikawa, F., Sano, M. and Tanaka, C.: In: Endocrine Gut and Pancreas. Fujita, T. (ed), Elsevier Scientific Publishing Co., Amsterdam, 371-380 (1976)

95. Eklund, S., Fahrenkrug, J., Jodal, M., Lundgren, O., Schaffalitzky De Muckadell, O.B. and Sjöqvist, A.: J. Physiol. (London) 302, 549-557 (1980)

96. Petterson, G., Dahlström, A., Larsson, I., Lundberg, J.M., Ahlman, H. and Kewenter, J.: Acta Physiol. Scand. 103, 219-224 (1978)

97. Nilsson, O.: Gut 24, 542-548 (1983)

98. Nilsson, O., Cassuto, J., Larsson, P.-A., Dahlström, A., Lundgren, O., Jodal, M., Lidberg, P. and Ahlman, H.: Neuroscience L. (Suppl. 5), 418 (1980)

99. Bülbring, E. and Lin, R.C.Y.: J. Physiol. (London) 140, 381-407 (1958)

100. Toh, C.C.: J. Physiol. (London) 126, 248-254 (1954)

101. Ahlman, H., Bhargawa, H.N., Dahlström, A., Larsson, I., Newson, B., Das Gupta, T.K. and Nyhus, L.M.: Acta Physiol. Scand. 112, 263-269 (1981)

102. Ahlman, H., Bhargawa, H.N., Donahue, P.E., Newson, B., Das Gupta, T.K. and Nyhus, L.M.: Acta Physiol. Scand. 104, 262-270 (1978)

103. Ahlman, H.: Acta Physiol. Scand. suppl. 437, 1-30 (1976)

104. Larsson, I., Dahlström, A., Pettersson, G., Larsson, P.-A., Kewenter, J. and Ahlman, H.: J. Neural Transm. 47, 89-98 (1980)

105. Larsson, I.: Acta Physiol. Scand. suppl. 499, 1-43 (1981)

106. Pettersson, G., Ahlman, H., Bhargawa, H.N., Dahlström, A., Kewenter, J., Larsson, I. and Siepler, J.K.: Acta Physiol. Scand. 107, 327-331 (1979)

107. Tansy, M.F., Rothman, G., Bartlett, J., Farber, P. and Hohenlein, F.J.: J. Pharmacol. Sci. 60, 81-84 (1971)

108. Larsson, L.I., Ahlman, H., Bhargawa, H.N., Dahlström, A., Pettersson, G. and Kewenter, J.: J. Neural Transm. 46, 105-112 (1979)

109. Nanopoulos, D., Belin, M.F., Maitre, M., Vincendon, G. and Pujol, J.F.: Brain Res. 232, 375-389 (1982)

110. Burks, T.F.: J. Pharmacol. Exp. Therap. 185, 530-539 (1973)

111. Thompson, J.H.: J. Am. Med. Assoc. 207, 1883-1886 (1969)

112. Kamikawa, Y. and Shimo, Y.: Br. J. Pharmacol. 78, 103-110 (1983)

113. Gershon, M.D.: Gastroenterology 54, 453-456 (1968)

114. Talalaenko, A.N.: Bull. Eksper. Biol. Med. 68, 961-964 (1969)

115. Gerner, T., Ertresvaag, K., Haffner, J.F.W., Moen, H. and Norstein, J.: XVIIth Congress of the European Soc. Surg. Res. 14, 176 (1982)

116. Misiewicz, J.J., Waller, S.L. and Eisner, M.: Gut 7, 208-216 (1966)

117. Couture, R., Mizrahi, J., Regoli, D. and Devroede, G.: Can. J. Physiol. Pharmacol. 59, 957-964 (1981)

118. Grubb, M.N. and Burks, T.F.: J. Pharmacol. Exp. Therap. 189, 476-483 (1974)

119. Drakontides, A.B. and Gershon, M.D.: Br. J. Pharmacol. Chemother. 33, 480-492 (1968)

120. Adam-Vizi, V. and Vizi, E.S.: J. Neural Transm. 42, 127-138 (1978)

121. Ouyang, A.: Am. J. Physiol. 244, G426-G434 (1983)

122. Moen, H., Ertresvaag, K. and Gerner, T.: Scand. J. Gastroenterol. 18, 145-150 (1983)

123. Mukai, T. and Kubota, K.: Eur. J. Pharmacol. 65, 157-163 (1980)

124. Pruitt, D.B., Grubb, M.N., Jaquette, D.L. and Burks, T.F.: Eur. J. Pharmacol. 26, 248-305 (1974)

125. Huidobro-Toro, J.P. and Foree, B.: Eur. J. Pharmacol. 61, 335-345 (1980)

126. Costa, M. and Furness, J.B.: J. Pharmacol. 65, 237-248 (1979)

127. Ruckebusch, Y. and Ooms, L.: J. Vet. Pharmacol. Therap. 6, 127-132 (1983)

128. Sorraing, J.M., Fioramonti, J. and Bueno, L.: Am. J. Vet. Res. 45, 942-947 (1984)

129. Veenendaal, G.H., Woutersen-Van Nijnanten, F.M.A. and Van Miert, A.S.J.P.A.M.: Am. J. Vet. Res. 41, 479-483 (1980)

130. Arias, J.L., Zurich, L. and Bastias, J.: Pharmacol. Res. Commun. 12, 975-985 (1980)

131. Ratzenhofer, M.: Z. Gastroenterol. 7, 464-471 (1969)

132. Erspamer, V.: Fortschr. Arzneimittelforsch. 3, 351-376 (1961)

133. Donowitz, M., Charney, A.N. and Heffernan, J.M.: Am. J. Physiol. 231, E85-E94 (1977)

134. Gershon, M.D.: Enteric Serotoninergic Neurons, 27-41 (1982)

135. Costa, M. and Furness, J.B.: N-S Arch. Pharm. 294, 47-60 (1976)

136. North, R.A., Henderson, G., Katayama, Y. and Johnson, S.M.: Neuroscience 5, 581-586 (1980)

137. Gershon, M.D.: Science 149, 197-199 (1965)

138. Julé, Y.: J. Physiol. (London) 309, 487-498 (1980)

139. Wood, J.D.: Fed. Proc. 41, 1744 (1982)

140. Brownlee, G. and Johnson, E.S.: Br. J. Pharmacol. 21, 306-322 (1963)

141. Wood, J.D. and Mayer, C.J.: J. Neurophysiol. 42, 582-593 (1979)

142. Wood, J.D. and Mayer, C.J.: J. Neurophysiol. 42, 594-603 (1979)

143. Wood, J.D. and Mayer, C.J.: J. Neurophysiol. 42, 569-581 (1979)

144. Hirai, K. and Koketsu, K.: Br. J. Pharmacol. 70, 499-500 (1980)

145. Nijima, A.: Biomed. Res. 1, 95-97 (1980)

146. Sakai, K., Akima, M. and Shiraki, Y.: Jap. J. Pharmacol. 29, 223-233 (1979)

147. Dun, N.J. and Karczmar, A.G.: J. Pharmacol. Exp. Therap. 217, 714-718 (1981)

148. Glusman, S. and Kravitz, E.A.: J. Physiol. (London) 325, 223-241 (1982)

149. Akasu, T., Hirai, K. and Koketsu, K.: Brain Res. 211, 217-220 (1981)

150. Oderfeld-Nowak, B.: Gen. Pharmacol. 11, 37-45 (1979)

151. Gaginella, T.S., Rimele, T.J. and Wietecha, M.: J. Physiol. (London) 335, 101-111 (1983)

152. Grimmer, A.J. and Leathard, H.L.: Br. J. Pharmacol. 73, 190 (1981)

153. Humphrey, P.P.A.: Br. J. Pharmacol. 63, 671-675 (1978)

154. Majundar, A.P.N. and Nakhla, A.M.: Br. J. Pharmacol. 66, 211-215 (1979)

155. Grube, D.: Chromaffin, Enterochromaffin and related cells, 265-292 (1976)

156. Furness, J.B. and Costa, M.: Eur. J. Pharmacol. 56, 69-74 (1979)

157. Burnstock, G.: Arch. Int. Pharmacodyn. 280, suppl. 1-15 (1986)

158. Grube, D.: In: Endocrine Gut and Pancreas, Chapter 10. Coupland, R.E. and Fujita, T. (eds), Elsevier Scientific Publishing Company, 119-132 (1976)

References expecially on VIP

1. Polak, J.M. and Bloom, S.R.: In: Cell Basis of Chemical Messengers in the Digestive System. Grossman, M.I. et al. (eds), Acad. Press Inc., 267-282 (1981)

4. Polak, J.M. and Bloom, S.R.: In: Gut Peptides. Bloom, S.R. and Polak, J.M. (eds), 2nd ed., 487-494 (1981)

7. Sundler, F., Hakanson, R. and Leander, S.: Clin. Gastroenterol. 9, 517-543 (1980)

10. Jessen, K.R., Polak, J.M., Van Noorden, S., Bloom, S.R. and Burnstock, G.: Nature 283, 391-393 (1980)

12. Hakanson, R., Leander, S., Sundler, F. and Uddman, R.: In: Cell Basis of Chemical Messengers in the Digestive System. Grossman, M.I. et al. (eds), Acad. Press Inc., 169-199 (1981)

159. Alumets, J., Fahrenkrug, J., Hakanson, R., Schaffalitzky De Muckadell, O., Sundler, F. and Uddman, R.: Nature 280, 155-156 (1971)

160. Fahrenkrug, J.: In: Gut Peptides. Bloom, S.R. and Polak, J.M. (eds), 385-391 (1981)

161. Furness, J.B. and Costa, M.: In: Vasoactive Intestinal Peptides. Said, S.I. (ed), Raven Press NY, 391-406 (1982)

162. Uddman, R., Alumets, J., Edvinsson, L., Hakanson, R. and Sundler, F.: Gastroenterology 75, 5-8 (1978)

163. Fahrenkrug, J.: In: Vasoactive Intestinal Peptides. Said, S.I. (ed), Raven Press NY, 361-372 (1982)

164. Fahrenkrug, J.: Digestion 19, 149-169 (1979)

165. Hakanson, R., Sundler, F. and Uddman, R.: In: Vasoactive Intestinal Peptides. Said, S.I. (ed), Raven Press NY, 121-144 (1982)

166. Kachelhoffer, J., Mendel, C., Dauchel, J., Hohmatter, D., and Grenier, J.F.: Am. J. Dig. Dis. 21, 957-962 (1976)

167. Hokfelt, T., Schultzberg, M., Lundberg, J.M., Fuxe, K., Mutt, U., Fahrenkrug, J. and Said, S.I.: In: Vasoactive Intestinal Peptides. Said, S.I. (ed), Raven Press NY, 65-90 (1982)

168. Biancani, P., Walsh, Y.H. and Behar, J.: J. Clin. Invest. 73, 963-967 (1984)

169. Rosselin, G., Maletti, M., Besson, J. and Rostène, W.: Mol. Cell Endocrinol. 27, 243-262 (1982)

170. Cassuto, J., Fahrenkrug, J., Jodal, M., Tuttle, R. and Lundgren, O.: Gut 22, 958-963 (1981)

171. Edin, R., Lundberg, J.M., Ahlman, H., Dahlström, A., Fahrenkrug, J., Hökfelt, T. and Kewenter, J.: Acta Physiol. Scand. 17, 185-187 (1979)

172. Jessen, K.R., Polak, J.M., Van Noorden, S., Bryant, M.G., Bloom, S.R. and Burnstock, G.: Gastroenterology 76, 1161 (1979)

173. Kachelhoffer, J., Marescaux, J., Michel, F. and Grenier, J.-F.: Gastroenterology 3, 381-396 (1979)

174. Larsson, L.I., Polak, J.M., Buffa, R., Sundler, F. and Solcia, E.: J. Histochem. Cytochem. 27, 936 (1979)

175. Larsson, L.I., Fahrenkrug, J., Schaffalitzky de Muckadell, O., Sundler, F., Hakanson, R. and Rehfeld, J.F.: Proc. Natl. Acad. Sci. U.S.A. 73, 3197-3200 (1976)

176. Matsuo, Y., Yanaihara, N., Seki, A. and Fukuda, S.: In: Gut Peptides. Biomedical Press Kodanska/Elsevier, 275-280 (1979)

177. Miller, R.J.: Med. Biology 58, 179-181 (1980)

178. Schultzberg, M., Hökfelt, T., Terenius, L., Elfvin, L.G., Lundberg, J.M. and Brand, J.: Neuroscience 4, 249-270 (1979)

179. Morgan, K.G., Schmalz, P.F. and Szurszewski, J.H.: J. Physiol. (London) 282, 437-450 (1978)

180. Cooke, H.J., Carey, H.V. and Walsh, J.: Gastroenterology 86, 1053 (1984)

181. Laburthe, M. and Dupont, C.: In: Vasoactive Int. Pept. Said, S.I. (ed), Raven Press NY, 407-423 (1982)

182. Bishop, A.E., Blank, M.A., Christofides, N.D., Bloom, S.R., Tatemoto, K. and Polak, J.M.: Regul. Pept. 6, 287 (1983)

183. Bishop, A.E., Ferri, G.L., Probert, L., Bloom, S.R. and Polak, J.M.: Scand. J. Gastroenterol. 17(S72), 43-59 (1982)

184. Polak, J.M. and Bloom, S.R.: In: Vasoactive Int. Pept. Said, S.I. (ed), Raven Press NY, 107-120 (1982)

185. Leander, S., Hakanson, R. and Sundler, F.: Cell Tissue Res. 215, 21-39 (1981)

186. Bakker, R. and Groot, J.A.: Gastro Cl B 7, 496 (1983)

187. Barbezat, G.O. and Grossman, M.I.: Science 174, 422-424 (1971)

188. Fahrenkrug, J.: Biomed. Res. 1 (Suppl.), 84-87 (1980)

189. Polak, J.M., Pearse, A.G.E., Garaud, J.-C. and Bloom, S.R.: Gut 15, 720-724 (1974)

190. Lundberg, J.M., Hökfelt, T., Kewenter, J., Pettersson, G., Ahlman, H., Edin, R., Dahlström, A., Nilsson, G., Terenius, L., Uvnäs-Wallensten, K. and Said, S.I.: Gastroenterology 77, 468-471 (1979)

191. Said, S.I.: In: Gastrointestinal Hormones. Jerzy Glass, G.B. (ed), Raven Press NY, 245-273 (1980)

192. Vagne, M., Konturek, S.J. and Chayvialle, J.A.: Gastroenterology 83, 250-255 (1982)

193. Domschke, S. and Domschke, W.: In: Vasoactive Int. Pept. Said, S.I. (ed), Raven Press NY, 201-209 (1982)

194. Chayvialle, J.A., Miyata, M., Rayford, P.L. and Thompson, J.C.:

Gastroenterology 79, 844-852 (1980)

195. Makhlouf, G.M.: In: Vasoactive Int. Pept. Said, S.I. (ed), Raven Press NY, 425-446 (1982)

196. Turnberg, L.A.: Scand. J. Gastroenterol. (symposium book) 18, 85-89 (1983)

197. Andersson, P.O., Bloom, S.R. and Järhult, J.: J. Physiol. (London) 334, 293-307 (1983)

198. Neya, T., Yamasato, T., Takaki, M., Mizutani, M. and Nakayama, S.: Biomed. Res. 2, 398-403 (1981)

199. Fahrenkrug, J., Schaffalitzky De Muckadell, O.B., Holst, J.J. and Lindkaer Jensen, S.: Am. J. Physiol. 237, E535-E540 (1979)

200. Holst, J.J., Fahrenkrug, J., Jensen, S.I., Nielsen, O.V. and Knuhtsen, S.: Digestion 25, 37 (1982)

201. Schrauwen, E. and Houvenaghel, A.: IRCS Medical Science 10, 997-998 (1982)

202. Berridge, M.J.: Scand. J. Gastroenterol. (symposium book) 18, 43-49 (1983)

203. Gespach, C., Hui Bon Hoa, D. and Rosselin, G.: Endocrinol. 112, 1597-1606 (1983)

204. Kirkegaard, P., Skov Olsen, P., Poulsen, S.S. and Nexo, E.: Regul. Pept. 7, 367-372 (1983)

205. Siegel, S.R., Brown, F.C., Castell, D.O., Johnson, L.F. and Said, S.I.: Dig. Dis. Sci. 24, 345-349 (1979)

206. Grider, J.R., Said, S.I. and Makhlouf, G.M.: Gastroenterology 82, 1075 (1982)

207. Grider, J.R., Bitar, K.N. and Makhlouf, G.M.: Regul. Pept. 6, 316 (1983)

208. Gustavsson, S., Johansson, H., Lundqvist, G. and Nilsson, F.: Scand. J. Gastroenterol. 12, 993-997 (1977)

209. Grider, J.R., Bitar, K.N., Said, S.I. and Makhlouf, G.M.: Gastroenterology 84, 1175 (1983)

210. Bishop, A.E., Polak, J.M. and Lake, B.D.: Histopathol. 5, 679-688 (1981)

211. Holstein, B. and Humphrey, C.S.: Acta Physiol. Scand. 109, 217-223 (1980)

212. Konturek, S.J., Dembinski, A., Thor, P. and Krol, R.: Pflügers Archiv 361, 175-181 (1976)

213. Makhlouf, G.M., Zfass, A.M., Said, S.I. and Schebalin, M.: Proc. Soc. Exp. Biol. Med. 157, 565-568 (1978)

214. Anteunis, A., Gespach, C., Astesano, A., Emani, S., Robineaux, R. and Rosselin, G.: Regul. Pept. 6, 285 (1983)

215. Anteunis, A., Gespach, C., Astesano, A., Emani, S., Robineaux, R. and Rosselin, G.: Peptides 5, 277-283 (1984)

216. Saffouri, B., Duval, J.W., Arimura, A. and Makhlouf, G.M.: Gastroenterology 86, 839-842 (1984)

217. Waldman, D.B., Gardner, J.D., Zfass, A.M. and Makhlouf, G.M.: Gastroenterology 73, 518-523 (1977)

218. Mainoya, J.R. and Bern, H.A.: Zool. Sci. 1, 100-105 (1984)

219. Krejs, G.J.: In: Vasoactive Int. Pept. Said, S.I. (ed), Raven Press, NY, 193-200 (1982)

220. Gaginella, T.S., Hubel, K.A. and O'Dorisio, T.M.: In: Vasoactive Int. Pept. Said, S.I. (ed), Raven Press, NY, 211-222 (1982)

221. Camilleri, M., Cooper, B.T., Adrian, T.E., Bloom, S.R. and Chadwick, V.S.: Gut 22, 14-18 (1981)

222. Sninsky, C.A., Wolfe, M.M., Martin, J.L., Howe, B.A., O'Dorisio, T.M., McGuigan, J.E. and Mathias, J.R.: Am. J. Physiol. 244, G46-G51 (1983)

223. Krejs, G.J., Barkley, R.M., Read, N.W. and Fordtran, J.S.: J. Clin. Invest. 61, 1337-1345 (1978)

224. Krejs, G.J., O'Dorisio, T.M., Shulkes, A.A., Walsh, J.H., Said, S.I. and Fordtran, J.S.: Gastroenterology 76, 1177 (1979)

225. Krejs, G.J.: Regul. Pept. 6, 313 (1983)

226. Krejs, G.J.: Peptides 5, 271-276 (1984)

227. Kane, M.G., O'Dorisio, T.M. and Krejs, G.J.: Gastroenterology 84, 1202 (1983)

228. Krejs, G.J., Fordtran, J.S., Bloom, S.R., Fahrenkrug, Y., Schaffalitzky De Muckadell, O.B., Fischer, J.E., Humphrey, C.S., O'Dorisio, T.M., Said, S.I., Walsh, J.H. and Shulkes, A.A.: Gastroenterology 78, 722-727 (1980)

229. Isenberg, J.I., Wallin, B., Johansson, C., Smedfors, B., Mutt, V., Tatemoto, K. and Enas, S.: Regul. Pept. 8, 315-320 (1984)

230. Wu, Z.C., O'Dorisio, T.M., Cataland, S., Mekhjian, H.S. and Gaginella, T.S.: Dig. Dis. Sci. 24, 625-630 (1979)

231. Kanno, T. and Saito, A.: Endocrinol. Japon. S.R. 1, 51-57 (1980)

232. Ipp, E., Dobs, R.E. and Unger, R.H.: FEBS Letters 90, 76-78 (1978)

233. Nakaki, T., Nakadate, T., Yamamoto, S. and Kato, R.: J. Pharmacol. Exp. Therap. 220, 637-641 (1982)

234. Williams, J.T. and North, R.A.: Brain Res. 175, 174-177 (1979)

References especially on SP

1. Polak, J.M. and Bloom, S.R.: In: Cell Basis of Chemical Messengers in the Digestive System. Grossman, M.I. et al. (eds), Acad. Press Inc., 267-282 (1981)

4. Polak, J.M. and Bloom, S.R.: In: Gut Peptides. Bloom, S.R. and Polak, J.M. (eds), 2nd ed., 487-494 (1981)

7. Sundler, F., Hakanson, R. and Leander, S.: Clin. Gastroenterol. 9, 517-543 (1980)

8. Gabella, G.: In: Basic Science in Gastroenterology. Structure of the Gut. Polak, J.M. et al. (eds), Glaxo, 193-203 (1982)

12. Hakanson, R., Leander, S., Sundler, F. and Uddman, R.: In: Cell Basis of Chemical Messengers in the Digestive System. Grossman, M.I. et al. (eds), Acad. Press. Inc., 169-199 (1981)

14. Gershon, M.D.: Ann. Rev. Neurosci. 4, 227-272 (1981)

15. Blood, D.C., Henderson, J.A. and Radostits, O.M.: In: Veterinary Medicine. A Textbook of the Diseases of Cattle, Sheep, Pigs and Horses. London, B. Tindall (eds), 1135 (1981)

16. Baljet, B. and Drukker, J.: Stain Technology 50, 31-36 (1975)

17. Furness, J.B. and Costa, M.: Histochemistry 41, 335-352 (1975)

18. Forssmann, W.G., Pickel, V., Reinecke, M., Hock, D. and Metz, J.: In: Techniques in Neuroanatomical Research. Heym, Ch. and Forssmann, W.G. (eds), Springer Verlag, 171-205 (1981)

19. Sternberger, L.A.: Mikroscopy 25, 346-361 (1969)

20. Long, R.G. and Bryant, M.G.: In: Radioimmunoassay of Gut Regulatory Peptides. Bloom, S.R. and Long, R.G. (eds), W.B. Saunders Company Ltd., London (1982)

21. Malfors, G., Leander, S., Brodin, E., Hakanson, R., Holmin, T. and Sundler, F.: Cell Tiss. Res. 214, 225-238 (1981)

22. Marani, E.: Topographic enzyme histochemistry of the mammalian cerebellum 5-Nucleotidase and acetylcholinesterase. Thesis, Leiden (1982)

23. Silva, D.G., Farrell, K.E. and Smith, G.C.: Anat. Rec. 162, 157-175 (1968)

24. Furness, J.B. and Costa, M.: Ergebn. Physiol. 69, 1-51 (1974)

25. Jacobowitz, D.: J. Pharmacol. Exp. Therap. 149, 358-364 (1965)

26. Llewellyn-Smith, I.J., Furness, J.B., Wilson, A. J. and Costa, M.: In: Autonomic Ganglia. Lars Gösta Elfin (ed), 145-182 (1983)

27. Furness, J.B. and Costa, M.: Neuroscience 5, 1-20 (1980)

28. Costa, M. and Gabella, G.: Z. Zellforsch. 122, 357-377 (1971)

30. Burnstock, G.: In: Integrative Functions of the Autonomic Nervous System. Brooks, C. McC., Koizumu, K. and Sato, O. (eds), University of Tokyo Press Elsevier/North-Holland Biomedical Press, 145-158 (1979)

31. Degabriele, R.: Sciéntific American, 94-99 (1980)

32. Baumgarten, H.G., Holstein, A.-F. and Owman, Ch.: Zeitschrift Zellforsch. 106, 376-397 (1970)

33. Scheuermann, D.W. and Stach, W.: Histochemistry 77, 303-311 (1983)

34. Stach, W.: Z. Mikrosk. Ant. Forsch. Leipzig 95, 161-182 (1981)

35. Read, J.B. and Burnstock, G.: Comp. Biochem. Physiol. 27, 505-517 (1968)

36. Seno, N., Nakazato, Y. and Ohga, A.: Eur. J. Pharmacol. 51, 229-237 (1978)

62. Pearse, A.G.E., Polak, J.M., Bloom, S.R., Adams, C., Dryburgh, J.R. and Brown, J.D.: Histochemistry 41, 373-375 (1975)

178. Schultzberg, M., Hökfelt, T., Terenius, L., Elfvin, L.G., Lundberg, J.M. and Brand, J.: Neuroscience 4, 249-270 (1979)

183. Bishop, A.E., Ferri, G.L., Probert, L., Bloom, S.R. and Pôlak, J.M.: Scand. J. Gastroenterol. 17 (S72), 43-59 (1982)

235. Brodin, E., Alumets, J., Hakanson, R., Leander, S. and Sundler, F.: Cell Tiss. Res. 216, 455-469 (1981)

236. Donnerer, J., Bartho, L., Holzer, P. and Lembeck, F.: Neuroscience 11, 913-918 (1984)

237. Kamikawa, Y. and Shimo, Y.: Br. J. Pharmacol. 81, 143-149 (1984)

238. Ahlman, H., Dahlström, A., Lidberg, P. and Lundberg, J.: Gastroenterology 82, 1006 (1982)

239. Lidberg, P., Edin, R., Lundberg, J.M., Dahlström, A., Rosell, S., Folkers, K. and Ahlman, H.: Acta Physiol. Scand. 114, 307-309 (1982)

240. Rosell, S.: In: Peptides: Integrators of Cell & Tissue Function. Bloom, F.E. (ed), 147-162 (1980)

241. Bishop, A.E., Cole, G.A., Probert, L., Hodson, N.P., Bloom, S.R. and Polak, J.M.: Regul. Pept. 3, 65 (1982)

242. Cummings, J.F., Sellers, A.F. and Lowe, J.E.: Equine Vet. J. 71, 23-29 (1984)

243. Polak, J.M. and Pearse, A.G.E.: In: Endocrine Gut and Pancreas. Fujita, T. (ed), Elsevier Scientific Publishin Company Amsterdam, 103-111 (1976)

244. Hökfelt, T., Elde, R., Johansson, O., Luft, R., Nilsson, G. and Arimura, A.: Neuroscience 1, 131-136 (1976)

245. Sundler, F., Hakanson, R., Larsson, L.I., Brodin, E. and Nilsson, G.: In: Substance. Van Euler, U.S. and Pernow, B. (eds), Raven Press NY, 59-65 (1977)

246. Brimijoin, S., Lundberg, J.M., Brodin, E., Hökfelt, T. and Nilsson, G.: Brain Res. 191, 443-445 (1980)

247. Hökfelt, T., Elfvin, L.G., Elde, R., Schultzberg, N., Goldstein, N. and Luft, R.: Proc. Natl. Acad. Sci. 74, 3587-3591 (1977)

248. Hökfelt, T., Elfvin, L.G., Schultzberg, N., Goldstein, N. and Nilsson, G.: Brain Res. 128 , 29-41 (1977)

249. Reynolds, J.C., Ouyang, A. and Cohen, S.: Am. J. Physiol. 246, G346-G354 (1984)

250. Donnerer, J. et al.: Br. J. Pharmacol. 83, 919-925 (1984)

251. Delbro, D., Fändriks, L., Rosell, S. and Folkers, K.: Acta Physiol. Scand. 118, 309-316 (1983)

252. Lidberg, P., Dahlström, A., Lundberg, J.M. and Ahlman, H.: Regul. Pept. 7, 41-52 (1983)

253. Aggestrup, S. and Jensen, S.L.: Regul. Pept. 4, 155-162 (1982)

254. Fox, J.E.T., Daniel, E.E. and Jury, J.: Gastroenterology 84, 1158 (1983)

255. Hirning, L.D. and Burks, T.F.: Gastroenterology 84, 1188 (1983)

256. Mayer, E.A., Khawaja, S., Elashoff, J. and Walsh, J.H.: Gastroenterology 7, 715 (1983)

257. Mayer, E.A., Khawaja, S., Elashoff, J. and Walsh, J.H.: Gastroenterology 84, 1244 (1983)

258. Milenov, K. and Golenhofen, K.: Pflügers Arch. 397, 29-34 (1983)

259. Nieber, K., Oehme, P. and Milenov, K.: Pharmazie 37, 656-658 (1982)

260. Wali, F.A.: J. Physiol. (London) 351, 30 (1984)

261. Barber, W.D. and Burks, T.F.: Fed. Proc. 43, 895 (1984)

262. Fujisawa, K. and Ito, Y.: Br. J. Pharmacol. 76, 279-290 (1982)

263. Holzer, P. and Lembeck, F.: Neuroscience 17, 101-105 (1980)

110

263. Holzer, P. and Lembeck, F.: Eur. J. Pharmacol. 61, 303-307 (1980)
     Holzer, P. and Lembeck, F.: Neuroscience 6, 1433-1441 (1981)
264. Holzer, P.: N-S Arch. Pharmacol. 320, 217-220 (1982)
265. Krier, J. and Szurszewski, J.H.: Am. J. Physiol. 243, G259-G267
     (1982)
266. Mizrahi, J., D'Orléans-Juste, P. and Regoli, D.: Fed. Proc. 41, 457
     (1982)
267. Nieber, K., Milenov, K., Bergmann, J. and Oehme, P.: Acta Biol. Med.
     40, 209-216 (1981)
268. Yau, W.M.: Gastroenterology 74, 228-231 (1978)
269. Angel, F., Go, V.L.W. and Szurszewski, J.H.S.: Gut 25, 1327-1328
     (1984)
270. Huizinga, J.D., Chang, G., Diamant, N.E. and El-Sharkawy, T.Y.:
     J. Pharmacol. Exp. Therap. 231, 692-699 (1984)
271. Hedqvist, P. and Von Euler, U.S.: Acta Physiol. Scand. 95, 341-343
     (1975)
272. Katayama, Y. and North, R.A.: Nature 274, 387-388 (1978)
273. Benham, C.D. and Bolton, T.B.: Br. J. Pharmacol. 80, 409-420 (1983)
274. Holzer, P. and Lippe, I.T.: Br. J. Pharmacol. 82, 259-267 (1984)
275. Premen, A.J., Dobbins, D.E., Soika, C.Y. and Dabney, J.M.: Regul.
     Pept. 9, 119-127 (1984)
276. Angel, F., Go, V.L.W. and Dzurszewski, J.H.S.: Gastroenterology 82,
     1008 (1982)
277. Gabella, G.: Inter Review Cytology 59, 129-193 (1979)
278. Franco, R., Costa, M. and Furness, J.B.: Arch. Pharmacol. 3, 195-201
     (1979)
279. Ohkawa, H. and Tohoku, J.: J. Exp. Med. 142, 409-422 (1984)
280. Konturek, S.J., Jaworek, J., Tasler, J., Cieszkowski, M., Walus,
     K.M., Gustaw, P. and Thor, P.: In: Gut Peptides. Bloom, S.R. and
     Polak, J.M. (eds), 2nd ed., 402-406 (1981)
281. Andrews, N.J., Rinno-Barmada, S., Gurdett, K. and Elder, J.B.: Gut
     24, 326-332 (1983)
282. Kachur, J.F., Miller, R.J., Field, M. and Rivier, J.: J. Pharmacol.
     Exp. Therap. 220, 456-463 (1982)
283. Donowitz, M., Fogel, R., Battisti, L. and Asarkof, N.: Life Sci.
     31, 1929-1937 (1982)

References especially on functional approach

284. Bolton, T.B.: Physiol. Rev. 59, 606-718 (1979)

285. Weiss, G.B.: In: Advances in General and Cellular Pharmacology. Vol.
     II. Narahashi, T. and Bianchi, C.P. (eds), Plenum Press, NY, 71-154
     (1977)

286. Weiss, G.B.: In: New Perspectives on Calcium Antagonists. Weiss, G.B.
     (ed), Williams and Wilkins, Baltimore (1981)

287. Triggle, D.J.: In: New Perspectives on Calcium Antagonists. Weiss,
     G.B. (ed), Williams and Wilkins, Baltimore (1981)

288. Karaki, H. and Weiss, G.B.: Gastroenterology 87, 960-970 (1984)

289. Milanov, M.P., Stoyanov, N. and Boev, K.K.: Gen. Pharmacol. 15,
     99-105 (1984)

290. Ooms, L.A.A., Degryse, A.-D. and Weyns, A.: Presented at the
     Achtste Vergadering. FGWO Kontaktgroep "Sekreties en Motiliteit van
     het Spijsverteringsstelsel". Leuven. In Press (1985)

291. Ruckebusch, Y., Fargeas, J. and Bueno, L.: Annales de Recherches
     Vétérinaires 3, 131-148 (1969)

292. Fioramonti, J., Bueno, L., Ooms, L. and Ruckebusch, Y.: J. Vet.
     Pharmacol. Therap. 5, 213-215 (1982)

293. Ooms, L.A.A., Degryse, A.-D.A.Y., Weyns, A. and Ruckebusch, Y.: In:
     The Ruminant Stomach. Ooms, L.A.A., Degryse, A.D. and Marsboom, R.
     (eds), Proc. of an Intern. Workshop, Antwerp, 324-353 (1985)

4. RETICULO-RUMEN MOTILITY: IN VITRO AND IN VIVO EFFECTS OF ENDOGENOUS SUBSTANCES

A.S.J.P.A.M. van Miert

I. Introduction

II. Agents and their Actions

   1. alpha- en beta-sympathomimetic agents

   2. parasympathomimetics

   3. bradykinin and substance P

   4. prostaglandins

   5. histamine

   6. serotonin

   7. opioid agonists and antagonists

III. Conclusions

I. INTRODUCTION

The organizers had intended that my review for this workshop should cover a discussion of the current status in the field of pharmacological research, rather than encyclopedic coverage of many papers, dealing with drug-induced changes in forestomach motility. I have attempted to comply with this idea. Fortunately, many of the areas not discussed here have been given extensive coverage in related reviews (29,30,41,45,58).

Studies of isolated reticulo-ruminal muscle can yield a vast amount of information about motility. Of course, a complete understanding of the behaviour of the forestomach system must involve studies in intact animals. The use of drugs and techniques *in vivo*, however, is often limited on technical grounds. Furthermore, reticulo-rumen motility *in vivo* is complicated by many variable factors. Some of these, such as stress, are relatively easy to control. Others, such as the regulatory effects of the extrinsic nerves and of enterogastric reflexes, can be only partly eliminated by denervation and by other means. Even more difficult to control are the effects of circulating hormones such as ACTH, glucocorticosteroids, gastrin and cholecystokinin, physiologic and drug-induced changes in reticulo-ruminal blood flow, and the effects of drugs on the hypothalamus and on the cerebral cortex. Both areas may exert a controlling influence over those regions of the medulla oblongata in which the basis reflex centres are believed to be situated.

Isolation of reticulo-ruminal tissue from the body overcomes these problems. At the same time it introduces other important factors. First, contraction of an isolated strip does not necessarily correlate with mixing and propulsion of contents *in vivo*. Second, problems arise if the isolated strip has no blood supply. The central part of thick tissues then becomes hypoxic. A further consequence is that any drug administered *in vitro* must diffuse into the tissue in an abnormal manner. This point may account for differences in sensitivity and in the way the muscle responds. Diffusion into isolated strips may, on the other hand, be an advantage in some experiments. It may simulate more closely the conditions *in vivo*, when a substance is released inside the tissue instead of being carried there by the bloodstream. Advantages of studying isolated tissues are that only direct effects on the muscle or intrinsic nerves are measured, that many of the variable factors *in vivo* are eliminated, and that the techniques are relatively easy and are unlimited in scope. However, as many of the following examples will show, results *in vivo* and *in vitro* are often different. *In vitro*, many agents such as $alpha_1$-sympathomimetics, para-sympathomimetics, substance P, bradykinin, serotonin and PGE_1, induce dose-dependent increases in smooth muscle tone, whereas *in vivo* these substances cause a dose-dependent inhibition of the extrinsic contraction sequences (16,19,22,39,47,51,59-61). On the other hand, vasopressin and octapressin are potent inhibitors of forestomach motility *in situ*, although these substances are rather inactive on isolated ruminal smooth muscle (46,58). Therefore, other mechanisms, like local changes in gastric blood flow, may be involved. A more detailed investigation concerning the influence of changes in local blood flow on reticulo-rumen motility has to be done. Furthermore, the reticulo-rumen hypomotility induced by vasopressin administered either centrally or peripherally was associated with increased gastro-duodenal motor activity (30). This effect may be, in turn, at the origin of the changes in forestomach motility. Another example is ACTH. Administered i.v. at a dose of 10 µg kg^{-1}, this hormone induces hyperglycaemia and a moderate inhibition of the extrinsic rumen contractions in the goat (Fig. 1). Changes in the motility of the

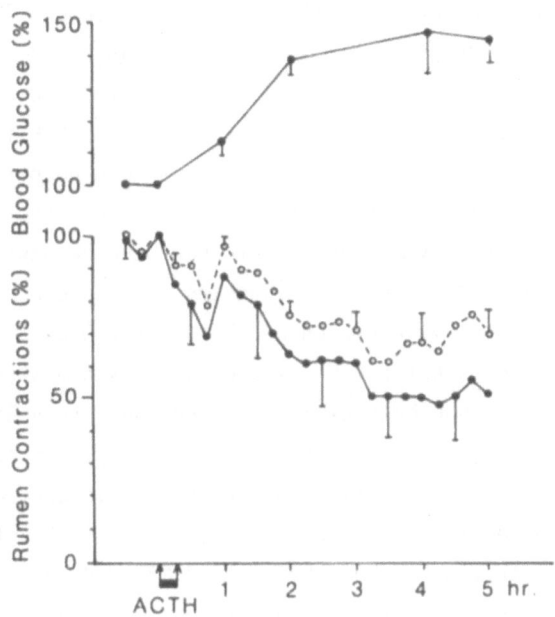

FIGURE 1. The effect of ACTH (Cortrosyn[R], 10 µg kg^{-1} body weight i.v. given in 15 min) on blood glucose levels (base line values $\pm$ SEM: 3.3 $\pm$ 0.1 mMol) and extrinsic rumen contractions in conscious goats (n=4). The contractions and blood glucose levels are expressed as percentages of base line value; o = frequency of contractions per 15 min; ● = summation derived from 15 min intervals of amplitude. All values are given as mean $\pm$ SEM (bars)

reticulum and rumen associated with hyperglycaemia have been reported by others as well (15,44,45). Where and how hyperglycaemia exerts its influence has not been defined. These examples demonstrate the complex nature of pharmacological research on reticulo-ruminal motor functions. The most obvious examples of correlation *in vivo* and *in vitro* are the effects of the beta-adrenergic drug isoprenaline and the gastro-intestinal hormone eledoisin, which respectively relax and contract reticulo-ruminal smooth muscles both *in situ* and in the organ bath (9,47,51).

How to analyse these complex responses? First of all, there exist different types of reticulo-ruminal contractions. There are characteristic, powerful *extrinsic* contraction sequences, termed primary and secondary cycle movements, which occur once per minute approximately, and which are wholy dependent upon reflex mechanisms involving *afferent* and *efferent* pathways in vagal nerves and bilaterally paired "gastric centres" in the medulla oblongata (12,13,18,41). These contractions cease after the vagus nerves have been cut or after administration of parasympatholytic agents and ganglionic-blocking drugs (2,5,6,11,45). These and other observations support the conclusion that the rumen and reticulum receive a cholinergic excitatory innervation via the vagus nerves. However, inhibitory effects of *efferent* vagus nerve stimulation on the reticulum have been recognized under certain experimental conditions (41). Furthermore, the presence of substance P-fibers in the bovine vagus nerve has been demonstrated, whereas in the gastro-intestinal tract of other species substance P has been found in neurons of the plexuses of Auerbach and Meissner (10,25,27,62). There-fore, the possibility of substance P being a vagal transmitter substance must be considered. Although both excitatory and inhibitory effects of sympathomimetic agents on reticulum and rumen motility have been reported, bilateral splanchnectomy has no effect on the extrinsic contractions (5,11, 49). Furthermore, there are weak, localized *intrinsic* contractions occurring 6-9 times per minute, both before and after denervation of the reticulo-rumen. They can be felt as "ripples" during manual exploration of the mucosal surfaces, being particularly evident in the cranial sac (17). These contractions give rise to electrical discharges, which - in long-term vagotomized sheep - can be blocked by atropine or hexamethonium (12,36). Therefore, Gregory concluded that the intrinsic contractions have a cholinergic nature, which depends on the activity of the myenteric plexus. Distension increases the intrinsic motor activity (8). In the *afferent* vagal nerves the number of spikes per discharge is greater and the interval between each discharge is smaller. Agents which cause an increase in smooth muscle tone have similar effects (17,19,48). It has been suggested that the *intrinsic* contractions play a role in the regulation of the *extrinsic* contractions by causing an excitatory *afferent* input to the gastric centres (8,16,18). The isolated rumen and reticulum strips were found to be simple and reproducible *in vitro* preparations for studying direct effects of agents on smooth muscle tone and motility. The spontaneous contractions of these strips, occurring 8 to 14 times per minute, are not affected by atropine (1,48) or tetrodotoxin (39), which suggests that they have a myogenic nature, rather than a neurogenic one. This point, which has been overlooked by many investigators, may mean that the *intrinsic* contractions *in situ* and the spontaneous contractions *in vitro* are not similar.

The *intrinsic* innervation of the bovine reticulo-rumen was investigated by Taneike and Ohga (40), analyzing the responses of isolated smooth muscle preparations to transmural electrical stimulation. Transmural stimulation caused a contraction, or a contraction followed by relaxation, in longitudinal muscle strips from the anterior and dorsal sacs of rumen, and from the greater curvature of the reticulum. The excitatory component of the biphasic response was enhanced by cholinesterase inhibitors. After atropine administration, it was converted into a relaxation, which was entirely resistent to $alpha_1$-and beta-sympatholytic agents. Tetrodotoxin and cocaine inhibited or abolished both excitatory and inhibitory responses evoked by transmural stimulation, whereas hexamethonium had a feeble effect on them. These results suggest that the smooth muscles of the reticulo-rumen are supplied by postganglionic excitatory cholinergic nerves and by nonadrenergic inhibitory nerves. There is some evidence that VIP may be the neurotransmitter involved in these nonadrenergic inhibitory nerves (28). The increase in smooth muscle tone induced by $alpha_1$-sympathomimetic agents, acetylcholine and histamine are probably due to an increase of Ca^{2+} permeability in both the plasma membrane and the membranes of the stores (4). However, there is only limited information about the excitation-contraction coupling in reticulo-ruminal smooth muscles. These examples demonstrate that, some basic features of fore-stomach motility have not yet been clearly elucidated. Therefore, more detailed studies of these processes are still required.

II. AGENTS AND THEIR ACTIONS

II.1. alpha- and beta-sympathomimetic agents

An i.v. injection of adrenaline in the conscious ruminant always gives an inhibition of the *extrinsic* reticulo-ruminal contractions (45,47,55), whereas in spinal and decerebrate preparations, and in anaesthetized animals, with and without the vagus nerves intact, adrenaline evokes contractions of the reticulum (41). Contractions of the reticulum also have been produced by *efferent* stimulation of the left splanchnic and right thoracic sympathetic nerve trunks (41). This led us to a study of the adrenergic receptors in the isolated ruminal smooth muscle (51,56). *In vitro*, spontaneous contractions were reduced in tension and in amplitude by beta-adrenergic agents, effects which could be blocked by beta-blockers but not by $alpha_1$-blockers. Noradrenaline and oxymetazoline caused a sharp rise in tone, sometimes associated with a reduction of the amplitude of the contractions. These effects could be blocked by $alpha_1$-blockers, but not by beta-sympatholytic agents. Some strips reacted with a strong contraction, others with a relaxation after exposure to adrenaline. The rise in tone could be antagonized by an $alpha_1$-blocker; thereafter, a second dose of adrenaline gave a relaxation, which in turn could be blocked by a beta-sympatholytic agent. Strips which reacted first with a relaxation, gave a contraction to a second dose of adrenaline after a beta-blocker.

From these results we concluded that, in the ruminal smooth muscle preparations, there exist $alpha_1$-excitatory and beta-inhibitory receptors. Others (38) have suggested that these receptors are located in both smooth muscle layers, with possibly $alpha_1$-receptors predominating in the circular layer of the reticulum. The observed effects after dopamine were a brief relaxation followed by an increase in smooth muscle tone, or a contraction not preceded by a short inhibition. These effects could be blocked by $alpha_1$-sympatholytic agents and the dopaminergic receptor blocking agent domperidone (23,55) but not by beta-sympatholytic agents. It is of interest that, in terms of producing stimulatory effects, dopamine was about 50 to 100 times less potent than l.adrenaline, whereas the latter appeared to be about 1.5 times as active as l.noradrenaline. *In situ*, dopamine and $alpha_1$- and beta-sympathominetics induce inhibition of the *extrinsic* reticulo-ruminal contractions. Only $alpha_1$-blockers were able to antagonize the effects induced by $alpha_1$-sympathomimetics, where-as only beta-blockers abolished the effects of beta-adrenergic drugs (47). The effects of dopamine were completely prevented by domperidone (23).

By using an electrophysiological "single fibre" technique to record the nervous activity present in *efferent* vagal preganglionic fibres and in the *afferent* vagal fibres innervating the reticulo-ruminal tension perceptors, it became clear that, in halothane anaesthetized sheep, isoprenaline decreased tension perceptor activity through a relaxation of the smooth muscle cells, which in turn caused a reduced activity in the *efferent* fibres (Fig. 2); $alpha_1$-sympathomimetic agents - such as phenylephrine - increased tension perceptor activity through an increase in smooth muscle tone. The supranormal stimulatory input to the gastric centres, caused a short-acting inhibition of the *extrinsic* contractions, followed by an increase in frequency of these contractions (Fig. 3).

The effect of adrenaline, in both conscious goats and anaesthetized and conscious sheep, seemed to be primarily due to stimulation of $alpha_1$-

adrenergic receptors (32,42,47,48). All these observations suggest that changes in smooth muscle tone can cause reflex inhibition of the extrinsic movements of the forestomach system.

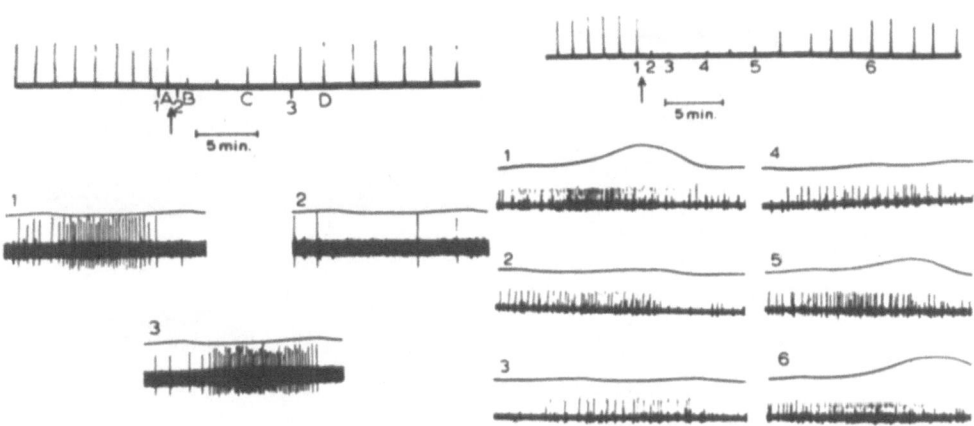

FIGURE 2. The effect of isoprenaline (↑ 10 µg kg^{-1} b.w. i.v.) on the extrinsic reticulum contractions (upper tracings) in halothane anaesthetized sheep. Left side: 1-3 resting discharges in an *afferent* vagal unit innervating reticular tension perceptors, associated with *intrinsic* contractions. The drug caused a reduction in the number of spikes probably due to a relaxation of the smooth muscles. Right side: 1-6 recordings showing the discharge patterns in an *efferent* gastric vagal unit, when the reticulum contracted under isometric conditions. The reflex inhibition caused by isoprenaline is shown by a decrease in the total number of spikes.

Hyperglycaemia is another effect which can be induced by adrenaline. When given i.v. for 15 minutes at a dose rate of 0.3 µg kg^{-1}min^{-1}, adrenaline increased blood glucose levels approximately 100 per cent from base line values. However, in these experiments with goats, no significant changes in forestomach motility were observed (48).

Although adrenaline and dopamine do not cross the blood-brain barrier to any significant extent, both agents do inhibit the *extrinsic* reticulo-rumen contractions after administration by the intracerebroventricular (ICV) route (3,33). Moreover, Ruckebusch and his co-workers have demonstrated that stimulation of centrally located alpha$_2$-adrenergic receptors cause a dose-dependent reduction of the frequency of these

120

contractions (43). This effect can be antagonized by alpha$_2$-sympatholytic agents such as tolazoline.

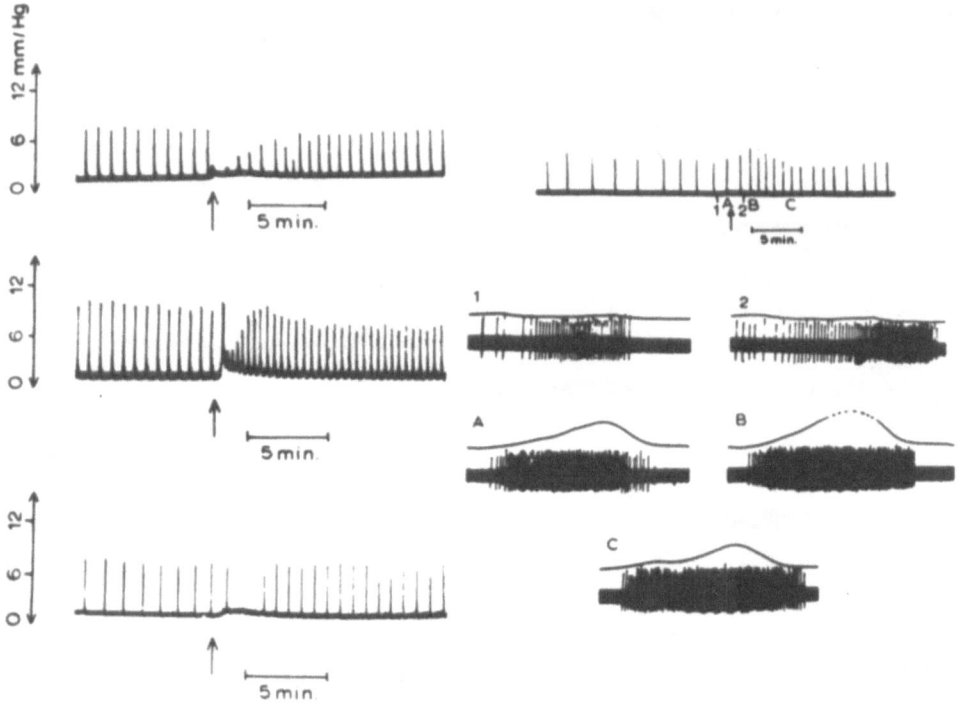

FIGURE 3. Left side: the effects of phenylephrine (↑ 50 μg kg^{-1} b.w. i.v.) on the extrinsic reticulum contractions in halothane anaesthetized sheep. Right side: 1-2 resting discharges in an *afferent* vagal unit innervating reticular tension perceptors associated with *intrinsic* contractions. The drug caused an increase in the number of spikes, due to an increase in smooth muscle tone (see also left side). A-C: records showing the discharge patterns associated with *extrinsic* contractions. The drug-induced increase in smooth muscle tone caused an increase in the frequency of the extrinsic contractions or (left side) a short period of inhibition, followed by an increase in frequency of these contractions.

II.2. Parasympathomimetics

In vitro, the threshold concentrations of acetylcholine and carbachol for increases in smooth muscle tone depend on the type of strips used (39,57). However, in comparison with other spasmogenic agents, such as serotonin, prostaglandin F$_{2alpha}$ and histamine, both substances are more potent. Pilocarpine and arecoline also induce sharp rises in tone, which can be blocked by atropine or other parasympatholytic drugs like homatropine and scopolamine (1). In anaesthetized sheep, carbachol increased tension perceptor activity through a contracture of the smooth

muscle cells, causing reflex inhibition of the *extrinsic* reticulum
contractions (16). Interestingly, in conscious sheep and goats bethanechol
and aceclidine (Fig. 4) increased the muscular tone of the forestomach
system without marked effects on the rate of the extrinsic contractions (29).

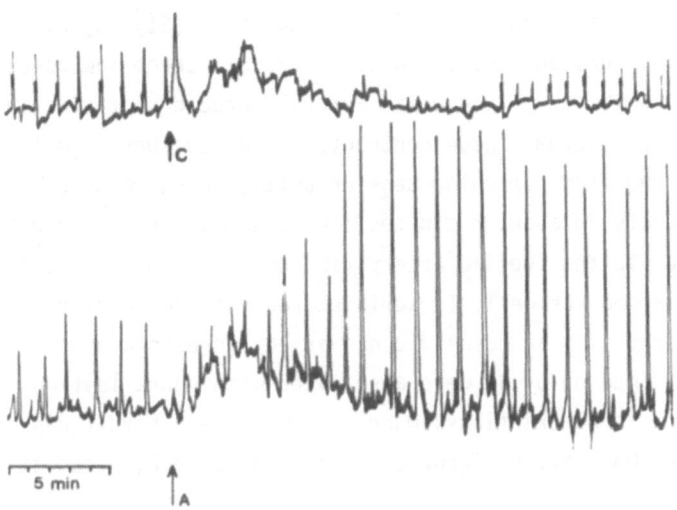

FIGURE 4. The effect of carbachol ($\uparrow$ C = 5 µg kg^{-1} b.w. i.v.) and
aceclidine ($\uparrow$ A = 50 µg kg^{-1} b.w. i.v.) on extrinsic reticulo-rumen
contractions in conscious goats. Upper tracing: reticulum contractions
recorded by an implanted transducer; lower tracing: intraruminal pressure
changes caused by rumen contractions.

Furthermore, it has been suggested that the inhibitory effects of acetylcholine and other parasympathomimetic agents are related to a central
action (7), to a vasodepressor effect (29) and to the inhibitory action
of adrenaline released by the adrenal medulla stimulated by it (6).

II.3. Bradykinin and Substance P
    Bradykinin (BK) and other tissue hormones like histamine and
prostaglandins are involved in inflammatory processes, immediate hyper-
sensitivity reactions and in endotoxin-induced shock (50). The isolated
rumen strip of goats was found to react with a sharp rise in tone after
exposure to BK. Sodium meclofenamate antagonized the stimulating action of
BK, but the shape of the concentration-response curve for BK in the
presence of this nonsteroidal anti-imflammatory agent indicated that the
antagonism was noncompetitive in nature (60). The EC_{50} values for

substance P on both goat ruminal strips and sheep reticular strips were approximately 15×10^{-9}M, which demonstrates its high intrinsic activity (22,61). *In vitro* the molar efficacy of substance P is of the same order as that of acetylcholine. As mentioned before, the presence of substance P within ruminant vagal fibres, and the release of this agent into the antral lumen of cats caused by vagal stimulation (21) suggest a physiological role for substance P. In an *anaesthetized* sheep low doses of BK and substance P (> 10 ng kg^{-1}, coeliac artery) induced short-lasting contractures of the reticulum. These contractures caused supranormal *afferent* vagal discharge from reticular tension units, which returned to resting discharge levels in about 5 minutes. In *conscious* sheep, both agents administered via the coeliac artery (100 ng kg^{-1}) induced contractures of the reticulo-rumen as well. If administered via the jugular vein or carotid artery, similar doses did not affect forestomach motility. The contractures induced by BK were associated with short-lasting inhibition of the extrinsic contractions, whereas substance P hardly depressed these contractions. Only after higher doses of substance P, hypomotility was

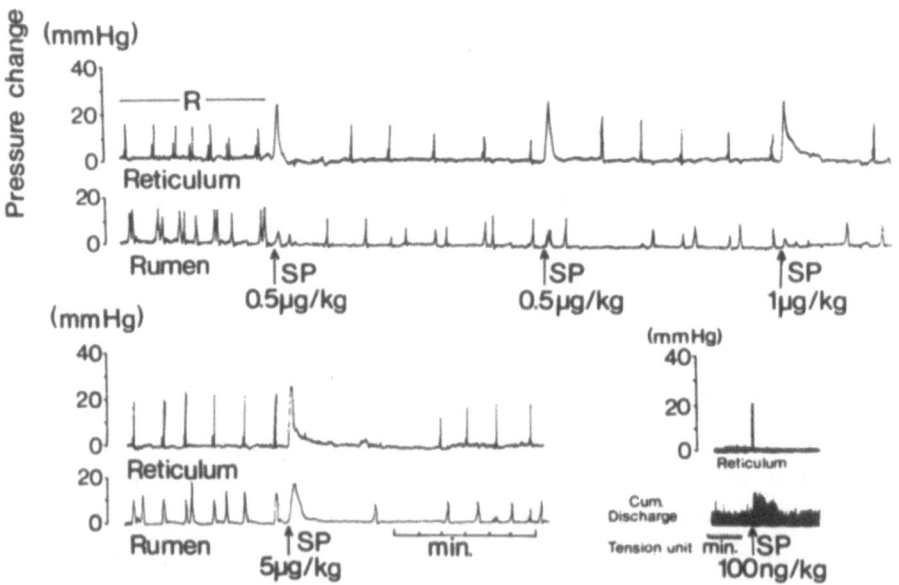

FIGURE 5. The effect of sub. P (given via the coeliac artery) on the extrinsic reticulo-rumen contractions in a conscious sheep. Lower tracing, right side: the effect of a sub. P induced contracture on the cumulative discharge of a reticular tension perceptor unit in a halothane anaesthetized sheep (the drug was given via the coeliac artery) (ref. 22).

observed, mainly due to the longer lasting contractures (Fig. 5). In conscious goats, a dose dependent inhibition of the rumen contraction sequences could also be induced by BK and substance P. Both hormones caused short-lasting effects, probably due to rapid inactivation by enzyme systems such as carboxypeptidases (60,61).

II.4. Prostaglandins

Concentration-response curves obtained for contraction of goat rumen strips *in vitro* showed that PGE_1 (with an activity equal to that of PGE_2) was more potent in inducing an increase in smooth muscle tone than PGF_{2alpha}. Polyphloretin-phosphate antagonized the excitatory effects of both PGE_1 and PGF_{2alpha}. The shift to the right, apparently in parallel, of the concentration-response curve for PGF_{2alpha} in the presence of polyphloretin-phosphate suggested that the antagonism was competitive in nature (59).

In *conscious* goats, both PGs caused a dose-dependent inhibition of the *extrinsic* rumen contraction sequences, PGE_1 being more potent than PGF_{2alpha}. These effects were short-lasting, probably due to rapid inactivation by enzyme systems, especially within the lung (59). The pharmacological effects of PGs are partly dependent on the mode of administration. The *intracerebroventricular* injection of PGE_2 (about 6 to 8 μg kg^{-1}) caused a sharp increase in body temperature, a lower heart rate and a long lasting and moderate inhibition of the extrinsic rumen contractions (54). Leakage of PGE_2 from the ventricular system into the central compartment was unlikely to be the cause of these effects since i.v. infusion of 0.4 μg $kg^{-1}min^{-1}$ for 20 minutes caused tachycardia, less inhibition of forestomach motility and no change in body temperature. Furthermore, a single i.v. dose of 8 μg kg^{-1} induced a short-lasting inhibition of the extrinsic contractions, tachycardia and no change in rectal temperature (58,59).

Another interesting observation was made by Maas and Leek (22). In conscious sheep, they injected a small dose of PGE_2 (100 ng kg^{-1}) into the coeliac artery, the jugular vein or into the carotid artery. Only after administration via the coeliac artery, a short-lasting contracture of the reticulo-rumen was seen, associated with a temporary stasis and a relatively long-lasting depression of the extrinsic contractions, which had a small amplitude but normal frequency (Fig. 6).

124

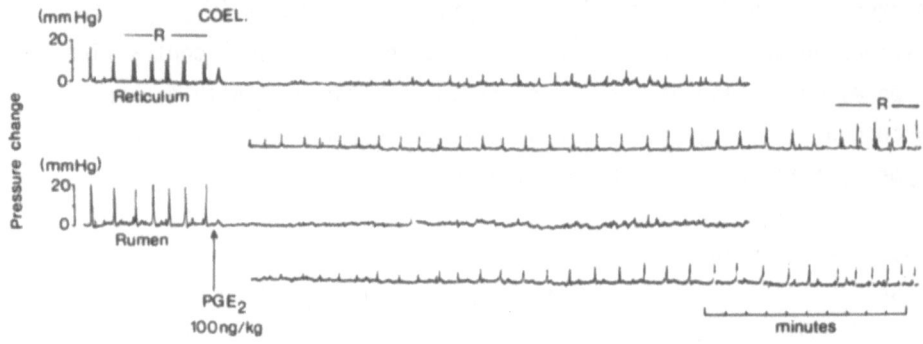

FIGURE 6. The effect of prostaglandin E_2 (given via the coeliac artery) on the *extrinsic* reticulo-rumen contractions in a conscious sheep. If administered via the jugular vein or carotid artery, 100 ng kg^{-1} b.w. of PGE_2 did not affect these contractions (ref. 22).

II.5. Histamine

Intravenous administration of histamine always causes a prompt and complete cessation of the *extrinsic* forestomach contractions, without affecting intraruminal pressure (53). This effect can be prevented by H_1-histaminergic receptor blocking agents such as clemastine, promethazine and mepyramine (35,58). The administration of cimetidine, a H_2-histaminergic receptor blocking agent, only had a partial antagonistic effect, whereas the H_2-blocker oxmetidine had no effect at all (35,58). Moreover, the frequency of the extrinsic reticulum contractions was not modified by impromidine, an H_2-receptor agonist (35). These observations suggest that H_2-receptors are not directly involved in the control of the extrinsic forestomach contractions.

In vitro experiments, using strips of the longitudinal and circular smooth muscles from the bovine reticulo-rumen, showed that histamine can induce different types of responses: contraction (H_1-receptor) relaxation (H_2-receptor) or contraction followed by relaxation (26). However, in our hands the goat ruminal strip preparation proved tp be very *insensitive* to histamine, the threshold concentration being about 12.8 µg ml^{-1} (58). Furthermore, there is some evidence, which suggests that other histamine-induced responses may be involved in the observed ruminal stasis. For example, it is well known that histamine stimulates abomasal secretion, has excitatory and inhibitory effects on the duodenal bulb and induces an increase in intestinal smooth muscle tone associated with diarrhoea (35,

45). Moreover, this agent has an effect on blood pressure and local blood flow. Interestingly, the histamine-induced tachycardia, probably of a reflex nature, was potentiated by H_1 or H_2-receptor blocking agents (53, 58).

II.6. Serotonin (5-HT)

In vitro, the spasmogenic agent serotonin was less potent than acetylcholine, substance P or PGE_1. The mean concentrations ($\pm$ SEM) of 5-HT and PGE_1 required for half maximal contraction of goat ruminal strips were respectively 0.14 ± 0.02 μg ml^{-1} and 9.8 ± 2.8 ng ml^{-1} (60). The serotonergic receptor blocking agents xylamidine and methysergide diminished the excitatory effects of 5-HT. However, the shape of the concentration-response curves for 5-HT in the presence of these 5-HT$_1$-receptor blocking agents, indicated that the antagonism was noncompetitive in nature (60). The effects of 5-HT on longitudinal smooth muscle strips from bovine rumen and reticulum were studied by Taneike (39). 5-HT caused a contraction and a relaxation of the ruminal strips, while it induced only an excitatory effect on reticular strips. These effects were not affected by tetrodotoxin, hexamethonium, atropine or morphine, but were blocked by 5-HT$_1$-receptor blocking agents. Furthermore, 5-HT potentiated the contraction evoked by transmural stimulation but did not show any effect on the relaxation produced by non-adrenergic inhibitory nerves stimulation. The author concluded that contractions or relaxations induced by serotonin were mediated through activation of D-receptors in the smooth muscle, and that the 5-HT-induced potentiation of the electrically evoked contraction might be induced through neural receptors present in the intramural cholinergic nervous pathway. However, it remains unclear whether a possible neural site of action of 5-HT is either identical with the proposed M-receptor or not. Therefore, a more detailed analysis would be necessary to confirm the existence of D- and M-receptors in the reticulo-ruminal smooth muscle layers.

In *conscious* goats, i.v. injection of 5-HT caused a dose-dependent and short-lasting inhibition of the rumen contraction sequences, which were partly prevented by 5-HT$_1$-receptor blocking agents (60), whereas ketanserin, a 5-HT$_2$-receptor blocking agent had no protective effect (fig. 7). In conscious sheep serotonin induced a short lasting contraction, which could be blocked by atropine, and a sustained increase in smooth muscle tone with a concomitant inhibition of the extrinsic forestomach

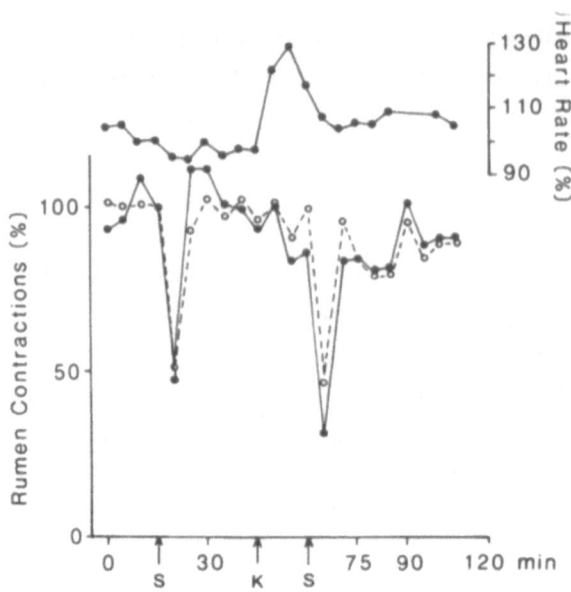

FIGURE 7. The effects of ketanserine (K, 0.1 mg kg^{-1} b.w. i.v.) on serotonin (S, 20 µg kg^{-1} b.w. i.v.)-induced changes in heart rate and rumen motility in a group of 4 conscious goats. Heart rate and contractions are expressed as percentages of base line values; o = frequency of contractions per 10 min; ● = summation derived from 10 min intervals of amplitude. Mean values are shown.

contractions. These latter effects could be antagonized by both a 5-HT$_1$- and 5-HT$_2$-receptor blocking agent (34). Moreover, chemical sympathectomy induced by 6-OH-dopamine abolished the inhibitory effect of 5-HT on the extrinsic contractions, which suggests the involvement of a central adrenergic mechanism (34). Interestingly the injection of 5-HT (6-8 µg kg^{-1}) into the *third cerebral ventricle* of conscious goats caused a marked inhibitory effect on the extrinsic ruminal contractions (54). Leakage of 5-HT from the ventricular system into the circulation was unlikely to be the cause of this effect, since i.v. infusion of 0.5 µg kg^{-1} min^{-1} of 5-HT for 5 hours did not cause changes in rumen motility. Moreover, single i.v. doses of at least 30 µg kg^{-1} had to be given to induce comparable effects on the extrinsic contractions, whereas these effects returned to preinjection values within 45 minutes, in contrast to those observed after intracerebroventricular administration (60).

II.7. Opioid agonists and antagonists

Morphine and other opioids are known to inhibit the *extrinsic* fore-stomach motility in different ruminant species (20,29,52). However, opiate antagonists, like naloxone and naltrexone, have been shown to stimulate the frequency of these contractions in conscious goats (20,22,23), indicating an inhibitory role for endogenous opioids in the control of forestomach motility. Using normorphine, pentazocine and etorphine, which have been reported to be rather selective for the proposed mu, kappa and delta opioid receptors respectively, Maas (21) examined whether the opioid action on the extrinsic ruminal contractions in conscious goats was mediated exclusively through one of these subtypes of receptors. After *i.v.* administration, these opioids induced qualitatively a similar inhibition of the frequency and amplitude of the contractions, whereas the agonists were similarly sensitive to pretreatment with naltrexone.

In contrast, Ruckebusch and his coworkers found that the reticular contractions in conscious sheep were enhanced by subcutaneous or intracerebroventricular administration of kappa type agonists such as ethylketazocine (31). In conscious goats, *intracerebroventricular* administration of loperamide (1 µg kg^{-1}) significantly depressed ruminal frequency, whereas *i.v.* injection of 10 µg kg^{-1} did not affect rumen motility (22,24). The *intracerebroventricular* injection of normorphine caused a longer lasting inhibition of the extrinsic contractions than *i.v.* infusion of a 30 times higher dose. Moreover, ICV administered naltrexone completely prevented the inhibitory effects of *i.v.* injected normorphine (21,52). Furthermore, the inhibitory effects of the opioid agonists given by the ICV route were abolished by *i.v.* naloxone, but not by the quaternary compound methylnaloxone (31). These observations in conscious sheep and goats, indicate a central opioid action depressing frequency and amplitude of the extrinsic forestomach contractions. The time course of the effects induced by ICV administered naltrexone, loperamide or normorphine was different from that after *i.v.* injection: the stimulatory effect of naltrexone and the inhibitory effect of loperamide has a slower onset after ICV injection than after *i.v.* administration (21,24), whereas normorphine caused a longer lasting inhibition after ICV injection. These differences can be explained by the postulated contribution of the lipophilicity of morphine-like compounds to the efficiency of their penetration into and clearance from the brain, following *i.v.* or ICV administration (14,37). Maas and Leek (22) administered opioids and their antagonists via selective routes in sheep: the *carotid artery* to challenge central mechanisms, the *aortic arch* as a general systemic route, the *jugular vein* as a systemic route after passing the pulmonary circulation, the *left gastric artery* serving the abomasum, and the *coeliac artery* cannulated in such a way that administration was mainly leading to reticulum and rumen. In conscious sheep, low doses of normorphine and loperamide inhibited frequency and amplitude centrally (given via the carotid artery), whereas locally (given via the coeliac artery) higher dose levels only affected the amplitude of the extrinsic contractions. The opioid peptides Leu- and Met-enkephalin preferentially depressed the amplitude of these contractions most efficiently if administered via the coeliac artery (22).

In anaesthetized sheep, opioids depressed in an identical manner both the amplitude of spontaneous extrinsic contractions and contractions evoked by electrical stimulation of the distal end of the cut cervical vagus nerve (22).

However, opioids did not alter the resting discharge of *afferent* tension units and similarly failed to modulate the smooth muscle tension of the longitudinal reticular strips or circular ruminal strips *in vitro*, suggesting that the opioids act locally on the intramural neuronal plexus, possibly by diminishing the output of excitatory transmitter (22,24,52).

In conclusion, these results indicate the presence both of a central opioid action depressing frequency and amplitude, and of a local opioid action depressing only the amplitude of the extrinsic reticulo-rumen contractions.

III. CONCLUSIONS

All the examples given demonstrate that, although the study of reticulo-rumen motility has had a long and distinguished history, many questions have not yet been clearly answered. For example, with respect to transmitters, receptors and motor activity, several aspects remain unresolved, such as: (a) what is the physiological role of substance P, VIP and serotonin? (b) What is the physiological role of beta-adrenergic and dopaminergic receptors in the reticulo-ruminal smooth muscle cells? Do there exist M-serotonergic receptors and if so, are they identical with $5-HT_2$-receptors? Is there a selective mediation of opioid depression of forestomach motility through one of the proposed subtypes of opioid receptors? (c) What is the physiological significance of the nonadrenergic inhibitory nerves? These and other intriguing questions deserve more detailed studies which certainly shall influence future concepts of reticulo-ruminal control mechanisms.

REFERENCES

1. Berecky, I.: Folia Veterinaria 12, 121-129 (1968)
2. Brunaud, M. and Navarro, J.: J. Physiol. (Paris) 46, 272-276 (1954)
3. Bueno, L., Sorraing, J.M. and Fioramonti, J.: J. Vet. Pharmacol. Therap. 6, 93-98 (1983)
4. Burgin, H.: J. Vet. Pharmacol. Therap. 2, 305-311 (1979)
5. Duncan, D.L.: J. Physiol. (London) 119, 157-169 (1953)
6. Duncan. D.L.: J. Physiol. (London) 125, 475-487 (1954)
7. Dussardier, M.: J. Physiol. (Paris) 46, 777-797 (1954)
8. Dussardier, M.: Recherches sur la contrôle bulbaire de la motricité gastrique chez les ruminants. Ph.D. Thesis, Paris, Institut Nationale de la Recherche Agronomique (1960)
9. Faustini, R., Ormas, P., Galbiati, A. and Beretta, C.: In: Trends in Veterinary Pharmacology and Toxicology, Proc. 1st EAVPT Congress, Van Miert, A.S.J.P.A.M., Frens, J. and Van der Kreek, F.W. (eds): Elsevier Sci. Publ. Company, Amsterdam, 175-183 (1980)
10. Gamse, R., Lembeck, F. and Cuello, A.C.: Naunyn-Schmiedeberg's Arch. Pharmacol. 306, 37-44 (1979)
11. Gregory, P.C.: J. Physiol. (London) 328, 431-447 (1982)
12. Gregory, P.C.: J. Physiol. (London) 346, 379-393 (1984)
13. Habel, R.E.: Cornell Vet. 46, 555-628 (1956)
14. Kutter, E., Herz, A., Techemacher, H.J. and Hess, R.: J. Med. Chem. 13, 801-805 (1970)
15. Le Bars, H., Nitescu, R. and Simonnet, H.: Bull. l'Acad. Vét. de France 27, 53-67 (1954)
16. Leek. B.F.: An electrophysiological analysis of the reflex regulation of reticulo-ruminal movements. Ph.D. Thesis, Edinburgh (1967)
17. Leek. B.F.: J. Physiol. (London) 202, 585-609 (1969)
18. Leek, B.F. and Harding, R.H.: In: Digestion and Metabolism in the Ruminant. McDonald, I.W. and Warner, A.C.I. (eds), The University of

New England Publishing Unit, Armidale, Australia, 60-76 (1975)

19. Leek, B.F. and Van Miert, A.S.J.P.A.M.: Rendiconti Rom. Gastroenterol. 3, 163-167 (1971)

20. Maas, C.L.: Eur. J. Pharmacol. 77, 71-74 (1982)

21. Maas, C.L.: Modulation of forestomach motility in small ruminants: Opioid and nonopioid mechanisms. Ph.D. Thesis, Utrecht (1984)

22. Maas, C.L. and Leek, B.F.: Vet. Res. Commun. 9, 89-113 (1985)

23. Maas, C.L., Van Duin, C.T.M. and Van Miert, A.S.J.P.A.M.: J. Vet. Pharmacol. Therap. 5, 191-194 (1982)

24. Maas, C.L., Van Duin, C.T.M. and Van Miert, A.S.J.P.A.M.: J. Vet. Pharmacol. Therap. 9, 63-70 (1986)

25. Nilsson, G., Larsson, L.I., Hakanson, R., Brodin, E., Pernow, B. and Sundler, F.: Histochem. 43, 97-99 (1975)

26. Ohga, A. and Taneike, T.: Brit. J. Pharmacol. 62, 333-337 (1978)

27. Pearse, A.G.E. and Polak, J.M.: Histochem. 41, 373-375 (1975)

28. Reid, A.M. and Titchen, D.A.: Can. J. Anim. Sci. 64 (suppl.), 91-92 (1984)

29. Ruckebusch, Y.: J. Vet. Pharmacol. Therap. 6, 245-272 (1983)

30. Ruckebusch, Y.: In: Control of Digestion and Metabolism in Ruminants. Milligan, L.P., Grovum, W.L. and Dobson, A. (eds), A Reston Book, Prentice Hall, Englewood Cliffs, N.J., pp. 60-78 (1986)

31. Ruckebusch, Y., Bardon, T. and Pairet, M.: Life Sci. 35, 1731-1738 (1984)

32. Ruckebusch, Y., Fargeas, J. and Bueno, L.: Ann. Rech. Vét. 3, 131-148 (1969)

33. Ruckebusch, Y., Grivel, M.L. and Laplace, J.P.: Thérapie 21, 483-491 (1966)

34. Ruckebusch, Y. and Ooms, L.: J. Vet. Pharmacol. Therap. 6, 127-131 (1983)

35. Ruckebusch, Y. and Soldani, G.: J. Vet. Pharmacol. Therap. 6, 229-232 (1983)

36. Ruckebusch, Y., Tsiamitas, Ch. and Bueno, L.: Life Sci. 11, 55-64 (1972)

37. Seydel, J.K. and Schaper, K.J.: Pharmacol. Therap. 15, 131-182 (1982)

38. Stoyanov, I.N., Loukanov, Y.B., Vassileva, P.V. and Vassilev, V.I.: Gen. Pharmacol. 7, 399-404 (1976)

39. Taneike, T.: J. Vet. Pharmacol. Therap. 2, 59-68 (1979)

40. Taneike, T. and Ohga, A.: Jap. J. Vet. Sci. 37, 301-311 (1975)

41. Titchen, D.A.: In: Handbook of Physiology, section 6 vol. 5. Heidel, W. (ed), Williams and Wilkins, Baltimore, 2705-2724 (1968)

42. Titchen, D.A. and Newhook, J.C.: J. Pharm. Pharmacol. 20, 948-950 (1968)

43. Toutain, P.L., Zingoni, M.R. and Ruckebusch, Y.: J. Pharmacol. Exp. Therap. 223, 215-218 (1982)

44. Vallenas, G.A.: Am. J. Vet. Res. 17, 78-89 (1956)

45. Van Genderen, H.: Tijdschr. Diergeneesk. 93, 1392-1401 (1968)

46. Van Miert, A.S.J.P.A.M.: Tijdschr. Diergeneesk. 93, 1402-1410 (1968)

47. Van Miert, A.S.J.P.A.M.: J. Pharm. Pharmacol. 21, 697-699 (1969)

48. Van Miert, A.S.J.P.A.M.: Inhibition of the reticulo-rumen motility during fever induced by bacterial pyrogen - lipopolysaccharides from Gram-negative bacteria - in sheep and goats. Ph.D. Thesis, Utrecht (1970)

49. Van Miert, A.S.J.P.A.M.: Arch. int. Pharmacodyn. Thérap. 193, 405-414 (1971)

50. Van Miert, A.S.J.P.A.M.: In: Fever. Lipton, J.M. (ed), Raven Press, New York, 57-70 (1980)

51. Van Miert, A.S.J.P.A.M. and Huisman, E.A.: J. Pharm. Pharmacol. 20, 495-496 (1968)

52. Van Miert, A.S.J.P.A.M. and Maas, C.L.: Can. J. Anim. Sci. 64 (suppl.), 8-10 (1984)

53. Van Miert, A.S.J.P.A.M., Van Duin, C.T.M. and Veenendaal, G.H.: Zbl. Vet. med. A23, 819-826 (1976)

54. Van Miert, A.S.J.P.A.M., Van Duin, C.T.M. and Woutersen-van Nijnanten, F.M.A.: Eur. J. Pharmacol. 92, 143-146 (1983)

55. Van Miert, A.S.J.P.A.M. van Van Vugt, F.: Zbl. Vet. med. A21, 96-104 (1974)

56. Van Miert, A.S.J.P.A.M., Veenendaal, G.H. and Van Genderen, H.: Dtch. Tierärztl. Wschr. 83, 188-192 (1976)

57. Vassilev, V., Stoyanov, I.N., Lukanov, Y. and Vassileva, P.: Agressologie 16, 101-106 (1975)

58. Veenendaal, G.H.: In: Trends in Veterinary Pharmacology and Toxicology. Proc. 1st EAVPT Congress. Van Miert, A.S.J.P.A.M., Frens, J. and Van der Kreek, F.W. (eds), Elsevier Sci. Publ. Company, Amsterdam, 193-199 (1980)

59. Veenendaal, G.H., Woutersen-Van Nijnanten, F.M.A., Van Duin, C.T.M. and Van Miert, A.S.J.P.A.M.: J. Vet. Pharmacol. Therap. 3, 59-68 (1980)
60. Veenendaal, G.H., Woutersen-Van Nijnanten, F.M.A. and Van Miert, A.S.J.P.A.M.: Am. J. Vet. Res. 41, 479-483 (1980)
61. Veenendaal, G.H., Woutersen-Van Nijnanten, F.M.A. and Van Miert, A.S.J.P.A.M.: Vet. Res. Commun. 5, 363-367 (1982)
62. Von Euler, U.S.: Ann. New York Acad. Sci. 104, 449-461 (1963)

5. FORESTOMACH: CONTROL OF DIGESTA FLOW

A.G. DESWYSEN

I   INTRODUCTION

Utilization of roughage diets by ruminants involves complex relationships among diet components, microorganisms in the reticulo-rumen and the
animal. Ingesting roughages requires from ruminants to complete an extensive
physiological work: the feed particles breakdown. Particle size reduction
is mostly achieved by mastication during eating and rumination. The
functional adaptations in the ruminant system to meet the challenge are
however extensive. This is relevant to the productivity of ruminants in
grazing situations and other intensive production systems based on silage

feeding and concentrates.

Many aspects of the appetite and passage system in ruminants are currently investigated. This paper will be limited to aspects of rumen function and to physical processes (degradation, movement, outflow) that occur as a result of the ingestion of roughages by ruminants.
Some of the factors affecting these processes, especially rumination, will also be considered.

II FUNCTIONAL MORPHOLOGY AND DIGESTIVE ADAPTATION OF THE FORESTOMACHS

As extensively described by Hofmann (38) and Hofmann and Schnorr (39), actual ruminants can be classified as roughage eaters, intermediate feeders or concentrate selectors with only 3 domesticated species out of 142 recent ruminants.

From comparative anatomical studies it appears that ruminants have all evolved from primitive selectors of a "concentrate diet" to a "grass diet". Grasses, in their various seasonal stages, are the natural diet for which the bovine stomach (*Bos taurus, Bos indicus, Bubalus bubalis*) is optimally suited. According to Hofmann (38), sheep and especially goats are not highly advanced "intermediate feeders",relying on a mixed diet of grass, herbs and foliage (browse material) which infers adaptability of their stomach.

Cattle are classified as non-selective roughage eaters with the most developed stomach whereas sheep are selective roughage eaters. The goat, classified as intermediate feeder, is more adaptable to changing habits and vegetation than most of the selectors and grazers. When fed highly digestible material the stomach structure is similar to a concentrate selector whereas similar to a roughage eater when fed poor roughage (39).

Concentrate selectors vs roughage eaters are characterized by a relatively smaller rumen, larger reticulum, smaller omasum and abomasum, larger caecum-colon. The "ostium ruminoreticulare" forms in all concentrate selectors a remarkable wide communication opening, up to 70% larger than in roughage grazers. The "ostium intraruminale" and "reticulo-omasicum" also are relatively large allowing a rapid passage of ingesta within the forestomachs (38). Since more fermentable food would leave the rumen of animals having a faster turnover, the fermentation in subsequent parts of the alimentary tract should be higher if turnover rate is the only difference. The completeness of food utilization in the rumen could however additionally

be affected by a higher fermentation rate and a considerable enlargment of
the absorptive surface (40). A high dense and more uniform distribution of
ruminal papillae even on pillars was clearly shown in concentrates selectors
vs roughage eaters (38).

Topographical studies of the thoracic and abdominal organs of a cow (47)
and of a sheep (63) showed clear differences especially in the area of the
reticulo-ruminal fold, cranial pillar and "ostium ruminoreticulare" as
illustrated in Figure 1.

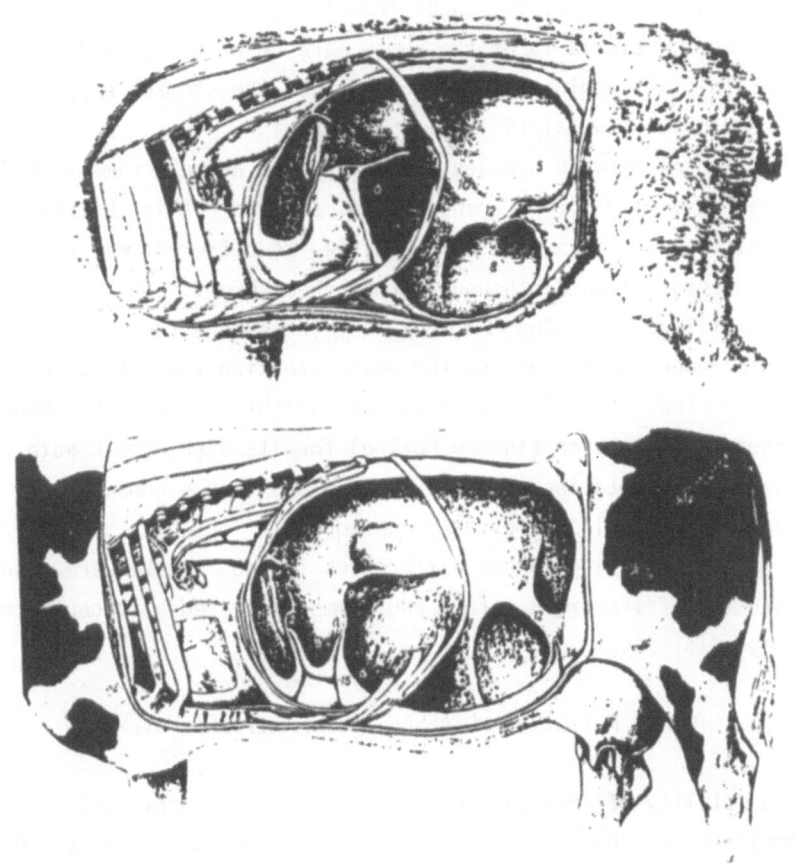

1. Reticular groove, 1' its lips; 2, 2' Ruminoreticular fold,
enclosing ruminoreticular opening; 3, 3' cranial sac, 4. dorsal
sac, 5. caudodorsal blind sac, 6. recessus ruminis, 7. ventral
sac, 8. caudoventral blind sac, 9. cranial pillar, 10, 10' right
longitudinal pillar, 11. insula ruminis, 12. caudal pillar,
13. dorsal coronary pillar, 14. ventral coronary pillar, 15.
cranial groove. 16. caudal groove.

FIGURE 1. Topography of the thoracic and abdominal organs of a sheep
(ref. 63) and an adult cow (ref. 47).

In sheep vs cattle, the reticulum is relatively large and well separated from the rumen possibly impairing the backflow of small particles from the ventral sac of the rumen into the cranial sac and reticulum. Relative capacities of the four compartments in cattle and sheep are respectively for the rumen 52% and 62%, the reticulum 6% and 11%, the omasum 28% and 5%, the abomasum 14% and 22% (9). The smaller omasum present in sheep is a typical similarity with the intermediate feeders as described by Hofmann and Schnorr (39). The capacity of the stomach of adult cattle depends on the size and the breed. It ranges from 110-235 liters. This stated absolute capacities, particularly of the rumen, are never fully utilized in the live animal. In small ruminants, the capacity of the stomach depends largely on the breed of the animal (48).

Differences between species are thus clear and experiments made on goats and even sheep may not be transposed as such to cattle. Within species, large differences in adaptation abilities to different diets exist. Heidschnucken, an autochthonous German sheep breed, and Merino sheep were able to utilize a low digestible diet by increasing the volume of the reticulo-rumen and increasing the mean retention time of fluid and particles. They maintained initial body weight. On the other hand, the Blackhead sheep chosen (as the Merino) for its high growth rate potential, was neither able to increase the rumen fluid volume considerably nor to prolong the retention time. They consequently lost body weight rapidly (62). In cattle, large breed differences in food intake were also found between the Afrikaner, Hereford and Simmentaler fed a concentrate or a roughage diet (44).

III FORESTOMACH MOTILITY AND ASSOCIATED PARTICLES MOVEMENT

The motility of forestomachs in different ruminants has been examined in many studies and presented in reviews (55,54) and films (27,64).

III.1. Motility and movement of particles within the reticulo-rumen
III.1.1. In general

Radiographic studies during eating of grass and grass silage have shown that each swallowed bolus was projected into the reticulo-rumen with considerable force and deposited in the upper part of the reticulum near the reticulo-ruminal fold. Two or three swallowed boli accumulated there before the reticulum contracted biphasically. During the second contraction the reticulum shrinks almost completely; food is forced caudally into the cranial sac of the rumen. During subsequent contraction of the cranial sac the floor lifts up and the liquid or pulpy contents are ejected from the lower parts of the cranial sac via the reticulo-ruminal fold into the relaxing reticulum.With further contraction of the cranial sac the light food is forced upwards and passes slowly over the cranial pillar of the rumen into the dorsal sac (26). The alternating contraction of the reticulum and the cranial sac of the rumen separate the ingested food from the liquid contents; liquid and heavy particles arrive in the reticulum, light food arrives in the dorsal sac of the rumen.

Dulphy and Demarquilly (18,19) found in sheep that the DM intake of silages with different qualities and different chop length was much lower during the two daily main meals than that of corresponding hay or fresh grass. They suggested that this rapid satiety specific to silage rations could be due to an obstruction of the cardiac region by the swallowed silage. Radiographic studies made on sheep fed wilted grass silage revealed no accumulation of swallowed material in the cardiac area (13). Therefore it seems doubtful that the lower voluntary intake level of silage over 24 hours and during the main meals is caused by an obstruction of the cardiac area.

During a meal, ingested coarse particles are progressively accumulated in the dorsal sac, in the middle of the rumen and in the caudoventral blindsac of the rumen. With the dorsal sac contraction the ruminal wall takes hold of the solid contents, squeezes them and imparts a slow rotation. The cranial pillar of the rumen, the longitudinal pillars and the caudal pillar undergo an annular contraction and move dorsally. This action kneads contents thoroughly in the central region of the rumen, the finer particles of food are probably washed out and forced into the liquid of the ventral sac of the rumen. During the following contraction of the ventral sac of the rumen, liquid and suspended particles are forced upwards so that they can return over the cranial pillar into the cranial sac. During subsequent reticulo-ruminal cycle and associated with the contraction of the cranial sac, particles will flow into the reticulum (Figure 2). From the reticulum, particles sufficiently small pass into the omasum whilst larger and lighter particles are ruminated (28).

138

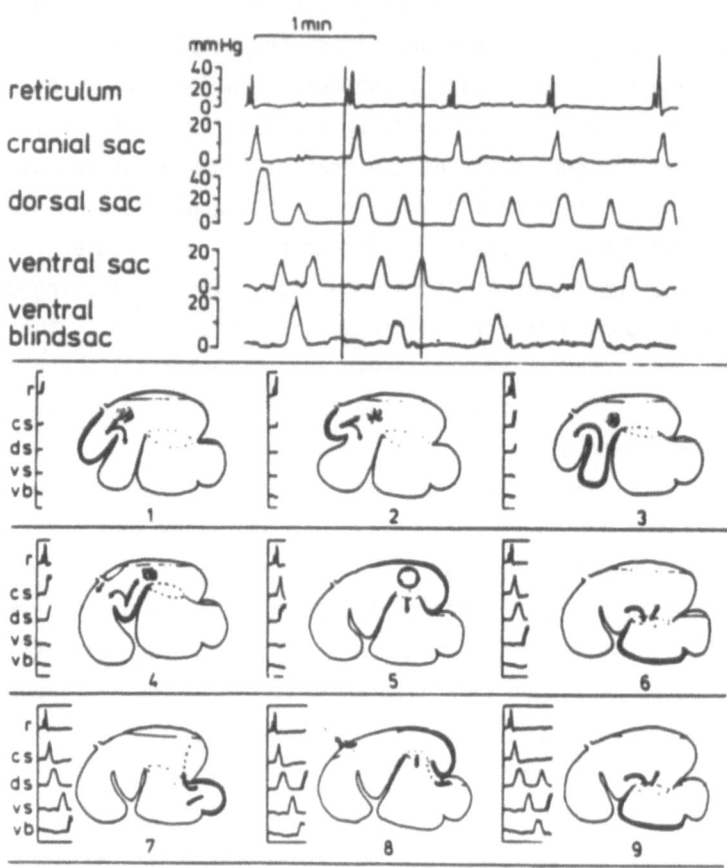

FIGURE 2. Motility tracings of the reticulum, cranial sac, dorsal sac,
ventral sac and ventral blind sac of the rumen. The sequence
of contractions during a reticulo-ruminal cycle (vertical
lines) is divided into 9 phases and shown by the diagrams
(ref. 28).
Key: r = reticulum; cs = cranial sac; ds = dorsal sac;
vs = ventral sac; vb = ventral blind sac.

III.1.2. Feeding long- vs short-chopped grass silage

By feeding long- vs short-chopped grass silage, it has been found (7,
20,12) that the particles in the rumen were longer and more interwoven.
Probably as a result of this, the separation and mechanical breakdown of
the particles is made difficult, so that the transfer of small particles
from the dorsal sac into the ventral sac of the rumen and the backflow
into the cranial sac and reticulum is delayed. Therefore, during the earlier
period after food intake,not enough solid particles are present in the

reticulum, where the most potent reflexogenic zones for rumination are localized (41,42). Consequently, and especially with the long grass silage, the beginning of the rumination activity following a main meal is delayed (longer latency time) and it presents a large number of pseudo-rumination boli especially for the first rumination periods during the day (Figure 3) (12).

Figure 3. With long silage compared to short chopped silage (Deswysen, 1980).

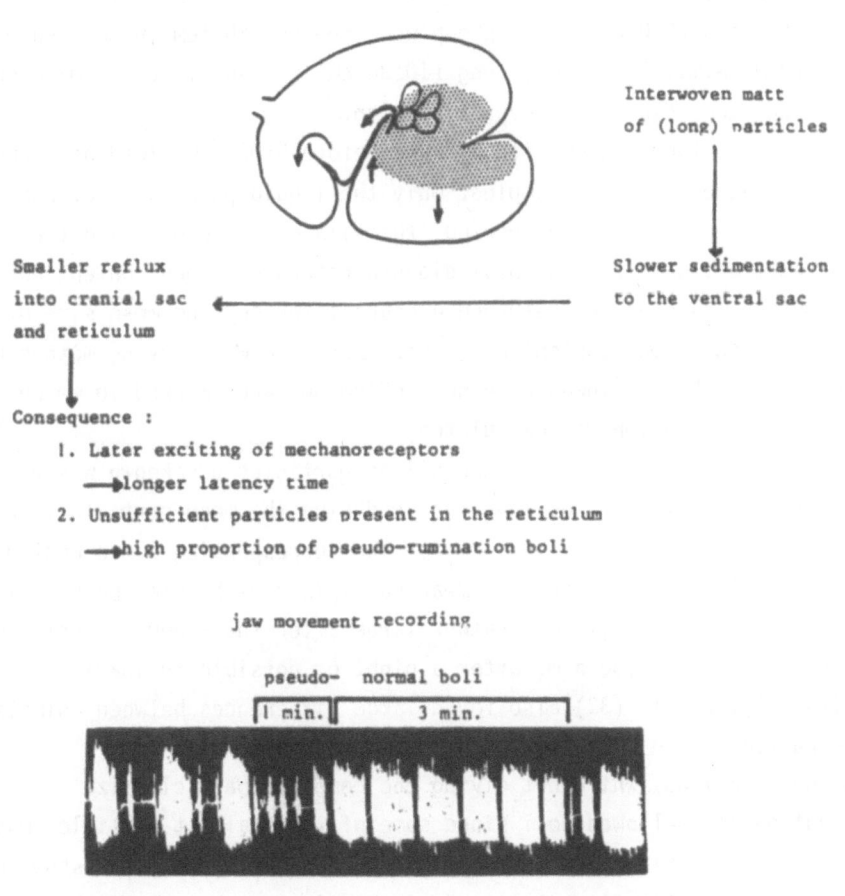

FIGURE 3. With long silage compared to short chopped silage (ref. 12).

The delayed and less efficient mechanical breakdown of the particles by the pseudo-rumination activity is a partial explanation of the underlying physiological basis for the lower voluntary intake of long- versus short-chopped grass silage (13).

III.1.3. Individual variations

Individual variations and species (sheep vs cattle) differences in sensitivity to chop length, silage fermentation quality, ... are evident for voluntary intake, associated eating and ruminating behaviour, particle size reduction and movement of digesta within the reticulo-rumen.

To investigate why some sheep, irrespective of the live weight, made much more pseudo-rumination boli when fed long grass silage, two adult rumen fistulated (9.0 cm, I.D.) sheep were fed ad libitum in two 2-h eating periods (9:00 a.m., 3:30 p.m.) long (10.30 cm) and short (2.28 cm) chopped grass silage according to a reversal design.

The rumen content was emptied by hand before 9:00 a.m. feeding, squeezed through a cheese layer and sampled. Only the liquid phase was returned into the rumen. After a 2-h eating period, the silage was removed and the rumen content emptied, sampled and total digesta returned. Rumen content was again emptied, sampled and returned 4 hours later on. The mean size of particles in the rumen content was determined by a wet sieving method using a mechanical shaker followed by hand-picking on paper marked in mm and the mean particle dimension was calculated.

During the 2 hours a.m. meal the silage particles breakdown was very efficient especially for the long form reducing the mean particle size from 10.3 cm for silage to 1.578 cm for the corresponding rumen content (Table 1) (12). The difference in mean particle size between both animals with similar intake levels was rather large after the 2 hours morning meal but much smaller at 8:30 a.m. after a night of possible rumination activity. Gill et al. (33) also found large differences between animals in the particle size distribution of swallowed boli.

Our observations, while not giving the complete particle size distribution of swallowed boli since some of the smallest particles may already pass the orifice reticulo-omasal during eating (53), do show that differences in mastication quality during eating may be one of the reasons for later on differences in rumination quality, turnover rates and voluntary intake.

TABLE 1. The voluntary dry matter (DM) intake, the mean particle size
and the percentage particles superior to 5 cm length in
reticulo-ruminal contents of two sheep fed long- and
short-chopped grass silage (ref. 12).

Sheep	Long			Short		
	# 5	# 6	Mean	# 5	# 6	Mean
Intake in a 2-h eating period (g DM/kg $W^{0.75}$/d)						
9:00 a.m.	14.42	13.14	13.78	15.83	14.68	15.25
3:30 p.m.	17.05	16.33	16.69	14.88	18.35	16.61
Mean particle size (cm) - in the silage - in the reticulo-rumen			10.30			2.28
8:30 a.m.	0.468	0.524	0.496	0.490	0.347	0.419
11:00 a.m.	2.055	1.100	1.567	1.419	0.961	1.190
3:00 p.m.	1.969	0.840	1.405	1.344	0.474	0.909
Particles superior to 5 cm - in the silage (%/total weight) - in the reticulo-rumen (%/total weight over 160mu)			67.60			9.27
8:30 a.m.	0.92	1.53	1.23	0.61	0.08	0.35
11:00 a.m.	11.06	2.55	6.81	3.46	2.08	2.77
3:00 p.m.	10.25	1.50	5.88	3.25	0.54	1.90

III.1.4. Species differences

Sheep vs cattle are much more sensitive to silage chop length (12,11,
21,22). Short chopping long grass silage just before feeding improved
significantly voluntary dry matter intake by 13.5-32% in sheep and
6.14-10.4% in heifers, probably through the significantly better rumination
quality (12).

These results raised the question of why cattle rumination behaviour vs
sheep was only slightly affected by chop length? In both species swallowed
silage particles are accumulated in the dorsal sac and the middle of the
rumen, and form an interwoven matt. Following ruminal contractions, the
smaller particles are washed out and sediment to the ventral sac. Because
of a better stratification (solid - liquid phase) and the more powerful
contractions of the rumen in cattle vs sheep (Ehrlein, personal
communication), the sedimentation into the ventral sac should be faster.
The backflow of small particles from the ventral sac to the cranial sac and

reticulum should be more easy in cattle since the cranial pillar and reticulo-ruminal fold do not separate the reticulum and rumen as strongly as in sheep and goats (48).

The movement of particles within the reticulo-rumen of cattle should thus be more easy, so that the rumination quality throughout the day is better in cattle vs sheep (15). This may partially explain the higher level of intake in cattle versus sheep when expressed in g per kg metabolic weight.

III.2. Omasal motility and passage of digesta through the orifice
      reticulo-omasal
III.2.1. Sequential motility and passage

From previous investigations (6,24,57),it is known that the omasum constitutes a pump which transfers digesta of the reticulum into the abomasum. Endoscopic observations made by Ehrlein and Lebzien (25) have elucidated the processes by which the digesta from the reticulum are aspirated into the omasal canal; and the time at which this takes place. During the regurgitation contraction and/or the first phase of the double contraction of the reticulum the reticular groove seals the omasal orifice, and lighter coarse food particles from the reticular contents are forced into the cranial sac of the rumen. During the second, and more powerful contraction of the reticulum, small particles with higher specific gravity are thrown from the floor of the reticulum directly towards the omasal orifice. The omasal body relaxes at this moment, the lowest portion of the reticular groove and the omasal orifice opens for a short moment and the omasal canal dilates so that the reticular contents which have been forced into the omasal orifice are aspirated into the omasal canal. The orifice reticulo-omasal (O.R.O.) is closed and by contraction of the omasal canal the reticular contents which have just been aspirated are compressed between the leaves of the omasal body. This process may be repeated a second time during a reticulo-rumino-omasal cycle, when the dorsal sac of the rumen contracts for a second time (Figure 4) (28).

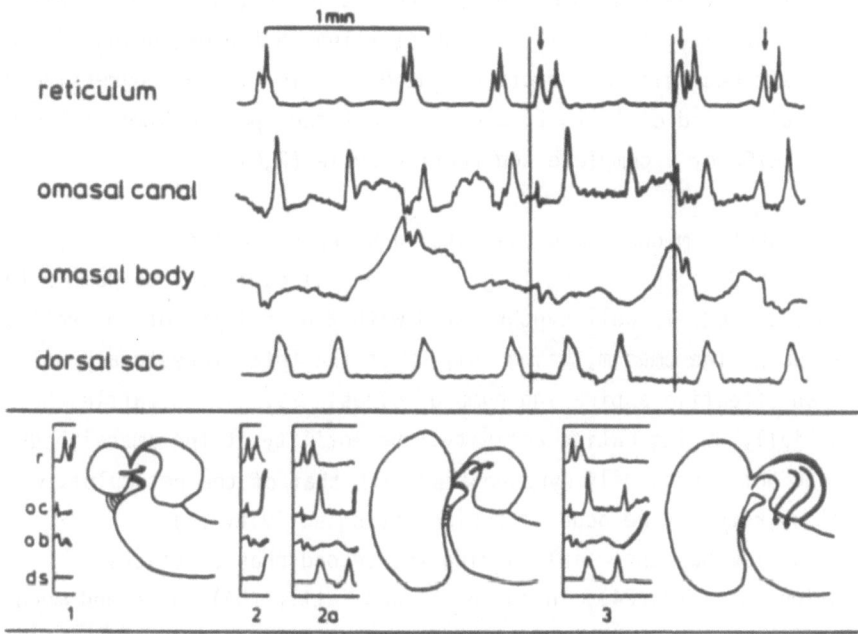

FIGURE 4. Motility tracings of the reticulum, omasal canal, the omasal
body and dorsal sac of the rumen. The sequence of contractions
during a reticulo-rumino-omasal cycle (vertical lines) is
divided into contraction phases and is shown by the diagrams.
Regurgitation occurred at the reticular contractions shown
by the arrows (ref. 28).
Key: r = reticulum; oc = omasal canal; ob = omasal body;
ds = dorsal sac of the rumen.

III.2.2. O.R.O. diameter and opening time in sheep vs cattle

The maximal diameter and the duration of large openings of the orifice
reticulo-omasal (O.R.O.) have been studied in details in sheep and cattle
by Bueno (6).

In sheep during a reticulo-rumino-omasal contraction cycle, the O.R.O.
is opened suddenly to its maximal size: 14 ± 6 mm for 0.76 ± 0.12 sec.
(0.85 ± 0.15 sec. during rumination activity) starting 0.25-0.30 seconds
after the beginning of the second phasic reticular contraction. The orifice
is opened and the associated flow of digesta is possible during 2.0-2.6
seconds for each contraction cycle. According to Bueno and Ruckebusch (5)
and Bueno (6) the total time of the O.R.O. opening does not exceed 15-20%
of the time of a complete reticulo-ruminal contraction cycle.

Similar studies made in cattle (6) showed that the O.R.O. is opened to its maximal size: 37 ± 6 mm during eating and idling, 28 ± 4 mm during rumination activity, for 10-12 seconds starting on the beginning of the second phasic reticular contraction. The O.R.O. is closed progressively over a total period of 15 to 25 sec., so that the opening time of the O.R.O. is about 60-70% of a complete contraction cycle (3,6).

III.2.3. Transfer mechanism of digesta in sheep vs cattle

In sheep and goats the motility of the omasal canal and to some extent of the omasal body is well synchronized with the motility of the reticulum and the rumen. The omasum, being only 5% of the total forestomach volume (9), is an effective aspirating pump of digesta (6,24). In cattle, however, and especially during eating activity, the motility of the omasal body is stable and not necessarily synchronized with that of the reticulum, which contraction rate may be doubled during eating activity (6).

Digesta flow happens mainly during the second phasic reticular contraction in goats (24), in sheep (6) and cattle (54). A second much smaller flow was observed in goats before the dorsal sac of the rumen contracts for a second time (24). In sheep and cattle the digesta flow through the O.R.O. is 30% higher during eating and ruminating activity compared to idling. During eating activity, the increase in frequency of reticular contractions is associated with an increased number of effluxes of digesta per unit time. During rumination, the duration of each digesta passage through the O.R.O. is short, the volume evacuated is however important (6).

The transfer of digesta from the reticulum into the omasum is obtained in sheep and goats by the synchronized contraction of the reticulum, opening of the O.R.O. and aspiration by the omasum. In cattle, however, because of the non-synchronization of the omasal body and its large dimension: 28% of the total forestomach volume (9), the omasum does not act as an aspirating pump. The transfer of digesta from the reticulum into the omasum is achieved by a 50% higher pressure in the reticulo-rumen compared to the abomasum, at the end of the second phasic contraction of the reticulum when the O.R.O. is largely opened for 10-12 sec. (6).

The differences between species in motility and associated transfer mechanism of digesta clearly demonstrate that the control of digesta flow, turnover rate and associated voluntary intake will not be identical in

sheep and cattle fed the same diet. Sheep are much more sensitive to chop
length and quality of silage fermentation than cattle (12).

III.3. Reflux of digesta from the omasum into the reticulum

The reflux of omasal digesta into the reticulum occurred mostly during
the omasal body contraction as shown in cattle (57) and goats (24).
Endoscopic studies made by Ehrlein and Lebzien (25) showed two types of
refluxes: a slow, continuous streaming and a strong, short reflux. The
function of those refluxes is to clean the papillae around the O.R.O. and
to reflux too long particles in order to prevent any obstruction of the
orifice reticulo-omasal, omaso-abomasal and the omasal canal. 10 mm
particles deposited *"de manu"* in the oral part of the omasum of sheep
refluxed back into the reticulum several hours later on. The maximal
dimension of particles flowing through the O.R.O. and omasum in sheep
was 6 mm (37).

IV COMPARTMENT FLOW METHODS AND LIMITATIONS

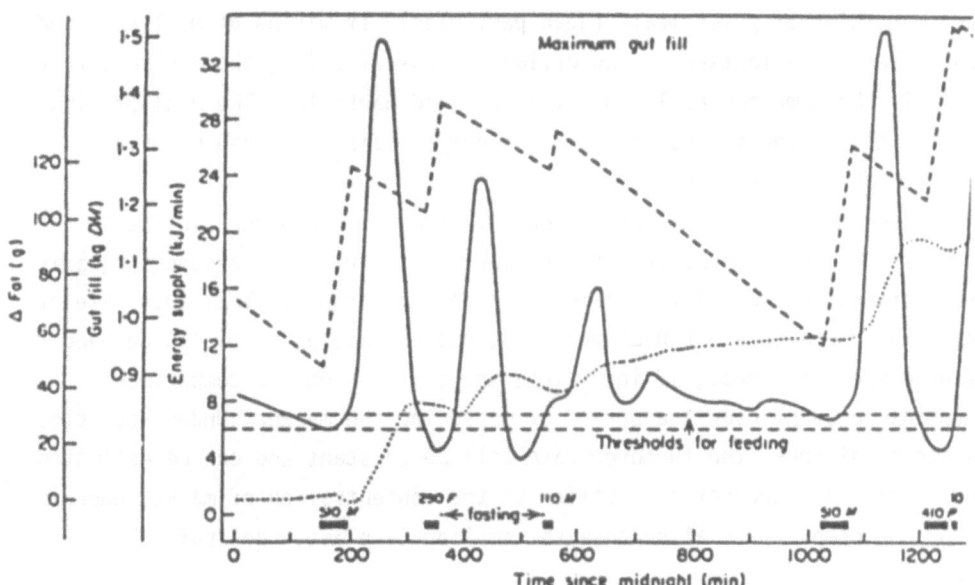

FIGURE 5. Predicted meals (▬), rates of absorption of energy-yielding
substrates (——), gut fill (----) and body fat content (....)
throughout a 24h period for a thin sheep offered a feed of 65%
DM digestibility. Meals are terminated metabolically (M),
physically (P) or by the start of a fasting period (F) and the
number above each meal gives its size (g) (ref. 32).

The reticulo-rumen is the dominant gastrointestinal turnover
compartment in cattle, sheep and goats. Variations in the digestive
capacity and flow rate of digesta are of great nutritional importance since
ruminant diets are often rich in roughage. Forage diets are relatively
indigestible (30-60%) and bulky compared to concentrates, and the voluntary
intake will be mostly physically limited by the reticulo-ruminal volume
depending on the time during the day, as proposed by a model of the short
term control of feeding (Figure 5) (32).

Compartmental flow models have been extensively used in estimating
volume and flow in compartments of many different biological systems.
Reviews are available concerning the basis of the approach and the relevant
mathematics involved (50,56,59). Illustration of some specific problems
when compartment models are applied to estimate the volume (mass) and flow
of feedstuff particles, was given by Ellis et al. (30). A compartment may
exist in any segment of the gastrointestinal (G.I.) tract where entering
particles mix with existing particles. Due to such mixing, particles which
exit the compartment represent a mixture of freshly ingested meal particles
and particles of prior meals (aged particles). If mixing of meal and aged
particles is instantaneous and efflux is non-selective, the probability for
exis is the same for newly ingested and aged particles. The meal origin of
particles exiting the compartment can only be distinguished by using
appropriate markers (29).

Measurement of the amount or concentration of the marker in the
compartment or emerging from the compartment over time provides the basis
for estimating the dilution rate and pool size of particles. This rate of
dilution represents a replacement or turnover rate of particles derived
from a specified meal, if input into and efflux from the compartment
remains constant over the period of measuring the marker. Under such steady
state conditions, the turnover rate will be constant and can be estimated
by fitting an exponential equation to the concentration of marker emerging
from the compartment at successive sampling time after dosing:

$$Ce(t) = Co \ e^{-kt}$$

where

$Ce(t)$ = concentration of marker on particles emerging from the
compartment at sampling time t.

Co = concentration of marker on all particles in the compartment the
instant after dosing and instantaneously mixing.

k = constant rate coefficient or turnover rate giving the fractional
   replacement per unit of time.

The pool size of particles or fill can be calculated from the dose of
marker (D) and its initial concentration:

Fill = D/C_o.

The assumptions involved in this approach are rarely met ideally in
biological systems and especially in the reticulo-rumen on a daily basis.
Major problems involve (30):

1) deviations from steady state,

2) slow mixing of particles,

3) selective rather than passive efflux of particles.

Deviations from steady state can be sustained by the circadian
evolution of the eating and ruminating activity as well as of the
rumination quality and associated particles size distribution in the
reticulo-rumen of sheep and cattle (12,16). In both species, the digesta
flow through the O.R.O. is 30% higher during eating and rumination
activity compared to idling (6).

The presence of a strong interwoven matt of particles in the middle of
the rumen especially with long grass silage and the delayed backflow of
small particles in the cranio-reticular area causing pseudo-rumination in
sheep (13) illustrates the slow movement or mixing of particles. Measurements of rate of passage through the G.I. tract obtained by a single dose
of marker administered via esophageal cannulae at the beginning or end of
a 3.5 hours available hay meal showed a 20.5% shorter time delay but a 42%
longer mean retention time for post-meal dosing. Mixing and rate of passage
of particles is thus meal and time dependent (14).

The efflux of particles from the reticulo-rumen is rather selective. The
mean size of omasal particles determined by sieving was 0.25 mm in sheep
fed hay (58) and 0.50 mm in cattle fed grass, hay, corn silage (34).
Particles with a mean length of 10 mm placed *"de manu"* in the omasum of
sheep refluxed whereas maximal 6 mm length particles flowed through the
orifice omaso-abomasal (37).

The practive of classifying particles into arbitrary size fractions,
while allowing deterministic descriptions, should not obscure the fact that
there is a continuum of particle sizes giving rise to a discontinuous range
of probabilities of removal from the reticulo-rumen (31). Poppi et al. (51)
proposed to use a standard sieve with a pore size of 1.18 mm in order to

separate particles into those with a low probability of removal from those with a high probability of removal from the rumen.

Indigestible plastic particles (.5x .16 cm) with different specific gravities (.90, .96, 1.17, 1.42, 1.77, 2.15) were fed in single doses to jersey steers and cows (10). The turnover rate and the proportion of ruminated particles was highest for those with a specific gravity of 1.17. The 0.90 and 0.96 specific gravity particles presented the highest proportion of ruminated particles but the lowest cumulative recovery percentage 10 days after dosing. This could be attributed to a slow escape rate from the floating interwoven matt normally found in the rumen of forage-fed ruminants. Particles with higher specific gravities (1.42, 1.77, 2.15) were poorly ruminated and cumulative recoveries were lower than for 1.17 specific gravity particles. This study clearly suggests that rumination and passage of indigestible particles is influenced by specific gravity.

Turnover rate of alfalfa cell wall particles (2.07 mm mean sieved particle size) mordanted with 2, 4, 8, 18, 32% chromium solutions was highest (0.0228%/h) for the 16% Cr-1.396 g/ml cell wall density and lowest (0.0072%/h) for the 4% Cr-1.165 g/ml cell wall density (23). Particle density and chromium concentration may be important factors biasing and/or affecting rate of particles turnover in the reticulo-rumen.

Compartmental flow might be expected to occur in those segments of G.I. tract having entrance and exit in close proximity and presenting thereby the opportunity for mixing particles of different meal origins. Examples include the reticulum, rumen, omasum, abomasum, caecum and colon. Digesta flow through other segments of the G.I. tract is largely unidirectional or polar or displacement in nature, with however some opportunity to mixing following "antiperistalty". Retention time due to displacement flow was referred by Ellis et al. (30) as time delay,or, Tau as proposed by Blaxter et al. (4). The concentration of marker in material emerging from the G.I. tract after flowing through a compartment and displacement segment can be described as:

$$Ce(t) = Co\ e^{-k(t-Tau)}$$

The mean retention time due to the turnover is the reciprocal of k (1/k) and the mean overall retention time is 1/k + Tau as proposed by Matis and Tolley (43).

V IMPROVING ROUGHAGE INTAKE BY SELECTING FOR EFFICIENT CHEWING AND RATE
   OF PASSAGE

The major part of particle size reduction is accomplished by chewing
during both eating and rumination activity when fed forages (2,46,49,60,
61) or whole grains (45). Communication via rumination is significantly
related to the level of voluntary intake and particles turnover rate
within the reticulo-rumen of sheep and cattle fed long- and short-chopped
grass silage (12).

Large variations occur among animals in the time, rate and quality of
eating and ruminating activities (1,13,65),in the weight of digesta in the
reticulo-rumen (35,52), in the rate of passage of digesta and intake (8,
12,35,36). Differences between animals is a recognized source of variation
in experiments. It will be removed from error term in most experimental
designs in order to improve chances of getting significant treatment
effects. These variations are however essential for genetical research.

Assuming that chewing quality, rumen motility, frequency of opening and
size of the orifice reticulo-omasal, gut fill, rate of passage are
heritable characteristics, animals could be selected for a fast or slow
rate of passage of particulate matter through the reticulo-rumen and for a
higher or lower voluntary intake level.

Grovum (35) suggested selection of animals at a given restricted level
of roughage intake. Those selected for a fast rate of passage through the
reticulo-rumen should have relatively small amounts of digesta in the
reticulo-rumen. They might be very efficient at fermenting and degrading
roughage to small particles and/or at removing small particles from the
reticulo-rumen. Those selected for a slow rate of passage would presumably
have relatively larger amounts of digesta in the reticulo-rumen and become
tolerant to reticulo-ruminal distension. They would have relatively high
ad libitum intakes of roughages and digest more of the food than
unselected animals.

Rate of passage is a constant giving the fractional replacement per
unit time. Higher intake levels by *ad libitum* feeding may be achieved
through a larger reticulo-ruminal pool size without any change in
fractional outflow rate. Maximal intake however should require a
combination of enlarging pool size and increasing rate of passage of
particles through the reticulo-rumen. As a possible consequence,

digestibility will decrease unless compensated in the caecum-colon.

In order to clarify the reasons for variability between animals in level of voluntary intake, six 1/4 Brahman 1/4 Jersey 1/2 Angus heifers each fitted with a rumen and T-duodenal cannula were fed *ad libitum* corn silage and daily 454 g cotton seed meal with or without 100 mg of monensin. The level of voluntary intake was highly related (p ≤ 0.001) to eating and ruminating rate, and quality of mastication. Fast eaters and ruminators had the highest intake level (p ≤ 0.001), the lowest unitary number (n/g DM/kg $W^{0.75}$) of reticulo-ruminal contractions and associated openings of the orifice reticulo-omasal (Table 2), and the lowest reticulo-ruminal NDF digestibility and particles degradation.

TABLE 2. Regression coefficient of the covariable and level of significance.

| Variable | Covariable | | | |
	(2)	(3)	(4)	(5)
Unitary time (min/g DM/kg $W^{0.75}$)				
1 - eating	0.062 NS	0.347***	0.093***	-0.023**
2 - rumination		0.660***	0.151***	-0.066***
3 - mastication			0.267***	-0.081***
4 Number of ruminal contractions per g DM/kg $W^{0.75}$				n.d.
5 Voluntary intake (g DM/kg $W^{0.75}$/d)				

n = 84; NS = non-significant; **p< 0.01; ***p< 0.001; n.d. = not determined following a significant interaction involving the DM intake

They compensated however partially by a better NDF digestion in the lower digestive tract so that total NDF digestibility was similar to the slow eaters, respectively 53.7% vs 54.3% (17). This indicates potential for identifying individuals with better than average mastication and flow capabilities, and possibly for selection of superior roughage eaters.

REFERENCES

1. Bae, D.H., Welch, J.G. and Smith, A.M.: J. Anim. Sci. 49, 1292-1299 (1979)
2. Balch, C.C. and Campling, R.C.: Nutr. Abstr. and Rev., 32, 669-686 (1962)
3. Balch, C.C., Kelly, A. and Heim, G.: Brit. J. Nutr. 5, 207-216 (1951)
4. Blaxter, K.L., Graham, N.M. and Wainman, F.W.: Brit. J. Nutr. 10, 69-91 (1956)
5. Bueno, L. and Ruckebusch, Y.: J. Physiol. (London) 238, 295-312 (1974)
6. Bueno, L.: Les fonctions motrices et digestives du feuillet. Thèse de Dr. Es-Sciences Naturelles, Université de Toulouse, 206 p. (1975)
7. Campling, R.C.: J. Brit. Grassld. Soc., 21, 41-48 (1966)
8. Campling, R.C., Freer, M. and Blach, C.C.: Brit. J. Nutr. 15, 531-540 (1961)
9. Church, D.C.: In: Digestive physiology and nutrition of ruminants, Vol. 1. (Ed), Corvallis, OSU Book Stores, Oregon, USA, 5-25 (1969)
10. Des Bordes, C.K. and Welch, J.G.: J. Anim. Sci. 59, 470-475 (1984)
11. Deswysen, A. and Vanbelle, M.: Proc. 7th Gen. Meet. Europ. Grassld. Fed., Gent, 6, 19-26 (1978)
12. Deswysen, A.G.: Influence de la longueur des brins et de la concentration en acides organiques des silages sur l'ingestion volontaire chez les ovins et bovins. Ph.D. dissertation, Université Catholique de Louvain, Belgium, 266 p. (1980)
13. Deswysen, A.G. and Ehrlein, H.J.: Brit. J. Nutr. 46, 327-355 (1981)
14. Deswysen, A.G., Pond, K.R. and Ellis, W.C.: Proc. Sixth Silage Conference, the Edinburgh School of Agriculture Scotland, 1-3 September, 29-30 (1981)
15. Deswysen, A.G., Bruyer, D.C. and Vanbelle, M.: Can. J. Anim. Sci. 64 (suppl.), 341-342 (1984)
16. Deswysen, A.G., Ellis, W.C. and Pond, K.R.: In: Techniques in particle size analysis of feed and digesta in ruminants. Kennedy, P.M. (ed), Canadian Soc. Anim. Sci., occasional publication 1, Edmonton, p. 172 (1984)
17. Deswysen, A.G., Ellis, W.C. and Pond, K.R.: Reprod. Nutr. Dēvelop., 26(1B), 271-272 (1986)
18. Dulphy, J.P. and Demarquilly, C.: Ann. Zootech. 21, 443-449 (1972)

152

19. Dulphy, J.P. and Demarquilly, C.: Ann. Zootech. 22, 199-217 (1973)
20. Dulphy, J.P., Bechet, G. and Thomson, E.: Ann. Zootech. 24, 81-94
    (1975)
21. Dulphy, J.P. and Michalet, B.: Ann. Zootech. 24, 757-763 (1975)
22. Dulphy, J.P., Michalet-Doreau, B. and Demarquilly, C.: Ann. Zootech.
    33, 291-320 (1984)
23. Ehle, F.R.: J. Dairy Sci. 67, 693-697 (1984)
24. Ehrlein, H.J. and Hill, H.: Zbl. Vet. Med. A. 16, 573-596 (1969)
25. Ehrlein, H.J. and Lebzien, : Proc. 20st. World Veterinary Congress,
    Saloniki, 1, 96-98 (1975)
26. Ehrlein, H.J.: Ann. Rech. Vet. 10, 173-175 (1979)
27. Ehrlein, H.J., Inst. Wiss. Film: Vormagenmotorik bei Wiederkäuern.
    Film C. 1328 des I.W.F., Göttingen, W. Germany (1979)
28. Ehrlein, H.J.: Forestomach motility in ruminants. Publ. Wiss. Film,
    Sekt. Med., Ser. 5, Nr. 9/C 1328, 29 p. (1980)
29. Ellis, W.C., Lascano, C., Teeter, R. and Owen, F.N.: Proc. of
    Symposium on Ruminant Protein Nutrition, Oklahoma State Univ.,
    MP-109, 37-56 (1980)
30. Ellis, W.C., Matis, J.H., Pond, K.R., Lascano, C.E. and Telford, J.P.:
    Proc. of Symposium on Herbivore Nutrition in the Sub-Tropics and
    Tropics. Gilchrist, F.M.C. and Mackie, R.I. (eds), The Science Press,
    Pretoria, p. 269-293 (1984)
31. Faichney, G.J.: The kinetics of particulate matter in the rumen.
    Modelling Meeting, Univ. of California, Davis, USA, Sept. 1984
32. Forbes, J.M.: Appetite 1, 21-41 (1980)
33. Gill, J., Campling, R.C. and Westgarth, D.R.: Brit. J. Nutr. 20,
    13-23 (1966)
34. Grenet, E.: Ann. Biol. Anim. Bioch. Biophys. 10, 643-657 (1970)
35. Grovum, W.L.: Proc. of Symposium on Herbivore Nutrition in the
    Sub-Tropics and Tropics. Gilchrist, F.M.C. and Mackie, R.I. (eds),
    The Science Press, Pretoria, p. 244-268 (1984)
36. Hartnell, G.F. and Satter, L.D.: J. Anim. Sci. 48, 381-392 (1979)
37. Hauffe, R. and Von Engelhardt, W.: Zbl. Vet. Med. A, 22, 149-163 (1975)
38. Hofmann, R.R.: The ruminant stomach: stomach structure and feeding
    habits of East African Game ruminants. E.A. Monogr. Biol., Kenya
    Literature, Box 30022, Nairobi, Vol. 2, 1-354 (1973)
39. Hofmann, R.R. and Schnorr, B.: In: Die funktionelle Morphologie des

Wiederkäuer-Magens. Ferdinand Enke Verlag, Stuttgart, 1-170 (1982)

40. Hungate, R.E.: Amer. Assoc. for the Advancement of Science 130, 1192-1194 (1959)

41. Iggo, A. and Leek, B.F.: In: Physiology of Digestion and Metabolism in the Ruminant. Phillipson, A.T. (ed), Oriel Press, Newcastle, 23-34 (1970)

42. Leek, B.F. and Harding, R.H.: In: Digestion and Metabolism in the Ruminant. Proc. 4th Int. Symp. Anim. Physiology, Sydney. McDonald,' I.W. and Warner, A.C.I. (eds), Univ. of New England Publ. Unit, 60-76 (1975)

43. Matis, J.H. and Tolley, H.D.: Fed. Proc. 39, 104-109 (1980)

44. Meissner, H.H., Van Staden, J.H. and Pretorius, E.: S. Afr. J. Anim. Sci. 12, 331-345 (1982)

45. Morgan, C.A. and Campling, R.C.: J. Agric. Sci. Camb. 91, 415-418 (1978)

46. Murphy, M.R. and Nicoletti, J.M.: J. Dairy Sci. 67, 1221-1226 (1984)

47. Nickel, R. and Wilkens, H.: Berl. Münch. Tierärztl. Wschr. 68, 264-277 (1955)

48. Nickel, R., Schummer, A. and Seiferle, E.: In: The Viscera of the Domestic Mammals. 2nd edition, Verlag Paul Parey, 1-403 (1979)

49. Pearce, G.R. and Moir, R.J.: Austr. J. Agric. Res. 15, 635-644 (1964)

50. Pond, K.R., Ellis, W.C. and Matis, J.H.: Development and application of compartmental models for estimating various parameters of digesta flow in animals. Modelling Meeting, Univ. of Calif., Davis, USA, September (1984)

51. Poppi, D.P., Norton, B.W., Minson, D.J. and Hendricksen, R.E.: J. Agric. Res., Camb. 94, 275-280 (1980)

52. Purser, D.B. and Moir, R.J.: J. Anim. Sci. 25, 509-515 (1970)

53. Reid, C.S.W., John, A., Ulyatt, M.J., Waghorn, G.G. and Milligan, L.P.: Ann. Rech. Vet. 10, 205-207 (1979)

54. Ruckebusch, Y. and Kay, R.N.B.: Ann. Rech. Vet. 2, 99-136 (1971)

55. Sellers, A.F. and Stevens, C.E.: Physiol. Rev. 46, 634-661 (1966)

56. Shipley, R.A. and Clark, R.E.: In: Tracer Methods for in vivo Kinetics: Theory and Applications. Academic Press (1972)

57. Stevens, C.E., Sellers, A.F. and Spurrell, F.A.: Am. J. Physiol. 198, 449-455 (1960)

58. Troelsen, J.E. and Campbell, J.B.: Anim. Prod. 9, 463-470 (1968)

59. Warner, A.C.I.: Nutr. Abstr. and Rev. 51, 789-820 (1981)

60. Welch, J.G.: J. Anim. Sci. 26, 849-854 (1967)

61. Welch, J.G.: J. Anim. Sci. 54, 885-894 (1982)

62. Weyreter, H. and Von Engelhardt, W.: Can. J. Anim. Sci. 64 (Suppl.), 152-153 (1984)

63. Wilkens, H.: Zbl. Vet. Med. 3, 803-816 (1956)

64. Wyburn, R.S.: In: Digestive Physiology and Metabolism of Ruminants. Ruckebusch, Y. and Thivend, P. (eds), Lancaster, England: MTP Press, p. 35-51 (1979)

65. Kennedy, P.M.: Austr. J. Agric. Res. 36, 819-828 (1986)

6. COMPARATIVE STUDIES OF FOOD PROPULSION IN RUMINANTS

R.N.B. KAY

I. INTRODUCTION

The ruminant mode of digestion has proved very successful. Ruminants can sustain themselves in most vegetative zones, from the arctic tundra to tropical forests, from deserts to swamps, and from mountain scrub to grassy plains. They range in weight by a thousandfold, from the lesser mousedeer (*Tragulus javanicus*) weighing little over 1 kg, to domestic cattle (*Bos taurus, B. indicus*), African buffalo (*Syncerus caffer*), eland (*Taurotragus oryx*) and giraffe (*Giraffa camelopardalis*) whose mature males may exceed 1000 kg.

The ruminant digestive tract and digestive process have to be remarkably adaptable in handling both quantity and quality of food. Nutrient requirement varies greatly with body weight. The fasting metabolic rate of adult mammals approximately reflects body weight raised to the power of 0.75, the inter-species mean for fasting heat loss being about 293 kJ/kg$^{0.75}$ (1). Consequently a 1.3 kg mousedeer needs to digest and absorb about 5 times as much energy per unit of body weight as a 1300 kg steer. Food intake/kg will also vary substantially within the life span of an individual, declining some two or three fold as the animal increases its weight some 10 to 20 times in growing to adult size. Females double or

triple their food intake at the onset of lactation, and in addition many
seasonal animals show a conspicuous cycle of voluntary food intake as a
consequence of metabolic and reproductive cycles entrained by daylength (2).

Between species, Hofmann has shown that functional characteristics of
the digestive tract can be related to differing food preferences which
allow various herbivores to occupy the same habitat without overmuch
competition for food (3,4). Different species are adapted to foods ranging
from the dry lignified grasses grazed by the buffalo to succulent shoots,
leaves and fruit selected by the smaller antelopes (5) and the mousedeer
(6,7). Almost as great a variation of diet may occur annually in many
species, especially in the seasonally adaptable, intermediate class
distinguished by Hofmann (3), as they adapt to seasons of plant growth and
dormancy - summer and winter, or wet and dry seasons.

Domesticated ruminants raised on unimproved pasture often face just as
great a seasonal variation in the quality of their diet as their wild
cousins. Those raised intensively at pasture or indoors may need to be
even more flexible, able to deal with diets foreign to them in nature
(grains, silage, molasses, byproducts), and to digest much greater amounts
to meet the nutrient demands of high productivity. We may therefore learn
much of value to our understanding and control of the digestive potential
and limitations of our domestic animals by comparing the ways in which
different ruminant species handle their dietary challenges.

II. RUMEN CAPACITY

If the energy requirements of different ruminant species were to be
met simply by alterations in rumen size, rumen capacity would have to vary
with body weight$^{0.75}$ and be five times greater in the smallest than the
largest species. Clearly, this does not happen. Indeed, data summarised
by Van Soest (8) shows that broadly speaking the weight of rumen contents
represents a fairly constant fraction of body weight across the full range
of species sizes. However, there is some variation in rumen capacity
between species that can be related to diet or metabolic requirement. The
more selective species that choose very digestible diets low in fibre tend
to have less rumen content (but more caecum-colon content) relative to
body weight than the less selective species (3,4,9,10). Among the less
selective grazers rumen content is rather greater in the smaller species
that have relatively high requirements to meet than the larger species (3.8).

Some domesticated breeds long dependent on very poor roughage diets
have remarkably large rumen capacities. Modern European breeds of cattle
do not grow at all well on diets of untreated straw, yet in Bangladesh
Bangali cattle are commonly reared on little but rice straw. Mould et al
(11) found that Bangali cattle had heavier digestive tracts than European
cattle, and that on a diet of untreated rice straw their rumen capacity
was enormous (rumen contents 24.5% of live weight). This allowed both the
intake and the digestibility of the straw to be high, leading to an
acceptable growth rate. Weyreter and Engelhardt (12) found that even larger
rumen volumes are found in the German Heidschnucken sheep, traditionally a
heathland breed. When given a diet of wheat straw for 6 months, they
increased their rumen fluid volume from 22 to 32% of live weight and were
able to maintain body weight.

III. RUMEN INGESTA VOLUME, RETENTION TIME AND DIGESTIBILITY

If the volume of rumen ingesta remains constant changes in food
intake or fluid input into the rumen are reciprocally related to retention
time and so to the extent to which the food is digested. In the short term
(periods of days or weeks) - which encompasses many feeding trials - it is
well known that an increase in the quantity of food eaten by an animal
does reduce the retention time of food in the gut and so depresses the
digestibility of the more slowly-digested fibrous components of the diet.
In red deer (*Cervus elaphus*), for instance, doubling the intake of a poor
hay diet reduced retention time by about 27% and dry matter digestibility
by 10% (13). Evidently gut capacity is unable to increase fast enough to
prevent a sudden change of intake from having a considerable influence on
retention time.

In the long term however (periods of months) ruminants show
considerable ability to adapt their gut to dietary needs. The changes in
the size and epithelial structure of the stomach compartments that occur
after weaning (14) and in response to increased food intake during
lactation (15) are well documented. The salivary glands, the source of
most of the fluid carrying food through the rumen, also mature and enlarge
considerably in response to weaning and consumption of fibre (16). Milne
et al (17) describe how Scottish red deer given diets of heather or
moorland grasses showed a large seasonal increase in intake between winter
and late spring that, surprisingly, was associated with longer retention

158

times in the rumen and gut and greater digestibility. A later study in
which the same deer were slaughtered when eating grass hay at one or other
season (18) showed that a 35% increase in food intake was accompanied by a
29% increase in weight of rumen contents, explaining how the deer avoided
the expected reductions in retention time and digestibility. The increased
rumen fluid volume shown by the Heidschnucken sheep maintained on a diet
of wheat straw was associated with an increased retention time of fluid in
the rumen and of particulate matter in the gut, which thus would enhance
digestion of the straw. Blackhead sheep showed lesser increases in rumen
fluid volume and retention time and lost 20% of body weight while
receiving this diet (12).

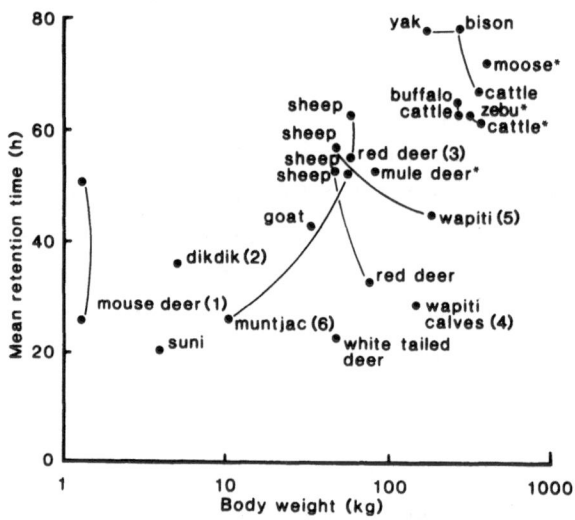

FIGURE 1. Mean retention times (MRT) of digesta in the digestive tract of
ruminants. Data from Warner (1981 Table 3) unless otherwise noted.
Lines link comparisons using a single diet.
(1) Morat & Nordin (1978). MRT for chromic oxide in mousedeer, 26.5 h, and
for stained sorghum, 52.8 h. (2) Hoppe (1977b). (3) Kay & Goodall (1976).
(4) Westra & Hudson (1981). (5) Kay & Hudson, unpublished. (6) Anderson
(1981).

Within species, then, gradually developing changes in the volume of
rumen contents may be utilised to help maintain retention time and so
digestibility in face of changes of intake and diet. Between species,
rumen volume is perhaps a less important variable than the inborn

differences in the structure and function of the digestive tract that directly affect retention time.

Ruminants seldom spend more than 10 h daily chewing their cud. Van Soest (8) argues that it is mainly this limit that restricts the efficient use of forage with high cell-wall content to the larger animals with their relatively low energy requirements. The small ruminants must either select less fibrous diets or manage to propel a fibrous diet rapidly through the forestomach, thus achieving a high intake at the expense of fibre digestibility. Figure 1 shown that mean retention times of food in the digestive tract tend to be related to body size. To the extent that whole gut retention reflects retention in the fermentation compartments of forestomach and caecum-colon this explains why the larger ruminants have the greater ability to digest poor quality roughage. One should be cautious in comparing such data, however, as they were obtained using a variety of diets and experimental conditions.

A few comparisons have been made between species that are similar enough in gut function to allow the same diet to be given to each without untoward effect. Sheep and cattle, weakly selective and non-selective grazers respectively, can readily be compared. The data summarised by Van Soest (Ref. 8, Fig, 20.6) indicate that a slightly higher dry matter digestibility is achieved by sheep for diets that are more than 66% digestible, and by cattle for less digestible diets. Cattle and sheep can also be compared with the larger deer, moderately selective but adaptable animals (4). Red deer showed shorter gut retention times and correspondingly poorer digestibility than sheep when a pelleted complete diet or diets of grass hay or dried grass were given, whether compared at equal absolute intakes or equal intake/kg body weight (13,23,24). This was true also when red deer and sheep were given diets of moorland grasses, though when heather was given the deer digested it better than sheep despite a higher intake and shorter retention time (17). A number of other wild browsing cervids (mule deer, *Odocoileus hemionus*, and wapiti, *Cervus canadensis*, but not barasingha, *C. duvauceli*) and bovids (such as eland), listed by Van Soest (Ref. 8, Table 20.7) show lower digestibility suggestive of shorter retention times when compared with cattle or sheep receiving the same diet.

The natural diets of the smallest ruminants do not overlap with those of cattle and sheep, so a controlled comparison of retention time and digestibility that is readily interpreted cannot easily be made between these groups. Nonetheless these small animals show clearly the ways in which a ruminant can adapt to a succulent, low-fibre diet. Nordin (6,7) provided captive mousedeer with diets of green kangkong leaves, seeds and fruit containing 10% or less cellulose in dry matter. The animals ate about 43 g of these diets daily (30 g/kg body weight) and spent very little time eating their food and ruminating. Mean retention time was not particularly short however (Fig. 1) perhaps explaining the high values (over 90%) for digestion of dry matter and cellulose (20). Like the mousedeer, Kirk's dikdik (*Madoqua kirki*) and the suni (*Nesotragus moschatus*) weighing 4 to 5 kg also select diets of green leaves and fruit from dicotyledenous plants. Rumen fermentation rate was found to be high, retention time short and digestion of fibre poor (5,25). In suni given lucerne hay, for example, mean retention time in the gut was also about 17 h (26). Farm ruminants given concentrated diets show changes in digestive function that generally are in the direction of those seen in the mousedeer, dikdik and suni, though they do not attain such rapid rates of propulsion and may not achieve satisfactory control of rumen fermentation and pH.

IV. DIGESTIVE TRACT ANATOMY AND FEEDING HABITS

Hofmann has made an admirably thorough study of the structure of the digestive tract of many wild and domesticated ruminants, first those of East Africa (3) and later those of Eurasia and North America (4). Dietary preferences and digestive anatomy could be inter-related so as to define three broad groups of ruminants. On the one hand are the non-selective grazers, medium to large in size, that consume coarse roughage and are adapted to the digestion of fibre. Cattle, sheep, African buffalo and musk-ox (*Ovibos moschatus*) belong to this group. The forestomach is large and muscular, the rumen being clearly divided by muscular pillars into sacs which retain the fibrous diet for prolonged fermentation. The rumen is well papillated only in its ventral parts, the dorsal wall and the pillars having a relatively smooth surface. The omasum is large with numerous well-developed laminae which may further filter and delay the passage of large particles as well as reabsorbing fluid and salts. The large intestine is relatively poorly developed, its fermentation chamber having only one thirtieth the volume of the rumino-reticulum for little is left for digestion once the food has undergone prolonged fermentation in the forestomach and has traversed the small intestine. On the other hand are the ruminants of all sizes that choose a more digestible diet with a low fibre content, selecting the shoots, green leaves and fruits of plants, eating frequently and ruminating relatively little. They include the dikdik and giraffe, roe deer (*Capreolus capreolus*) and moose (*Alces alces*). The rumino-reticulum is smaller and less muscular than that of the grazers and the pillars are poorly developed so that the wide ostia present little obstruction to the free movement of contents within the organ and towards the reticulo-omasal orifice. Ruminal papillae are well developed over the entire epithelium, greatly increasing the surface area available for absorption of volatile fatty acids from the rapidly fermenting contents. The omasum is small and has few leaves, presenting little obstruction to flow of contents. The mousedeer has almost no omasum at all, a small unlaminated portion at the anterior end of the abomasum perhaps representing the rudiment or vestige of an omasum (M. Nordin, personal communication). The fermentation chamber of the large intestine of the concentrate selectors is relatively voluminous, having one tenth of the capacity of the rumino-reticulum, suggesting that a considerable fraction of fermentable material survives the relatively short period it is retained in the foregut. Between the non-selective roughage eaters and the selective foliage and fruit eaters lies a flexible intermediate group, readily able to adapt their feeding habits and digestive functions to the forage available at different seasons and in different regions. Goat and chamois (*Rupicapra rupicapra*), red deer and caribou (*Rangifer tarandus*) belong to this group. Indeed, all ruminants are adaptable to a considerable degree, and the extent to which the digestive characteristics observed in an animal are determined genetically rather than as responses to the food the animal happens to be eating can only be determined by controlled feeding experiments.

The salivary glands, which provide both akaline salts to buffer the fermenting rumen contents and water to maintain the contents in fluid suspension, also tend to vary in size and so presumably in secretion rate with feeding habit. Fig. 2 summarises data tabulated by Kay et al. (10) and gives additional measurements. The latter provide further evidence that the salivary glands of the non-selective grazers are not very large. The slow continuous production of volatile fatty acids by fermentation of

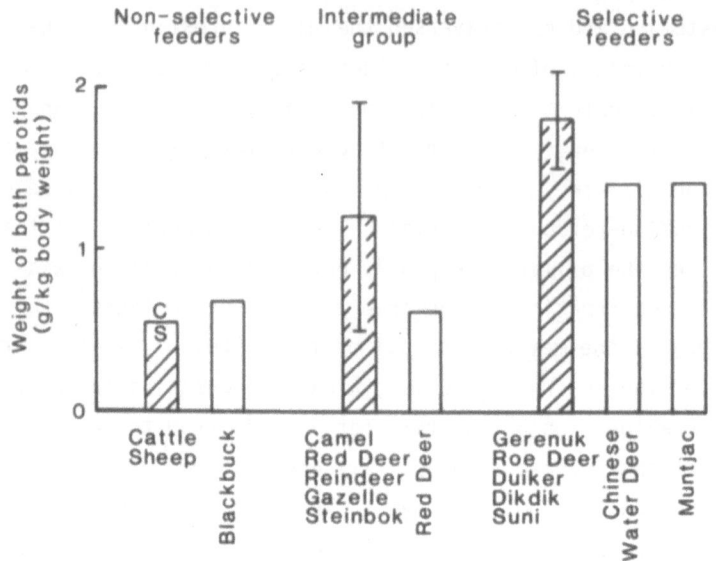

Parotid gland weight in ruminants having different feeding habits

FIGURE 2. The weight of both parotid salivary glands relative to body weight in ruminants of different feeding habits. Heads were kindly supplied for dissection by the Zoological Society of London (captive Chinese water deer, *Hydropotes inermis*, and blackbuck, *Antilope cervicapra*) and by Mrs Norma Chapman (wild English muntjac, *Muntiacus reevesi*).
(1) Mean for European ox and sheep (Kay et al 1980).
(2) Blackbuck (n=2; R.N.B. Kay, unpublished).
(3) Mean ± SD for camel, red deer, Norwegian and Svalbard reindeer, Grant's and Thomson's gazelle and steinbock (Kay et al 1980).
(4) Red deer (n=11; R.N.B. Kay, unpublished).
(5) Mean ± SD for gerenuk, roe deer, red duiker, dikdik and suni (Kay et al 1980).
(6) Chinese water deer (n=6; R.N.B. Kay, unpublished).
(7) Muntjac (n=6; R.N.B. Kay, unpublished).

fibre probably does not make exceptional demands on salivary buffers and prolonged retention of food reduces the need for fluid to suspend the ingesta. Those of the selective feeders are more than twice as heavy per kg body weight, able to supply the large amounts of alkali needed to buffer spurts of acid released from meals containing rapidly fermented carbohydrate and to provide the volumes of fluid required for rapid onward carriage of ingesta. Again, one needs to consider carefully how far these differences may be genetically determined and how far merely a response to the current diet. In the case of the red deer in Fig. 2, column 4, the weights of the parotid glands of two domesticated grazing animals, 1.05 and 0.85 g/kg, were much greater than those of nine pen-fed animals receiving hay and pelleted concentrates, mean 0.53 g/kg, range 0.49 to 0.68.

V. CONTROL OF DIGESTA FLOW

Hofmann (3,4) associates the feeding habits and digestive anatomy of ruminants in a manner that is attractively comprehensive and consistent, yet his account is mainly at a descriptive level: the precise links between anatomy and digestive function largely remain to be demonstrated by experiment. Of relevance to the subject of this review is the question of how far anatomical and physiological characteristics of various species influence the movement of fluids and solids through the forestomach.

Food is held in fluid suspension throughout most of the ruminant's gut. Exceptions are in the mouth where food is compressed into a mass until mastication and ensalivation render it into a sufficiently fluid slurry to allow it to be swallowed, within the dorsal and ventral sacs of the rumen where short roughage floats as a mat and long roughage forms tangled masses that are slowly rotated in the dorsal and the ventral sacs (27), and in the lower colon and rectum where residues are concentrated into solid faeces. While in fluid suspension the movement of food through the gut will be governed by pressure gradient, viscosity and resistance. Since resistance to fluid flow through an orifice is, as described by Poiseuille's Law, inversely proportional to the fourth power of the radius of the orifice, anatomical and physiological factors influencing the nature and behaviour of sphincter-like structures are of prime importance.

The pressure gradients causing movement of fluid around the forestomach and through to the abomasum are generated by muscular contractions of the wall of the organ. While contractions of the abdominal muscles are partly responsible for reflux of ingesta into the thoracic oesophagus during rumination, they can scarcely create differential pressures within the abdominal cavity. The effect of forestomach contractions on movements of ingesta will depend on their frequency, vigour and duration, on the way in which contractions progress around the wall of the stomach, and on the timing and duration of the opening of the orifices in relation to pressure gradients generated on either side. Few quantitative measurements have been made on a comparative basis.

VI. FORESTOMACH MOTILITY

In a study made in 1984 at the University of Alberta (R.N.B. Kay and

R.J. Hudson, unpublished) stomach motility and retention times were compared in two yearling wapiti and two adult sheep fitted with rumen cannulas. Brome grass hay was offered to both species at the same level of intake (56 g/kg$^{0.75}$).

The duration of primary rumino-reticulum contraction cycles in these wapiti and in other species, during rest, rumination and feeding, are compared in Table 1. The wapiti resembled sheep, and like most other deer

TABLE 1.

Duration of primary reticulo-ruminal contraction cycles in various species (sec)

	During rest	During rumination	During feeding	References
Wapiti	72	43	41	Kay & Hudson, unpublished
Sheep	66	54	41	(39)
Red deer	35	58	36	(40)
White-tailed deer	30	27	29	(41)
Bison	66	80	34	(42)
Cattle	60	72	35	(31)

they showed an accelerated contraction rate during rumination; bison (*Bison bison*) like cattle showed the reverse tendency. The wapiti also tended to have a longer cycle than the smaller red and white-tailed deer (*Odocoileus virginianus*). However, one should not interpret such comparisons too finely. Only two members of each wild species were studied; cycle durations are considerably influenced by the method of recording that is adopted (Ruckebusch and Kay 1971); they are also affected by diet and posture and by external events - when the wapiti were irritated by flies, for example, rumination cycles were nearly twice as long.

The llama (*Lama guanacoe*), despite being classified with the Tylopoda rather than the Ruminantia, has a forestomach analogous to the rumino-reticulum and omasum with a comparable pattern of contractions (29) and achieves equally effective digestion of fibre.

Mean retention times of a particulate marker (Dy-treated hay) and of a fluid marker (PEG) were rather less in the digestive tract of the wapiti studied by Kay and Hudson (unpublished), 46 and 27 h respectively, than in the sheep, 57 and 30 h, despite the fact that the level of food intake adopted proved insufficient for maintenance of body weight in the wapiti. Excretion of the particulate marker was largely complete in 4 days, indicating more rapid transit than was found by Dean et al. (30) in wapiti given baled alfalfa hay where 80% excretion times were 101-112 h. Much shorter mean retention times for Dy-hay, 21.4 and 28.7 h in October and February respectively, have been recorded in wapiti calves given a pelleted roughage-concentrate diet to appetite (21).

Contractions of the reticulo-omasal orifice and of the omasum were also recorded. A water-filled balloon, made from a 3 cm length of inelastic glove finger fixed between short soft cross-pieces which anchored the balloon in position, was inserted into the orifice or the omasum of the wapiti by hand to provide pressure records of contractions. The omasal balloon recorded strong contractions of the omasal body at about 16 sec intervals with relaxation during reticulum contractions, much as in cattle (28,31,32). The orifice balloon recorded a vigorous double rise of pressure that accompanied each double reticulum contraction. This is illustrated in Fig. 3. The first rise in pressure started with the first reticulum contraction but reached its peak about 0.8 sec later. The orifice pressure then rapidly fell before rising to a second peak about

Wapiti 8

Reticulum and reticulo-omasal orifice contractions

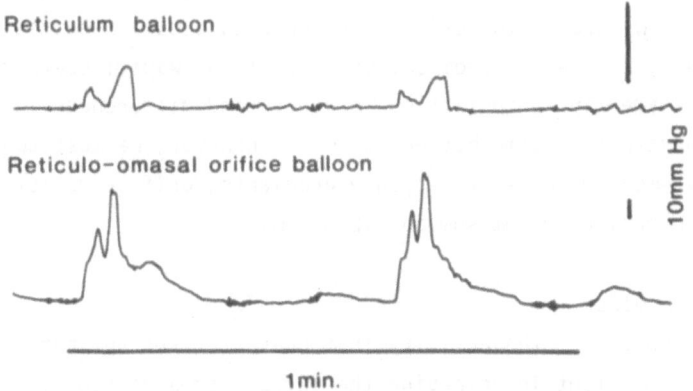

FIGURE 3. Contractions of the reticulum and the reticulo-omasal orifice recorded by balloon in a wapiti (*Cervus canadensis*) (R.N.B. Kay & R.J. Hudson, unpublished).

1.7 sec. before the second reticulum contraction. The orifice relaxed rapidly during the second reticulum contraction, and the balloon showed a weaker and less regular pressure rise a few seconds later, perhaps associated with contraction of the omasum.

In cattle Balch et al. (31) recorded by balloon a single contraction of the reticulo-omasal orifice during the first reticular contraction followed by another contraction after the second reticular contraction. Stevens et al. (32) recorded by palpation and open-ended catheters a closure of the reticular groove over the orifice during the first reticular contraction and a brief contraction of the orifice as the reticulum relaxed before its second contraction. During the second reticular contraction the orifice opened and a flow of fluid through it was recorded. These events correspond reasonably well with the pressure changes recorded at the reticulo-omasal orifice of the wapiti. However they do not correspond with records made by electromyography (e.m.g.) of the activity of the orifice in sheep (33,34) which show contractions recurring 3.5 to 10 times each minute. An orifice balloon is no doubt sensitive to contractions in surrounding tissues such as the lips of the reticular groove which are beyond the reach of e.m.g. electrodes in the orifice itself. Interpretation of e.m.g. records from an orifice is uncertain - muscular contraction might open rather than close the orifice - whereas compression of a balloon by whatever means presumably reflects the obstruction that would be offered to flow of fluid down a pressure gradient. It is during the second reticulum contraction, when pressure is high in the reticulum and low in the relaxed omasum, that the main phase of forward flow through the orifice is found to occur in cattle (28). Qualitatively, the reticulo-omasal orifice of the wapiti seems to function in much the same way as in cattle. To understand differences in forestomach retention time between species, however, we must await quantitative measurements of pressure gradients, orifice resistance and flow between reticulum, omasum and abomasum.

VII. PARTICLE SIZE

Chewing the cud is the activity that characterises ruminant animals. While it is important in enlarging the surface area of food particles that is accessible to microbial attack and in promoting salivary secretion, its main function is probably to reduce the size of particles so as to encourage their flow to the lower digestive tract. The reticulo-omasal orifice and the papillae within it have often been regarded as a filter preventing the onward passage of particles above a critical size. Uden (35) found that the particle size index in the faeces, a little less than abomasal particle size, was 0.89 mm in large cattle and 0.46 mm in sheep and goats; Nordin (7) records about 0.060 mm in the lesser mousedeer. Endoscopy has been used by McBride et al (36,37) to study the reticulo-omasal orifice in a mature steer. The orifice closed during the biphasic contraction of the reticulum, its margins rolling inwards to form a tight slit. It opened only as the reticulum relaxed, unfurling its margins to expose the interior of the omasum as the lips of the reticular groove stretched apart. When relaxed, the orifice measured 45 mm long by 10 mm wide (60 by 40 mm in the cows studied by Stevens et al., 32) and when the rumen was filled with saline solution stained alfalfa stems 10 mm long could be seen to move readily between reticulum and omasum. Similar observations have previously been made in goats. McBride et al. (37) argue that since the critical size for particle flow out of the bovine rumino-reticulum is so much less than 10 mm the orifice can have little of the filtering action that has been emphasised in the past. Perhaps attention should now be turned to the factors which may cause most particles above the critical size to remain trapped within the fibrous mass of ingesta that is retained in the centre of the rumen. The extent to which trapping occurs may well be affected by the differences in forestomach structure in selective and non-selective ruminants that are described by Hofmann (3). The studies on the wapiti suggest that further examination is warranted of the timing and duration of reticulo-omasal orifice opening in relation to reticulo-omasal pressure gradients and the to and fro movements of fluid ingesta between the reticulum and the cranial sac of the rumen at the onset of the reticulo-rumen contraction cycle, whether during rest, feeding or rumination.

VIII. CONCLUSION

Many behavioural, anatomical and physiological factors influence how much food a ruminant can eat and how well it is digested: food selection and mastication, microbial and enzymic activity within the gut, and as considered in this review, the capacity of the stomach and intestines and their anatomical structure, the size of the salivary glands, propulsive

168

motility and the rate of flow of food and fluid. These characteristics
are flexible, allowing the individual animal to meet changes in its
nutritional requirements and to adapt to short term or seasonal changes in
the nature, quality and availability of its diet. They also vary
genetically between species, allowing ruminants to exploit a wide range of
habitats and become fitted to different nutritional niches. Comparative
studies help us to understand how a ruminant can adapt, and so indicate
how we can select and best utilise domestic species suited to different
environments, nutritional conditions and productive performances.

REFERENCES

1. Kleiber, M.: The fire of life, Wiley, New York (1961).
2. Kay, R.N.B., In: Recent advances in animal nutrition - 1985, W.
   Haresign (ed.), Butterworths, London, 199-210 (1985).
3. Hofmann, R.R.: The ruminant stomach, East African Literature
   Bureau, Nairobi (1973).
4. Hofmann, R.R.: Roy. Soc. N.Z. Bull. 20: 51-58 (1983).
5. Hoppe, P.P.: Vet. Med. Rev. 1: 77-86 (1977).
6. Nordin, M. In: Symposium on animal population: wildlife management,
   1978, Bogor, Indonesia (1978).
7. Nordin, M.: J. Wildl. Mgmt 42: 185-187 (1978).
8. Van Soest, P.J.: Nutritional ecology of the ruminant, O & B Books,
   Corvallis, Oregon (1982).
9. Prins, R.A. and Geelen, M.J.H.: J. Wildl. Mgmt. 35: 673-680 (1971).
10. Kay, R.N.B., Engelhardt, W.V. and White, R.G., In: Digestive
    physiology metabolism in ruminants, Y. Ruckebusch and P. Thivend
    (eds) MTP Press, Lancaster (1980).
11. Mould, F.L., Saadullah, M., Haque, M., Davis, D., Dolberg, F. and
    Orskov, E.R.: Trop. Anim. Prod. 7: 174-181 (1982).
12. Weyreter, H. and Engelhardt, W.V.: Can. J. Anim. Sci. 64 (suppl):
    152-153 (1984).
13. Kay, R.N.B. and Goodall, E.D.: Proc. Nutr. Soc. 35: 98A (1976).
14. Warner, R.G. and Flatt, W.P., In: Physiology of digestion in the
    ruminant, R.W. Dougherty (ed.), Butterworths, London, 39-50 (1965).
15. Fell, B.F. and Weekes, T.E.C., In: Digestion and metabolism in the
    ruminant, I.W. McDonald and A.C.I. Warner (eds), University of New

England Publishing Unit, Armidale, Australia, 101-118 (1975).

16. Wilson, A.D.: Aust. J. agric. Res. 14: 226-238 (1963).

17. Milne, J.A., MacRae, J.C., Spence, A.M. and Wilson, S.: Br. J. Nutr. 40: 347-357 (1978).

18. Milne, J.A.: Proc. N.Z. Soc. Anim. Prod. 40: 151-157 (1980).

19. Warner, A.C.I.: Nutr. Abs. Rev. B 51: 789-820 (1981).

20. Morat, P. and Nordin, M.: Malay. Appl. Biol. 7: 11-17 (1978).

21. Westra, R. and Hudson, R.J.: J. Wildl. Mgmt 45: 148-155 (1981).

22. Anderson, J.M.: Studies on digestion in *Muntiacus reevesi*, M. Phil. thesis, University of Cambridge (1981).

23. Maloiy, G.M.O., Kay, R.N.B., Goodall, E.D. and Topps, J.H.: Br. J. Nutr. 24: 843-855 (1970).

24. Maloiy, G.M.O., and Kay, R.N.B.: Quart. J. Exp. Physiol. 56: 257-266 (1971).

25. Hoppe, P.P., In: Proceedings of 13th Congress of Game Biologists, Atlanta, 141-150 (1977).

26. Hoppe, P.P. and Gwynne, M.D.: Saugetierkundliche Mitteilungen 3: 236-237 (1978).

27. Wyburn, R.S., In: Digestive physiology and metabolism in ruminants, Y. Ruckebusch and P. Thivend (eds), MTP Press, Lancaster, 35-51 (1980).

28. Ruckebusch, Y. and Kay, R.N.B.: Ann. Rech. Vet. 2: 99-136 (1971).

29. Heller, R., Gregory, P.C. and Engelhardt, W.V.: J. Comp. Physiol. B 154: 529-533 (1984).

30. Dean, R.E., Thorne, T. and Moore, T.D.: J. Wildl. Mgmt 44:272-273 (1980).

31. Balch, C.C., Kelly, A. and Heim, G.: Br. J. Nutr. 5: 207-216 (1951).

32. Stevens, C.E., Sellars, A.F. and Spurrell, F.A.: Amer. J. Physiol. 198: 449-455 (1960).

33. Ruckebusch, Y.: J. Physiol. Lond. 210: 857-882 (1970).

34. Derrick, R.J., Patten, B.E. and Titchen, D.A.: Proc. Aust. Physiol. Pharmacol. Soc. 4: 137-138 (1973).

35. Uden, P.: PhD thesis, Cornell University, Ithaca, N.Y. (1978). Cited by Van Soest (8).

36. McBride, B.W., Milligan, L.P. and Turner, B.V.: J. Agric. Sci., Camb. 101: 749-750 (1983).

37. McBride, B.W., Milligan, L.P. and Turner, B.V.: Can. J. Anim. Sci. $\underline{64}$ (suppl): 84-85 (1984).

38. Ehrlein, H.J.: Ann. Rech. Vet. $\underline{10}$: 173-175 (1979).

39. Gordon, J.G.: Rumination in the sheep, PhD thesis, University of Aberdeen (1955).

40. Maloiy, G.M.O.: The physiology of digestion and metabolism in the red deer, PhD thesis, University of Aberdeen (1968).

41. Dziuk, H.E., Fashingbauer, B.A. and Idstrom, J.M.: Amer. J. Vet. Res. $\underline{24}$: 772-783 (1963).

42. Dziuk, H.E.: Amer. J. Physiol. $\underline{208}$: 343-346 (1965).

7. METABOLIC AND ENDOCRINE CONTROLS OF FOOD INTAKE IN RUMINANTS

A. de JONG

I. INTRODUCTION

Although the mechanism regulating feeding behavior of domestic ruminants has been the subject of intensive research for many years, it is not yet clearly understood. Components of this complex system are still being identified, and investigators are just beginning to unravel its intricate interrelationships. Although it has long been thought that ruminant animals have their feeding limited only by physical factors such as gastrointestinal fill (29), there is a large body of experimental evidence that they do regulate body energy content and food intake (10). This physiological regulation is probably achieved by negative feedback controls: feedback signals inform the central nervous system, in particular the ventromedial and the ventrolateral hypothalamus (10,111), but also other brain areas (16,22,111), regarding the nutritional state of the body.

Feed intake in the ruminant is a composite of meals, as is the case in most mammals. Size and/or frequency of the meals determine the amount food ingested. Many of the known metabolites and hormones have been ascribed roles in controlling meal patterns. In the past few decades remarkable shifts in interest have occurred, but the starting point has remained the same, i.e., for a substance in blood or rumen fluid to fulfill a regulatory function in meal size and meal frequency, at least two conditions must be met: first, ingestion of food must change the concentration of the component; second, changes in the concentration within the physiological range should result in an altered food intake.

This review will consider current concepts on the role of humoral components in this control in ruminants. The focus is on the regulation of spontaneous rather than scheduled meals as the former bring out the properties of the controlled system most clearly. Moreover, in current management practice there is a shift towards continuous availability of food to the animals. Firstly, the contribution of some metabolites will be reviewed, then the role of the major pancreatic hormones, and the influence of some peptides of the gastrointestinal tract and the brain will be described. Finally, I will elucidate means of chemically modify feeding behavior of healthy or diseased domestic ruminants to increase the motivation to eat, as in many practical situations livestock ruminants do not consume the amount of food required. In the metabolite-section only short-term factors will be considered whereas in the hormone-section both the short-term and long-term regulation of food intake will be discussed. The distinction between both types of regulation has been defined in a previous review (40).

Other aspects of the regulation of food intake and body weight such as the role of the nervous system or gastrointestinal distension are beyond the scope of this paper and have been reviewed elsewhere (6,7,29, 50,65,75). As the literature on the involvement of humoral feedback signals in controlling feeding is very extensive (for references see, e.g., 10,59,61,71,111), this chapter will be selective and in the text reviews covering important related material will sometimes be referenced, instead of the original papers.

II. METABOLITES

The importance of volatile fatty acids (VFA) in ruminant energy metabolism would indicate that VFA are likely to have a controlling function on food intake and, therefore, their role in the initiation and/or termination of meals will be extensively discussed.

II.1. Volatile fatty acids

In ruminants adapted to restricted access to feed, jugular VFA concentrations increase rapidly during and after eating (36,56,101). This is not only true for acetate - quantitatively the main VFA - but also for propionate and n-butyrate, whose systemic levels are very low due to their removal by the liver and the rumen wall. Similar findings were observed in the hepatic portal circulation. Generally, both peripheral and portal VFA increased within 15 min after the start of eating (30,36). In the free-feeding situation meals are much smaller and more frequent. For instance, sheep and goats usually take 7-14 meals per day with an average size of 50-300 g. To verify whether meals affect portal and peripheral VFA levels in this case, a remote sampling device was used, permitting frequent blood sampling without disturbing normal feeding behavior (31,37). In both studies spontaneous meals had no influence on either peripheral or portal VFA concentration. However, even at constant VFA concentrations, increased   blood flow might trigger VFA receptors. Increased portal blood flow has been observed in sheep and cattle fed infrequently, but no significant rise in net uptake of VFA was observed in sheep after spontaneous meals (1). Therefore, it is suggested that the onset of spontaneous meals is neither preceded nor followed by changes in blood VFA that could transmit feedback signals influencing the starting and ending of meals.

In the absence of changes in circulating VFA levels, the VFA in the rumen fluid might provide feedback cues. Here, too, in scheduled feeding, large meals induce marked increases in acetate, propionate and n-butyrate (97), but it still remains to be established whether spontaneous meals are related to   ruminal VFA concentrations. However, there is evidence that the ruminal VFA concentrations do not rise and fall with spontaneous meals either in sheep fed ad libitum. Hence, there is little hope that a relationship between spontaneous meals and ruminal VFA levels can be found although further studies are required.

If meal patterns are indeed governed by VFA levels (either in the circulation or in the rumen), feeding behavior should be prevented or postponed by infusion of VFA in amounts such that their normal concentration range is not exceeded. The effect of intrajugular infusions of

VFA has been studied by a large number of workers but only in a few cases a depressed intake by VFA has been reported (for references see 10,57 and 83). However, the interpretation of these results is open to question due to unphysiological conditions resulting from factors like the amount or the acidity. In addition, in some work the energy content of the VFA may have accounted for depressions in food intake.

The influence of VFA in the hepatic portal system on meal patterns has been studied by a few research groups. We investigated this on goats fed a concentrate diet in free access with intake being recorded continuously (41). Portal infusions of individual VFA or mixtures of VFA were given at a constant rate for 4 h and the effects thereof on feeding behavior and peripheral blood levels determined. In spite of high blood levels reached, infusion of acetate, propionate or butyrate failed to affect meal size, intermeal interval, latency to eat the first meal and total 4 h intake. Similarly, infusions of mixtures of these VFA did not affect meal patterns despite about 2-fold elevations in blood VFA levels (Table 1). Presumably the animals compensated the extraorally introduced energy over longer periods of time after the infusions. We conclude that, if circulating VFA play a role in the control of short-term feeding in the goat, the feedback signals are not generated from portal or peripheral blood. Baile (5) found that in goats and sheep, infusions of propionate during a spontaneous meal caused premature termination of that meal when made into the ruminal vein, but not into a mesenteric vein, the portal vein or the carotid artery. Therefore, it seems that portal infusion of VFA, even at very high rates as used by Baile, will not affect feeding. Infusion into the ruminal vein - upstream from the portal site - may be effective but Baile's work can be criticized on two points: unphysiological doses were used and the infusions were given during meals only, whereas the absorption of VFA produced after a meal takes place over a period of hours and spontenous meals are not related to blood VFA levels (31,37). As far as I know, the postulated proionate receptors in the ruminal vein wall have not been demonstrated by electrophysiological techniques.

In contrast to the intraportal infusions of Baile and ours, Anil & Forbes (3) and Elliot et al. (55) observed that the infusion of propionate into the hepatic portal region reduced feeding in sheep and steers respectively, using essentially the same approach as in our study.

TABLE 1

Lack of effect of volatile fatty acids on meal patterns of goats. Intra-portal infusions were made for 4 h. The ratio of a parameter is defined as the ratio of the mean of the parameter on the infusion day to that of the preinfusion day. Mean ± SEM (N=5) is presented. The food intake during the control and VFA infusions was 370 ± 50 and 341 ± 78 g, respectively.

behavior parameter

Treatment	meal size	ratio interval length	latency to first meal
control	1.09 ± 0.09	0.97 ± 0.12	1.11 ± 0.13
VFA-mixture	1.10 ± 0.12	1.26 ± 0.28	1.02 ± 0.09

blood parameter

Treatment	Dosis $(\mu g.kg^{-1}.min^{-1})$	concentration Preinfusion $(\mu mol.l^{-1})$	Infusion $(\mu mol.l^{-1})$
acetate	29	452 ± 80	815 ± 181
propionate mixture	7	11.5 ± 2.2	23.2 ± 5.4
n-butyrate	3	6.7 ± 1.9	16.5 ± 3.1

Although the induced changes in blood concentrations are not known in the sheep-study, in the steers a 2- to 4-fold increase in systemic propionate levels was acieved. In the latter study, however, the feeding responses to propionate were less consistent compared with Forbes' study, in spite of the clear increases in propionate. Elliot et al. (55) suggested that differences in the energy status of the animals, may account for part of the conflicting results. This may be true because, for instance, in sheep fed restricted amounts of food, infusions of propionate into the visceral circulation at a rate 20% lower than that used by Anil & Forbes (3), resulted in tripled propionate levels in systemic and portal blood but never caused a reduction in food intake (86). Similarly, in sheep fed a hay ration satiation of a hay meal was not affected by large increases in ruminal and (presumably) blood VFA concentrations by foregoing feeding of concentrates (54).

The Forbes group found evidence that the liver contains receptors sensitive to propionate and that nervous pathways are important links between liver and brain regarding the control of food intake (3,59,60). However, this does not imply that these receptors control food intake under physiological conditions; they may act as a safety mechanism. By way of comparison, evidence for glucoreceptors in the liver of monogastrics has been reported (for review see 93) but the physiological function of these receptors on food intake control is not yet clear (23,80).

To summarize the influence of blood VFA on meal patterning, intrajugular infusions did not affect food intake in the majority of the trials and, if a decrease was observed, unphysiological conditions may have been responsible. Our results suggest that VFA in hepatic portal blood do not govern either meal size or meal frequency. The literature on infusions into the hepatic portal drainage system, however, diverges more than can be explained by invoking differences in species, rates of infusion or energy status of the animal.

Much work on intraruminal infusions of VFA was carried out in the sixties in schedule-fed sheep and cattle (for references see 10,83); acetate usually, but not always, was shown to be a potent inhibitor of feed intake whereas propionate and n-butyrate had varying effects. However, experimental conditions often were unphysiological and changes in rumen fluid or blood composition were not measured even though large doses of chemicals were given. Less was done at that time on free-feeding ruminants. In goats, intraruminal infusions of acetate, propionate or n-butyrate depressed meal size (13; see also 57,58). Baile and McLaughlin (14) believe that, in the case of acetate, this effect is mediated by receptors in the wall of the dorsal sac of the ruminoreticulum. However, Leek and Harding (75) showed that these ruminal receptors are also sensitive to acids other than acetic acid. Some points of the investigations of Baile and co-workers are open to criticism. They gave infusions during meals only and the infusion rate greatly exceeded that of ruminal VFA production. The thereby occurring changes in the rumen fluid during and just after the infusions are unknown (13). Moreover, data on the effect of these infusions on blood VFA - presumed negative- are inconclusive as the infusions were limited to a 20 min period (12), and similar infusions caused a rise in blood acetate only after about 1 hour (39). It should also be stressed that infusions may cause extreme local changes in the rumen before mixing takes place. In sum, the above work does not adequately support the hypothesis under consideration.

Negative results on the other hand may be of interest. For instance, intraruminal infusions of large amounts of acetate had no effect on food intake in sheep (87). It was pointed out that changes in ruminal osmolality, but not in the pH, may play a role in short-term control of feeding under normal conditions (88). Similarly, in pigs compelling evidence was found regarding the role of intestinal osmoreception in the physiological control of feeding: Houpt (71) demonstrated that the rise in duodenal osmolality during a spontaneous meal was comparable with that produced by intraduodenal infusion of hypertonic solutions which effectively suppressed feeding. Other groups (54,57) also found that in sheep and goats ruminal VFA do not affect short-term feeding. For instance, in careful studies Focant (57) showed that intraruminal infusions of physiological doses of VFA did not affect meal patterns.

On the basis of one study it has been suggested that another.rumen microbial product, lactate, plays a role in the control of appetite in sheep (27,59), because intraduodenal infusions of DL-lactate effectively depressed feeding (27). However, it has not been investigated whether the concentration of duodenal lactate is related to a meal. Additionally, Bueno used pharmacological doses of lactate and did not determine the induced changes in duodenal or circulating lactate levels. Thus, the idea that the duodenal lactate concentration is one of the major regulators of normal ruminant feeding, seems doubtful. Bueno considered the latter concept in a later paper (53).

Generally, spontaneous meals and changes in plasma or ruminal VFA which may produce feedback signals, do not go hand in hand, and there is little evidence that manipulation of VFA concentrations influence the initiation or termination of a meal. It would appear appropriate to abandon the commonly held view that VFA levels to a major extent regulate meal patterns in free-feeding ruminants.

II.2. Other metabolites

Virtually every nutrient or metabolite has been proposed as a major signal whose surplus or deficit indicates satiety or hunger. Only some of these are covered by the following. Glucose does not seem to be a suitable cue for meal patterning in the ruminant because blood glucose levels are not related to spontaneous meals (31, 37; see also Fig. 1) and even severe, unphysiological hypoglycemia (38) and hyperglycemia (13) usually fail to affect meal patterns. Even in monogastrics, blood glucose is believed not to control normal feeding behavior (99), although lack of available glucose may trigger feeding in an emergency.

Changes in plasma concentrations of amino acids are unlikely to govern the initiation or the ending of a meal in the ruminant since amino acids are absorbed mainly from the small intestine several hours after ingestion. The effect of spontaneous meals on plasma amino acids is unknown but, in sheep, feeding once daily resulted in a gradual decrease lasting up to 4-6 h rather than an increase (19).

Plasma free fatty acids (FFA) present a varied picture. In steers they were clearly increased during spontaneous meals (31); in lactating cows the highest levels were seen during and shortly after such meals (107; in fasting ruminants they are elevated and feeding results in decreased concentrations (e.g., 101). In rats, plasma FFA levels augmented steeply during a meal and a few minutes afterwards, and then they declined to below premeal levels (A.B. Steffens; pers. comm.). Experimental elevation of FFA levels has been associated with a decreased food intake in both sheep and rats (73, 104). Thus, FFA may play some role in the control of meal size. In spite of these results, a major role of plasma FFA in meal patterning is questionable, if only because FFA levels are very erratic and starved animals are hungry despite their elevated plasma levels of FFA.

III. HORMONES

Hormones may be essential links in the physiological control of food intake in so far as they can act as messengers reporting to the brain either concentration reflecting the amounts of nutrient present at strategic points in the body, or rates of change in concentrations due to intake or metabolic expenditure. Below, we shall first consider the possible involvement of the pancreatic hormones insulin and glucagon in the regulation of food intake and body weight and then the role of the brain-gut hormones cholecystokinin and the opioid family will be elucidated. The role in meal patterning of other pancreatic hormones such as somatostatin and pancreatic polypeptide, and of the brain-gut hormones bombesin, gastrin, secretin has been discussed recently (40). Here, it

will suffice to mention that there is little evidence that these hormones
are involved in the regulation of ruminant food intake under normal
conditions. Although other neuropeptides have been shown to affect feeding
in both monogastric and ruminant animals (e.g., calcitonin, growth
hormone-releasing factor, thyrotropin-releasing hormone, neurotensin,
neuropeptide Y (e.g., 16,28a,69,91)), their physiological effects on food
intake are unknown.

III.1. Insulin

The pancreatic hormones are at the center of metabolic regulation in
ruminants and thus may be important for the regulation of energy balance
(20,26). The fact that the same area of the brain that is involved in the
regulation of food intake and body weight, i.e. the hypothalamus, is also
implicated in the regulation of the endocrine pancreas (42), emphasizes
the significance of insulin and glucagon. Two sources of evidence indicate
that insulin is involved in the physiological control of food intake.

Both in schedule-fed (19,56) and free-fed (20,31,37) ruminants, eating
induces a small, but significant increase in plasma insulin level. With
regard to spontaneous meals, this increase during meals frequently occurs
as rapidly as that seen in monogastric animals and man (Fig. 1). With

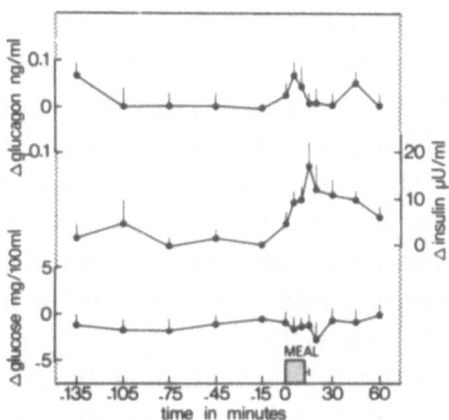

FIGURE 1. Effect of spontaneous meals on changes in blood glucose, and
plasma insulin and glucagon concentrations in goats. The concentrations
just before a meal are for glucose, insulin and glucagon 56.9 mg. 100 ml^{-1},
36.7 µU.ml^{-1} and 0.24 ng.ml^{-1}, respectively.
Mean $\pm$ SEM (N=5) is presented.

regard to schedule-fed ruminants, the increase in insulin may be due in part to meal-induced increases in VFA having 3 to 5 C-atoms (regarded as potent insulinogenic stimuli (20,39)), because peripheral insulinogenic VFA and insulin levels increase *pari passu* for some hours. Relative changes rather than absolute levels of peripheral VFA may be important here (39,86), so that in schedule-fed and perhaps also in *ad libitum* fed ruminants, VFA may, at least to some extent, control insulin secretion. For another part, the effect upon meal initiation in ruminants as well as in monogastrics (42) appears to be due to a vagal reflex triggered by oral stimulation during eating, as insulin is released - especially during spontaneous meals - almost as soon as eating starts, i.e., before there is any change in blood VFA levels (31,37). This was even seen in a sham-feeding sheep (20). On the other hand, it is unlikely that meal initiation is controlled by insulin as the plasma insulin level is not at its lowest immediately before a meal (Fig. 1).

An increase in insulin in response to a meal does not simply imply involvement in the control of feeding; the cause and effect relationships must be established. There is, indeed, some evidence that changes in insulin levels influence ruminant feeding behavior through short-term regulation. Intrajugular (34) or intraportal (35) administration of physiological amounts of insulin to sheep fed various diets resulted in depressions of food intake, even though plasma insulin levels were increased for half an hour at most and blood glucose remained unaffected. This increase in insulin level is possibly too short to cause an intra-cerebral change in insulin due to the slow passage of insulin through the blood-brain barrier (110,111). Hence, the reduced food intake after the intravascular insulin infusions may be mediated by hepatic receptors or by insulin receptors in brain areas devoid of the blood-brain barrier, e.g., in cerebral microvessels (105). Findings similar to those of the Wangsness group were made in pigs (2).

Although these facts advocate the function of insulin in the short-term regulation of food intake in ruminants (perhaps not in rats (99)), it is doubtful whether this could result in precise control since plasma insulin concentrations are subject to wide fluctuations due to factors such as exercise and stress. In contrast, these relatively rapid fluctuations may not interfere with a function of insulin in long-term regulation of intake. Woods and Porte (110,111) discovered that the insulin levels in the cerebrospinal fluid (CSF) serve as an integrator of plasma insulin levels over some interval of time. Specific insulin receptors identified in the brain (68, 105) are therefore exempt from the vagaries of plasma insulin. It is also well known that in ruminants, as in monogastrics including man, there is a strong positive correlation between the degree of adiposity and mean plasma insulin concentration (37, 103). To clinch the argument, proof is needed that chronic experimental elevation of CSF insulin level results in reduced food intake and consequently a decrease in body fat mass. Unfortunately, this evidence is lacking so far for ruminants, but it is available for baboons (109,111) and rats (25). The fact that in the rat the removal of insulin (by specific antibodies) from the ventromedial hypothalamus causes an acute increase of food intake, also fits (98). It should be emphasized that animals overeat after peripheral administration of unphysiologically high doses of insulin (4, 35), but this response is due to the resulting hypoglycemia and reduced glucose availability to the brain, and not to hyperinsulinemia *per se* In the case of ruminants, pending studies on the relationship between plasma and CSF insulin and adiposity, and on the effect of chronic changes of CSF insulin concentration on energy-balance, it would seem plausible that insulin may mediate the long-term control of food intake which causes ruminants to eat more when thin than when fat (24,84). It may also explain the fact that upon termination of a period of enforced over- or underfeeding, which results in a weight change, ruminants (as well as monogastrics) revert to their previous weight by eating less or more, respectively (10,111). The fact that there is an upward drift of adiposity with age does not negate this concept. It is true that information on the degree of adiposity reaching the brain through other humoral or neural messages, may also play a role in long-term control of food intake (e.g., 104,111). However, ruminal or circulating VFA can probably be excluded as direct regulators of body weight since, in cows and sheep, their concentrations in rumen fluid and blood plasma are not clearly correlated with the degree of adiposity (24).

III.2. Glucagon

Plasma glucagon levels increase clearly in response to feeding in schedule-fed sheep (19,82), but in lactating cows glucagon remained unchanged after feeding (18). Only moderate effects of spontaneous meals on glucagon levels were observed in goats (Fig. 1; 37). In monogastrics, the latter effects are much greater (42). Although secretion of glucagon, like that of insulin, can be stimulated by manipulating the gastrointestinal hormones, the autonomic nervous system and nutrients such as VFA having 3 to 5 C-atoms (20,39,86), it is still not clear to what extent these factors underlie the meal-induced release of glucagon.

A possible effect of pancreatic glucagon on feeding behavior of mono-gastric animals has recently received special attention. In rats, glucagon injected intraperitoneally prior to a meal reduces meal size and produces normal satiety behavior (62,63). Although changes in glucagon levels following glucagon injections have not been reported, the doses required for these effects are probably in the physiological range as they cause reductions in the liver glycogen content comparable to that at the end of normal meals (72). To bind plasma glucagon, Langhans et al. (74) injected pancreatic glucagon antibodies intraperitoneally to rats at the beginning of the first meal of the dark phase and observed a large increase in meal size and duration. This strongly indicates that glucagon is a satiety factor in the rat. The satiating of glucagon was attributed to its glycogenolytic action because the glucagon injections decreased the liver glycogen content whereas they only had very small lipolytic and ketogenic effects (62).

In sheep, intravenous injection of pancreatic glucagon during spontaneous meals reduced daily food intake (34). Although the induced changes in blood just after the administration were not measured, it is likely that they were within the physiological range. Simultaneous injection of propionate (a substrate for gluconeogenesis) did not enhance this reduced intake. In summary, particularly in monogastrics, but also in ruminants, there is evidence that glucagon acts as a short-term satiety signal. A long-term function for glucagon seems unlikely.

III.3. Cholecystokinin

It is now known that the gastrointestinal tract is a large reservoir of peptides whose physiological actions have yet to be completely defined. Many, if not all, of these gut peptides are also present in the brain, and therefore they are also classified as brain-gut peptides or neuro-peptides. For instance, at least five different forms of cholecystokinin (CCK) were found in the brains of sheep or other species (e.g., 94). The current concept is that CCK has two functions. Firstly, it tailors the digestive process to a meal eaten by stimulating the concentration of the gal bladder (e.g., 92) and by the secretion of enzymes from the pancreas, and secondly, it transmits, directly or indirectly, information to the CNS to indicate when a meal will terminate. This second function is elucidated below in more detail.

The best information on CCK is derived from monogastrics. Even here, no reliable data are available   on the effect eating has on circulating CCK concentrations. This is due to the difficulties of CCK assay. For at least a decade, now, more is known about the effects of CCK on eating. Intraperitoneal injection of CCK dose-dependently decreased the subsequent intake in fasted rats (for review see 96). In sham-fed rats this resulted in the consumption of a normal-sized meal, whereas without CCK eating would have gone on. In the subsequent years, various compatible findings were reported, using several forms of CCK, in monkeys, mice, cats, chicks, rabbits, pigs and humans (e.g., 9,45,96,111). Yet the interpretation of these data is still somewhat controversial: CCK may create a general malaise so that the reduction of food intake is secondary to the malaise (e.g., 17,51). Moreover, the difficulties of plasma CCK assay leave much uncertainty as to its physiological levels. It would seem unlikely that CCK plays a role in governing long-term food intake (108). The satiating effect of peripherally administered CCK is mediated by peripheral receptors in an abdominal organ and this visceral effect of the peptide activates vagal afferent fibers.

Much less is known about the involvement of CCK in feeding behavior in ruminants. Possible effects of eating on plasma CCK concentrations have not been established, whereas a few studies on the effect of CCK on food intake have been reported. Intravenous infusions of CCK or its analogues, CCK-octapeptide and the decapeptide ceruletide, for 1 h before and during feeding suppressed food intake in a dose-related manner in sheep (66). However, only for CCK significant decreases were observed. In a follow-up study Grovum (67) showed, by administering CCK at different intravascular sites, that the liver and the brain did not mediate the CCK-induced satiety. Intravenous injection of high doses of CCK-octapeptide were also effective in reducing intake in sheep (70). On the other hand, in sheep, briefly fasted or *ad libitum* fed, intrajugular (43) or intraportal (4) infusions of CCK for 3 h did not affect eating. Thus, the findings are not entirely consistent. Moreover, their physiological significance is uncertain as it is not known, firstly, whether eating causes an increase in plasma CCK levels and secondly, whether physiological doses were administered. On the latter point, determination of the gut motility in response to the infusions, may be of some help. Depression of food intake is probably non-specific if associated with a markedly disturbed motility pattern and this was in fact observed with doses of CCK that suppressed intake (66). In pharmacological studies using electrophysiological techniques the influence of CCK on duodenal motility has been confirmed (33). To clarify the possible role of CCK in feeding behavior more accurately, radioimmunoassays applicable to ruminants will be needed to answer the question of its physiological range. Taken together, CCK released from the intestinal tract of the sheep does not act as a satiety cue in the same way as in monogastrics. As in ruminants food is first held and digested in the reticulorumen, and then slowly passed into the intestines, so that the effect of a meal on intestinal absorption is not immediate, a minor role for plasma CCK can be anticipated.

On the other hand, the possible role of CCK as a satiety signal released by certain brain areas has been hypothesized. Continuous infusions of CCK-octapeptide, the predominant form, for 3 h into the lateral cerebral ventricles of sheep deprived of food for 2-24 h, decreased food intake in a dose-related manner (44). As little as 0.01 $pmol.min^{-1}$ depressed feeding significantly after 2 h of deprivation, and according to Della-Fera & Baile (44), this dose is approaching the physiological range. Sheep fasted for increasing periods required increasing doses of CCK-octapeptide to produce equivalent decreases in food intake. The depression of food intake was neither due to decreased water intake nor to an elevated body temperature, and the infusions elicited changes in rumen motility similar to those that normally accompany feeding (43). Similar findings were made in sheep fed restricted amounts of hay and infused via the same route for 1 h at slightly higher doses than used by Baile's group (28). It should be noted that in neither study CSF samples have been collected to determine the induced increase in the CCK concentration. Conversely, 2-h infusions of CCK-octapeptide antibodies into the lateral ventricles of satiated sheep caused an increase in intake of approximately 100 percent (48), presumably as a result of sequestration of endogenous CCK released during the meal. The observation that food intake increases upon removal of a factor normally present, is an important argument against generalised discomfort or illness as an explanation for the reduction of intake by its administration. Another approach of studying whether a putative satiety compound produces conditioned taste aversions, is to assess the complete behavioral sequence of satiety, and to determine the pattern of behavior that occur when the meal size is reduced by that compound. Unfortunately, both types of observations have not been made for CCK in the ruminant.

Based on these findings and similar ones in pigs (85), it can be hypothesized that CCK is released at specific brain sites, or released into the CSF in response to meal-related signals from the periphery and is then transported by CSF to receptor sites that elicit satiety behavior and possibly other changes occurring during a meal, e.g., gut motility (28). The facts that CCK is present in many areas in the brain (21), that CCK peptides are synthesized in neurons of the brain (45), that in sheep the hypothalamic CCK content declines after deprivation (45), and that specific CCK binding sites appear to be distributed among many of the same areas (94), are compatible with this hypothesis. In addition, an increased feeding has been observed after the injection of a CCK receptor blocker, dibutyryl cyclic GMP, into the CSF of sheep (45) and there is some evidence that CCK is actively taken up from the CSF (47). On the other hand, the possibility that CCK is being released directly at its receptor sites and thus, acting as a neurotransmitter, should also be given consideration. It is unlikely that the satiating effect of brain CCK is mediated by hormones such as insulin or glucagon, if only because CCK injected into the lateral ventricle depressed the plasma levels of these hormones (46). As long as it is not precisely known which changes take place in the ventricular system and in the surrounding brain areas during eating as well as during administration of compounds, the question of which mode of administration mimics the normal events, cannot be answered. Until then, some doubt will remain as to the role of CCK peptides in controlling the termination of a meal. Nevertheless, the hypothesis that CCK released during eating, both in monogastric animals and in ruminants, serves as a short-term satiety factor, is likely. While in monogastric animals the emphasis is on circulating CCK as a signal, in the ruminant a case can be made for a role of brain CCK in satiety.

III.4. Opioid peptides

Since the discovery of this family of neuropeptides about one decade ago,it has been found that they affect many physiological and behavioral functions (e.g., pain, stress, learning and memory processes) and certain neurological disorders (e.g., schizophrenia; for review see 81). More recently, evidence has shown that the endogenous opioid peptides are involved in the physiological regulation of eating (79,81,89). Central administration of endogenous opiates (β-endorphin, dynorphin, enkephalins) as well as peripheral or central administration of opiate agonists (e.g., morphine or ethylketocyclazocine) increase the amount of food eaten during a meal in a number of species, e.g., mice, rats and sheep, whereas peripheral or central administration of low doses of naloxone, an opiate receptor antagonist, decreases food intake or blocks the opiate-induced feeding (11,45,79). Moreover, the discovery of some types of opiate receptors and endogenous ligands in the hypothalamus (the major region controlling appetite), is in line with their postulated role in the initiation of feeding. Both κ and μ opiate receptors appear to play a role in the hyperphagia response. As opiates also inhibit gastrointestinal motility (77,90), it is possible that they control eating in this way. In sheep there is some evidence that opioids mediate the central-CCK elicited inhibition of food intake and/or ruminoreticular motility as naloxone abolished these effects (28). Although the brain is very likely to be the main site of action for the opioid peptides, it remains to be shown, where the intravenous-injected peptides are acting.

Regarding rats, there are data showing that the levels of opioid peptides are correlated to eating, for instance, a decline in the hypo-thalamic endorphin content was observed after starvation and the highest enkephalin levels have been shown to occur during the nocturnal feeding phase with the lowest levels during the light phase (78,81). Although suggestive, these data are not conclusive and, especially in the case of sheep, more work needs to be done. The role of endophinergic mechanisms in the physiological control of feeding remains unclear until changes in endogenous opiate release are measured and related to alterations in ingestive behavior. Additionally, some conflicting evidence on the opiatergic role in the physiological regulation of appetite does exist (111).

IV. STIMULATION OF FOOD INTAKE

In many practical situations, the daily food intake is a major factor limiting production in livestock ruminants. Increasing food intake results in larger amounts of nutrients being available for a productive function, because maintenance requirements do not increase proportionally when food intake increases. It should be pointed out that most food-producing animals, even in good health, establish a rate of intake substantially below the metabolic limitations. This results in suboptimal efficiency of production. On the other hand, many disease conditions, e.g., infectious and metabolic diseases, have an associated depressed intake. For example, in the lactating cow certain metabolic diseases could be prevented if food intake could be increased to provide the needed nutrients. Thus, methods of overcoming the disease-associated anorexias should also be examined. Therefore, means to chemically modify voluntary food intake of both healthy and diseased domestic ruminants to achieve maximal production, are of interest. In this section emphasis is places on the modification of feeding by centrally acting drugs. Below it will be apparent that the ideal centrally acting drug has not been found and, therefore, alteration of peripheral factors involved in governing intake, such as peripheral receptor number or sensitivity, should also be considered (100). There are a number of peripheral sites where pharmacological intervention is possible, as has already been described in the preceding sections of this chapter. Presently it is difficult to predict whether an agent that will interfere peripherally with a signal to the brain to stimulate feeding, will cause a sustained increase in food intake.

Although few chemical classes have been systematically investigated, several agents were found to increase the drive to overcome hunger. In cattle and sheep, various compounds injected into the brain can evoke feeding. Baile and associates found that intraventricular and intra-hypothalamic injection of some putative neural transmitters and ions increased food intake spectacularly in sheep (for review see 6). For instance, central administration of α- or β-adrenoceptor agonists (e.g., norepinephrine, epinephrine, isoproterenol), cholinergic agonists (e.g., carbachol), 5-hydroxytryptamine or ions (e.g., calcium or magnesium which depress neuronal activity) stimulated intake by sheep markedly. Conversely, feeding evoked by the above adrenergic and cholinergic agents was suppressed by their antagonists (6). In contrast, Driver et al. (52) found that injection of norepinephrine or 5-hydroxytryptamine into the lateral ventricle of sheep did not significantly affect feeding, whereas carbachol inhibited feeding. The fact that β-adrenoceptor agonists cause feeding in satiated sheep and cattle (6), suggests that in ruminants and rats the CNS control of feeding differs. In the latter species activation of β-adrenergic receptors of medial hypothalamic neurons inhibits feeding whereas activation of α-adrenergic receptors of the perifornical or lateral hypothalamic regions stimulates feeding (76). More recent work has indicated that changes in the concentration of some brain peptides may also stimulate feeding, as has been described above. In summary, certain monoaminergic and peptidergic transmission systems have been shown to be involved in the central control of feeding in the ruminant. Although compounds injected intracerebrally may cause large increases in short-term food intake, this route of administration appears of very little practical interest.

A variety of drugs has been found that also stimulate feeding in ruminants when given systemically or added to the diet, e.g., benzodiazepines, barbiturates, cannabinol-like chemicals, tertiary alcohols and phenylalkylsulfamides. Most studies have been focused on the former two classes. Elfazepam, an experimental benzodiazepine, has been extensively studied by Baile's group, and has been shown to be a potent feeding enhancer in ruminants as well as in many other species (for review see 15). Injected intravenously into satiated sheep and cattle, elfazepam immediately stimulated feeding. A several-fold increase in food intake was observed 30 to 120 minutes after injection of the compound; daily intake remained unaffected. The feeding response to intravenously injected elfazepam was at least as great as the response to any of over 100 analogues. Additional advantages of elfazepam are that it is effective over a wide dose range and that it has no undesirable side effects over much of the effective dose range (15). Furthermore, the daily food intake by sheep was significantly increased when elfazepam was administered for some days during each meal. The increase in daily intake was due to an increased meal size rather than to an increase in meal frequency. Elfazepam can also overcome loss of appetite due to gastrointestinal fill, aversive sensory cues or anorexias caused by chemicals, disease, heat stress or protein deficiency (15). For instance, hypophagia is frequently caused by monensin, a widely-used feed

additive the primary role of which is believed to be that of increasing
the ruminal percentage of propionate at the expense of methane, acetate
and butyrate. In some instances, but not all, the monensin-induced
hypophagia was corrected by elfazepam. Further, the profound anorexia
induced by amphetamine can be readily reversed by elfazepam. However,
studies with diazepam, another benzodiazepine, indicate that this drug is
indeed very effective in stimulating appetite of healthy goats but not
when fever is present (106).

Not enough is known about the site and mode of action of the feeding
response to benzodiazepines. Elfazepam is readily absorbed from the bovine
gastrointestinal tract so that it reaches threshold levels in the blood
and presumably also in the CNS. In rats, there are some data which would
indicate a hypothalamic mechanism in the benzodiazepine-induced hyperphagia (32). However, in sheep neither intracerebroventricular nor
intrahypothalamic injection of elfazepam could explain the feeding
responses after systemic administration (15). Further work is required to
define hypothalamic and extrahypothalamic involvement in benzodiazepine-
induced feeding. It has been suggested that benzodiazepines enhance the
activity of γ-aminobutyric acid (an inhibitory neurotransmitter synthesized
by hypothalamic neurons) which in turn reduces the serotonergic inhibitory
effects on feeding. Recent developments, mainly in monogastric animals,
show that the benzodiazepine-induced hyperphagia is also related to
central endophinergic mechanisms as low doses of naloxone or passive
immunoneutralization of endogenous opioid peptides abolished the benzodiazepine-induced feeding (e.g., 32,64). In sheep also, the elfazepam-
induced feeding response was completely suppressed by naloxone (8). Thus,
pending further research, it is possible that the mechanisms by which
benzodiazepines override the normal feeding control, involve the release
of endogenous opiates and their action on opiate receptors.

Elfazepam has an effect on a variety of gastrointestinal functions. It
can increase the digestibility in ruminants presumably because it
increases retention time of gastrointestinal tract content (15). Elfazepam
also increases the quantity of ingesta; it can decrease ruminal motility
(49,106) and abomasal physiology can be affected by elfazepam (15). It
does not affect ruminal fermentation. The cause of the changes in gastrointestinal functions is in all probability related to the effect of
elfazepam on the CNS which controls the activity of the gastrointestinal

tract.

The performance has been tested in a large number of feeding trials under a variety of conditions with cattle fed diets containing 0.5 to 2 ppm elfazepam (for summary see 15). Unfortunately, only small increases in food intake have been recorded. These feeding responses were much less than predicted from the already described 1- or 2-day tests. Unexpectedly, however, weight gain and feed efficiency were notably improved. The substance appears to be most effective in cattle on roughage diets. The improved growth rates cannot be explained by the subtle increase in food intake alone. Clearly, more research is required to explain these effects.

The long-term effects on feeding were also unsatisfactory in the case of another chemical class, the barbiturates including pento- and pheno-barbital. In experiments of short duration these drugs when administered centrally, intravenously or added to the diet, are very potent food intake stimulants in ruminants as well as in various other species (7). For instance, an increase of almost 20% in the daily intake was observed in sheep on phenobarbital given for two days. This increase was the result of increased meal size; such a meal pattern change is similar to that occurring in rats made hyperphagic by ventromedial hypothalamic lesions. In contrast, in a 9-week growth study sheep receiving a concentrate diet including 200, 400 or 800 mg phenobarbital per kg feed, quickly developed a tolerance to the drug (7). Much of the 5% increased feed intake occurred during the first month of the trial; feed efficiency remained unaltered. Such a development of tolerance to centrally acting agents has often been observed (100). Thus, although various drugs can be used to achieve clear increases in food intake in acute tests, in many cases this is of little practical use in performance trials. However, they often provide an invaluable experimental tool to study appetite control.

V. SUMMARY AND CONCLUSION

Feeding is a complex behavior finally controlled by the central nervous system. This control system is responsive to a variety of gastrointestinal, metabolic and sensory signals. The brain will coordinate this complex input and decide whether or not the organism needs food. Teleologically the existence of multiple feedback systems makes eminent sense. Thus, the over-zealous pursuit in the hunt for a particular nutrient, hormone or organ critical in governing eating, is not desirable; instead, the decision to start or stop eating depends on the balance of several cues. In the search for such feedback cues it is essential to correlate metabolic and hormonal changes with hunger and satiety; the simple demonstration that a compound reduces meal size is not sufficient to label it as a satiety factor.

Regarding the role of metabolites in short-term food intake regulation, volatile fatty acids presumably play a minor role in controlling meal duration and frequency in ruminants under normal conditions. They may operate as an emergency mechanism, e.g., under conditions such as fasting or in schedule-fed ruminants. This limited role is compatible with behavioral data in sheep and cattle since no correlation has been observed between meal size and either pre- or postmeal intervals. Of other metabolites, some evidence has revealed that free fatty acids are involved in the control of appetite, but here major questions are still open.

Hormones such as pancreatic and brain-gut hormones, have been considered as essential links in short-term satiety. Of these hormones, insulin, glucagon, cholecystokinin and opioid peptides have produced the most compelling evidence for a physiological role in the control of feeding. The opioid peptides have been reported to increase meal size whereas the other hormones reduce meal size. In the case of cholecysto-kinin, a reliable assay is urgently needed to clarify its role. Much still has to be learned about the mode of action of the brain-gut peptides. This field of science is still in its infancy and undoubtedly new neuropeptides will be discovered. It is obvious that a major field of research during the next decade will be the evaluation of the role of numerous neuro-peptides in the physiological regulation of feeding behavior. Of the hormones not discussed in this paper, one merits particular attention, namely growth hormone which may play a role in governing food intake (52,59,102,107).

Regarding long-term regulation, insulin levels in the cerebrospinal fluid, which reflect the mean plasma insulin levels over a long period, may control energy-balance and body weight. In monogastric animals this hypothesis is supported by the fact that experimentally elevated insulin levels in the cerebrospinal fluid reduce intake and body weight, and that insulin levels in plasma and in cerebrospinal fluid predict the degree of body fatness. For ruminants such experimental data are still limited.

192

To further improve ruminant performance in relation to food production for mankind, means of chemically increase voluntary food intake of healthy or diseased ruminants are of interest. Although many drugs have been found to be effective in stimulating intake, only few chemical classes are of any practical interest. The benzodiazepine elfazepam and some analogues are promising for some, but not all conditions. However, a definite judgement cannot be made until the developmental research of these drugs has been completed.

REFERENCES

1. Adams, G.B. & Forbes, J.M.: J. Physiol. 330: 47P-48P (1982).
2. Anika, S.M., Houpt, T.R. & Houpt, K.A.: Physiol. Behav. 25: 21-23 (1980).
3. Anil, M.H. & Forbes, J.M.: J. Physiol. 298: 407-414 (1980).
4. Anil, M.H. & Forbes, J.M.: Horm. Metabol. Res. 12: 234-236 (1980).
5. Baile, C.A.: Physiol. Behav. 7: 819-826 (1971).
6. Baile, C.A.: Fed. Proc. 33: 1166-1175 (1974).
7. Baile, C.A., In: Digestion and metabolism in the ruminant. I.W. McDonald & A.C.I. Warner (eds), University of New England Publishing Unit, Armidale, Aust., 333-350 (1975).
8. Baile, C.A., Della-Fera, M.A. & McLaughlin, C.L.: Proc. Int. Cong. Physiol. Sci. 14: 308 (1980).
9. Baile, C.A., Della-Fera. M.A. & McLaughlin, C.L.: Proc. Nutr. Soc. 42: 113-127 (1983).
10. Baile, C.A. & Forbes, J.M.: Physiol. Rev. 54: 160-214 (1974).
11. Baile, C.A., Keim, D.A., Della-Fera, M.A. & McLaughlin, C.L.: Physiol. Behav. 26: 1019-1023 (1981).
12. Baile, C.A. & Mayer, J.: J. Dairy Sci. 51: 1490-1494 (1968).
13. Baile, C.A. & Mayer, J.: Am. J. Physiol. 217: 1830-1836 (1969).
14. Baile, C.A. & McLaughlin, C.L.: J. Dairy Sci. 53: 1058-1063 (1970).
15. Baile, C.A. & McLaughlin, C.L.: J. Anim. Sci. 49: 1371-1395 (1979).
16. Baldwin, B.A.: Proc. Nutr. Soc. 44: 303-311 (1985).
17. Baldwin, B.A., Cooper, T.R. & Parrot, R.F.: Physiol. Behav. 30: 399-403 (1983).
18. Barnes, M.A., Kazmer, G.W., Akers, R.M. & Pearson, R.E.: J. Anim. Sci. 60: 271-284 (1985).

19. Bassett, J.M.: Austr. J. Biol. Sci. 25: 1277-1287 (1972).
20. Bassett, J.M., In: Digestion and metabolism in the ruminant. I.W.
    McDonald & A.C.I. Warner (eds), University of New England Publishing
    Unit, Armidale, Aust., 383-398 (1975).
21. Beinfeld, M.C.: Neuropeptides 3: 411-427 (1983).
22. Bell, F.R.: J. Anim. Sci. 59: 1396-1372 (1984).
23. Bellinger, L.L., Mendel, V.E., Williams, F.E. & Castonguay, T.W.:
    Physiol. Behav. 33: 661-667 (1984).
24. Bines, J.A. & Morant, S.V.: Br. J. Nutr. 50: 81-89 (1983).
25. Brief, D.J. & Davis, J.D.: Br. Res. Bull. 12: 571-575 (1984).
26. Brockman, R.P., In: Control of digestion and metabolism in ruminants.
    L.P. Milligan, W.L. Grovum & A. Dobson (eds), Reston Publishing Co.,
    Reston, U.S.A., 405-419 (1986).
27. Buéno, L.: Ann. Rech. Vétér. 6: 352-336 (1975).
28. Buéno, L., Duranton, A. & Ruckebusch, Y.: Life Sci. 32: 855-863
    (1983).
28a.Buéno, L., Fargeas, M.J. & Julie, P.: Physiol. Behav. 36: 907-911
    (1986).
29. Campling, R.C., In: Physiology of digestion and metabolism in the
    ruminant. A.T. Phillipson (ed), Oriel Press, Newcastle upon Tyne, U.K.,
    226-234 (1970).
30. Chase, L.E., Wangsness, P.J., Kavanaugh, J.F., Griel, L.C. Jr. &
    Gahagan, J.H.: J. Dairy Sci. 60: 403-409 (1977).
31. Chase, L.E., Wangsness, P.J. & Martin, R.J.: J. Dairy Sci. 60: 410-415
    (1977).
32. Cooper, S.J.: Life Sci. 32: 1043-1051 (1983).
33. Cottrell, D.F. & Iggo, A.: J. Physiol. 354: 477-495 (1984).
34. Deetz, L.E. & Wangsness, P.J.: J. Anim. Sci. 53: 427-433 (1981).
35. Deetz, L.E., Wangsness, P.J., Kavanaugh, J.F. & Griel, L.C. Jr.: J.
    Nutr. 110: 1983-1991 (1980).
36. De Jong, A.: J. Agr. Sci. Camb. 96: 643-657 (1981).
37. De Jong, A.: J. Agr. Sci. Camb. 96: 659-668 (1981).
38. De Jong, A.: Ph.D. Thesis, State University of Groningen (1981).
39. De Jong, A.: J. Endocr. 92: 357-370 (1982).
40. De Jong, A., In: Control of digestion and metabolism in ruminants.
    L.P. Milligan, W.L. Grovum & A. Dobson (eds), Reston Publishing Co,
    Reston, U.S.A., 459-478 (1986).

41. De Jong, A., Steffens, A.B. & De Ruiter, L.: Physiol. Behav. 27: 683-689 (1981).

42. De Jong, A., Strubbe, J.H. & Steffens, A.B.: Am. J. Physiol. 233: E380-E388 (1977).

43. Della-Fera, M.A. & Baile, C.A.: Ann. Rech. Vétér. 10: 234-236 (1979).

44. Della-Fera, M.A. & Baile, C.A.: Physiol. Behav. 24: 943-950 (1980).

45. Della-Fera, M.A. & Baile, C.A.: J. Anim. Sci. 59: 1362-1368 (1984).

46. Della-Fera, M.A. & Baile, C.A.: Physiol. Behav. 34: 283-289 (1985).

47. Della-Fera, M.A., Baile, C.A. & Beinfeld, M.C.: Peptides 3: 963-968 (1982).

48. Della-Fera, M.A., Baile, C.A., Schneider, B.S. & Grinker, J.A.: Science 212: 687-689 (1981).

49. Della-Fera, M.A., McLaughlin, C.L., Weston, R.H., Bender, P.E., Baile, C.A. & Chalupa, W.V.: Fed. Proc. 36: 1141 (1977).

50. Desweysen, A.G.: In: Physiological and Pharmacological Aspects of the Reticulo-Rumen. L.A.A. Ooms, A.D. Degryse and A.S.J.P.A.M. van Miert (eds), Martinus Nijhoff-Dr. W. Junk Publ., Boston-Dordrecht, 133 - 154 (1987).

51. Deutsch, J.A. & Hardy, W.T.: Nature 266: 196 (1977).

52. Driver, P.M., Forbes, J.M. & Scanes, C.G.: J. Physiol. (London) 290: 399-411 (1979).

53. Duranton, A. & Buéno, L.: Am. J. Vet. Res. 44: 802-805 (1983).

54. Duranton, A. & Buéno, L.: Physiol. Behav. 35: 105-108 (1985).

55. Elliot, J.M., Symonds, H.W. & Pike, B.: J. Dairy Sci. 68: 1165-1170 (1985).

56. Evans, E., Buchanan-Smith, J.G. & MacLeod, G.K.: J. Anim. Sci. 41: 1474-1479 (1975).

57. Focant, M.: Ph.D. Thesis, Université de Louvain-La Neuve (1986).

58. Focant, M., Gallouin, F. & Leclercq, M.: Ann. Rech. Vétér. 10: 226-228 (1979).

59. Forbes, J.M.: In: Digestive Physiology and Metabolism in Ruminants. Y. Ruckebusch & P. Thivend (eds), MTP Press, Lancaster, U.K., 145-160 (1980).

60. Forbes, J.M.: Proc. Nutr. Soc. 44: 331-338 (1985).

61. Forbes, J.M.: In: The Voluntary Food Intake of Farm Animals, Butterworths, London-Boston (1986).

62. Geary, N., Langhans, W. & Scharrer, E.: Am. J. Physiol. 21: R330-R335 (1981).

63. Geary, N. & Smith, G.P.: Physiol. Behav. 28: 313-322 (1982).

64. González, Y., Fernáncez-Tomé. M.P., Sánchez-Franco & del Rio, J.: Life Sci. 35: 1423-1429 (1984).

65. Grovum, W.L.: Br. J. Nutr. 42: 425-436 (1979).

66. Grovum, W.L.: Br. J. Nutr. 45: 183-201 (1981).

67. Grovum, W.L.: J. Physiol. 326: 55P-56P (1982).

68. Havrankova, J., Roth, J. & Brownstein, M.J.: Adv. Metab. Disord. 10: 259-268 (1983).

69. Hawkins, M.F.: Physiol. Behav. 36: 1-8 (1986).

70. Hondé, C. & Bueno, L.: Peptides 5: 81-83 (1984).

71. Houpt, T.R.: J. Anim. Sci. 59: 1345-1353 (1984).

72. Langhans, W., Geary, N. & Scharrer, E.: Am. J. Physiol. 243: R450-R453 (1982).

73. Langhans, W., Wiesenreiter, F. & Scharrer, E.: Physiol. Behav. 30: 113-119 (1983).

74. Langhans, W., Zieger, V., Scharrer, E. & Geary, N.: Science 218: 894-896 (1982).

75. Leek, B.F. & Harding, R.H., In: Digestion and metabolism in the ruminant. I.W. McDonald & A.C.I. Warner (eds), University of New England Publishing Unit, Armidale, Aust., 60-76 (1975).

76. Leibowitz, S.F.: Nature, 226: 963-964 (1970).

77. Maas, C.L.: Ph. D. Thesis, State University of Utrecht (1984).

78. Morley, J.E. & Levine, A.S.: Am. J. Clin. Nutr. 35: 757-761 (1982).

79. Morley, J.E., Levine, A.S., Yim, G.K. & Lowy, M.T.: Neurosci. Behav. Rev. 7: 281-305 (1983).

80. Novin, D., Robinson, K., Culbreth, L.A. & Tordoff, M.G.: Am. J. Clin. Nutr. 42: 1050-1062 (1985).

81. Olson, G.A., Olson, R.D. & Kastin, A.J.: Peptides 6: 769-791 (1985).

82. Ostaszewski, P. & Barej, W.: Ann. Rech. Vétér. 10: 385-387 (1979).

83. Papas, A. & Hatfield, E.E.: J. Anim. Sci. 46: 288-296 (1978).

84. Paquay, R., Doizé, F. & Bouchat, J-Cl.: Ann. Rech. Vétér. 10: 223-225 (1979).

85. Parrott, R.F. & Baldwin, B.A.: Physiol. Behav. 26: 419-422 (1981).

86. Peters, J.P., Bergman, E.N. & Elliot, J.M.: J. Nutr. 113: 1229-1240 (1983).

87. Phillip, L.E., Buchanan-Smith, J.G. & Grovum, W.L.: J. Agr. Sci. Camb. 96: 429-438 (1981).

88. Phillip, L.E., Buchanan-Smith, J.G. & Grovum, W.L.: J. Agr. Sci. Camb. 439-445 (1981).

89. Reid, L.D.: Am. J. Clin. Nutr. 42: 1099-1132 (1985).

90. Ruckebusch, Y., Bardon, Th. & Parret, M.: Life Sci. 35: 1731-1738 (1984).

91. Ruckebusch, Y. & Malbert, C.H.: Life Sci. 38: 929-934 (1986).

92. Ruckebusch, Y. & Soldani, G.: J. Vet. Pharmacol. Therap. 8: 263-269 (1985).

93. Russek, M.: Appetite 2: 137-143 (1981).

94. Saito, A., Sankaran, H., Goldfine, I.D. & Williams, J.A.: Science 208: 1155-1156 (1980).

95. Sanger, D.J.: Appetite 2: 193-208 (1981).

96. Smith, G.P., Gibbs, J. & Kulkosky, P.J., In: The neural basis of feeding and reward. B.G. Hoebel and D. Novin (eds), Haer Institute, Brunswick, ME, 149-165 (1982).

97. Sniffen, C.J. & Robinson, P.H.: Can. J. Anim. Sci. 64: 529-542 (1984).

98. Strubbe, J.H. & Mein, C.G.: Physiol. Behav. 19: 309-313 (1977).

99. Strubbe, J.H., Steffens, A.B. & De Ruiter, L.: Physiol. Behav. 18: 81-86 (1977).

100. Sullivan, A.C. & Gruen, R.K.: Fed. Proc. 44: 139-144 (1985).

101. Thye, F.W., Warner, R.G. & Miller, P.D.: J. Nutr. 100: 562-572 (1970).

102. Tindal, J.S., Blake, L.A., Simmonds, A.D. & Hart, I.C.: J. Endocr. 104: 159-163 (1985).

103. Van der Meerschen-Doizé. F., Bouchat, J-C., Bouckoms-Van der Meir, M-A, & Paquay, R.: Reprod. Nutr. Dévelop. 23: 51-63 (1983).

104. Van der Meerschen-Doizé, F. & Paquay, R.: Appetite 5: 137-146 (1984).

105. Van Houten, M. & Posner, B.I.: Diabetologia 20: 255-267 (1981).

106. Van Miert, A.S.J.P.A.M., Anika, S.M. and Van Duin, C.T.M. In: Comparative veterinary pharmacology, toxicology and therapy. Part I. Proc. 3rd EAVPT Congress, Ghent. A.S.J.P.A.M. van Miert, M.G. Bogaert and M. Debackere (eds), EAVPT, Utrecht, 174 (1985).

107. Vasilatos, R., & Wangsness, P.J.: J. Nutr. 110: 1479-1487 (1980).

108. West, D.B., Fey, D. & Woods, S.C.: Am. J. Physiol. 246: R776-R787 (1984).

109. Woods, S.C., Lotter, E.C., McKay, L.D. & Porte, D. Jr.: Nature 282: 503-505 (1979).

110. Woods, S.C. & Porte, D. Jr.: Am. J. Physiol. 233: E331-E334 (1977).

197

111. Woods, S.C., Taborsky, G.J. Jr. & Porte, D. Jr.: In: Handbook
     of Physiology. Intrinsic regulatory systems of the brain. F. Bloom
     (ed), Am. Physiol. Soc. (in press).

8. RUMEN MICROBIAL METABOLISM OF PLANT SECONDARY COMPOUNDS, XENOBIOTICS AND DRUGS

R.A. PRINS

I. Introduction
   1. The rumen as a digestive organ; basal discussion of the special position of polygastric animals.
   2. The rumen as an organ metabolizing foreign compounds.
II. Main types of biochemical reactions in rumen metabolism of foreign compounds.
   1. Hydrolytic reactions.
   2. Reduction reactions.
   3. Fission reactions.
III. Main categories of foreign compounds entering the rumen.
   1. Non-intentional (accidental) intake of foreign compounds in ruminants.
      1.1. Intake of feed contaminants (pesticides).
      1.2. Toxic principles formed in feed plants or soil before consumption (mycotoxins).
      1.3. Naturally formed toxic compounds in plants (secondary compounds).
      1.4. Toxicological consequences of rumen metabolism of toxic compounds from plants.
   2. Foreign compounds added to the feed or dosed orally.
      2.1. Drugs used in the treatment of rumen disorders or microbial diseases (antibiotics and chemotherapeutics).
      2.2. Additives used to improve animal production by manipulating the rumen fermentation (feed additives).
      2.3. Drugs in veterinary practice aimed at the treatment of non-rumen disorders.
      2.4. Nutritional and pharmacological consequences of drug-microbe interactions in the rumen.

I. INTRODUCTION

I.1. The rumen as a digestive organ; basal discussion of the special
      position of polygastric animals.

A tremendous amount of knowledge has been collected during the last 25
years on various aspects of the ruminant's digestive processes (1). Much of
the attention has been focussed on rumen function, especially on the role
of rumen microbes (2,3). It is generally believed that the major rumen
microorganisms have now been identified and a great many of these were
studied with respect to nutritional requirements, biochemical pathways and
physiological functions. However, most of these studies were confined to
the fermentation of the major nutrients such as cellulose and other
carbohydrates, proteins, non-protein nitrogen compounds, lipids and organic
acids. Much less attention has been given to rumen transformations of
compounds that do not seem to play an important direct nutritional role,
but which happen to be present in the ruminant's feed (feed contaminants,
mycotoxins, plant secondary compounds) or compounds which are administered
intentionally to the animal. Among the latter are feed additives or
therapeutics dosed orally in veterinary practice. In this chapter all of
these categories of compounds are designated as "foreign compounds",
although they are of quite different origin and structure.

Among the herbivores, ruminants have been very successfull in conquering
nutritionally hostile habitats. This is undoubtedly due to their
mutualistic association with bacteria, protozoa and anaerobic fungi, which
made it possible to make use of the plant cell walls in fibrous feeds and
to thrive on such feeds low in nitrogen and vitamins. The fermentation of
toxic principles would confer an additional advantage to the ruminant
animal. Interesting examples of the latter possibility are gradually
unveiled in studies e.g. in the United States, Canada and Australia. The
knowledge acquired will be of considerable importance also for our
understanding of the fate of drugs in the rumen.

I.2. The rumen as an organ metabolizing foreign compounds.

In considerations on plant compound or drug toxicity in the ruminant,
the role of the reticulo-rumen cannot be overlooked. Its action towards
certain compounds makes the reticulo-rumen quantitatively speaking an organ
of great importance, comparable with the role the liver plays in drug
metabolism. However, there are some major reasons why the role of the rumen

is a very specific and unique one.

First, the site of the rumen proximal to the major absorptive organs - the acidic stomach and small intestine is of special importance. When it occurs, rumen metabolism of foreign compounds profoundly changes the nature of the compounds before absorption. In the second place, even when no metabolism ensues in the rumen, physico-chemical interactions with the digesta mass and the kinetics of digesta transfer influence the rate of passage of the foreign compound and eventually influence absorption.

A very specific difference with liver and kidneys lies in the nature of the enzymes involved in foreign compound metabolism in the rumen. Hydrolytic and reducing reactions play major roles in the metabolism of foreign compounds in the rumen, in addition to a number of degradative reactions such as decarboxylation, dealkylation and dehalogenation.

A further difference concerns the changing nature of the microflora and -fauna and their enzymes as a result of changes in feeding practice or physiological conditions. Adaptation to a certain drug is possible, resulting in strongly enhanced metabolism of the drug in the rumen. One way adaptation may occur is connected with the role certain foreign compounds may play as (additional) energy sources. Feeding practices can have an influence on drug metabolism through changes in the composition of the microbial population or by altering the kinetics of rumen outflow. Level of feed intake, type of feed, frequency of feed intake are all of influence. A certain portion of the drugs offered orally - such as anthelmintics in veterinary medicine - may bypass the rumen, when closure of the oesophageal groove is stimulated. Because of the changing nature of the factors mentioned and because of the numerous interrelations between these factors, metabolism of foreign compounds in the rumen forms a very complex issue.

In the lower intestines of monogastric animals microbial metabolism of foreign compounds by the chiefly anaerobic intestinal microflora may occur, strongly resembling the nature of reactions in the rumen. In fact, much of the knowledge on the types of drug metabolizing reactions to be discussed here stems from research on monogastric animals (4,5,6). Since hydrolysis and reduction are among the chief reactions and since these reactions largely undo the detoxification reactions in liver and kidneys (where oxidation and conjugation reactions prevail), it is not surprising that enterohepatic cycling of drugs and drug detoxification products in bile occurs between liver and the intestines as a consequence.

Enterohepatic cycling between rumen and liver probably plays a limited role, since many of the products of rumen drug metabolism will not return to this organ once they are absorbed. However, not much is known about this aspect.

II. MAIN TYPES OF BIOCHEMICAL REACTIONS IN RUMEN METABOLISM OF FOREIGN COMPOUNDS.

Information on the metabolism of foreign compounds by intestinal and ruminal microorganisms has been reviewed in many places (e.g. 5,6,7,8). Some of the major types of reactions (Table 1) will be repeated briefly below, grouped according to Walker (9). It should be realized that examples were also drawn from the literature on gut flora metabolism in monogastric animals in the belief that, at least qualitatively speaking, rumen and intestinal flora perform similar reactions.

TABLE 1.

Metabolic reactions carried out by gastrointestinal microorganisms (adapted from Walker, 9 and Scheline, 4).

1. Hydrolysis:	glycosides
	glucuronides
	amides
	peptides
	esters
	ethereal sulfates
	sulfamates
2. Reduction:	C-C double bonds
	azo groups
	nitro groups
	N-oxides
	N-hydroxy groups
	aldehydes
	ketones
	arsonic acids
	epoxides
3. Fission reactions:	decarboxylation
	O-dealkylation
	N-dealkylation
	deamination
	heterocyclic ring fission
	reduction of benzene group
	dehalogenation

II.1. Hydrolytic reactions.

The mixed rumen microbial population shows a very broad array of

hydrolytic enzymes of which many are known to function in microbial
digestion of plant constituents. Enzymes that hydrolyze polysaccharides
(cellulose, hemicellulose, pectic polyuronides, plant storage
polysaccharides and many other types of carbohydrate polymers),
oligosaccharides, glycosides, proteins, peptides, amides, nucleic acids and
various esters including triacylglycerols are known to be present in the
rumen associated with the microbial cells or adsorbed to digesta
particles. In general, levels of free enzymes in the extracellular rumen
fluid are low.

A large number of plant secondary compounds are esters, notably
glycosides. The release of the aglycones from flavonoid glycosides, from
cyanogenic glycosides or release of 3-nitro-1-propanol from miserotoxin -
the toxic principle of *Astragalus miser* var. *serotina*- by rumen microbial
hydrolases have been demonstrated experimentally. Among the glycosidases in
the rumen, β-glucosidase - and β-galactosidase activity are most prominent.
Hydrolysis of glucuronides, ethereal sulfates and sulfamates take place in
the lower intestine and are catalyzed by the gut microbes.

II.2. Reduction reactions.

In the normal rumen, reducing conditions exist and a low redox
potential can be measured as a consequence of the presence of many reduced
compounds (sulfides, hydrogen). In the fermentation of carbohydrates, the
bulk of the plant food, several intracellular intermediates in the pathways
by which the acidic fermentation end products (propionate, butyrate,
valerate) are formed and the glycolytic intermediate pyruvate serve as
electron acceptors. In addition, several microorganisms are capable of
using certain extracellular compounds as electron acceptors. Bicarbonate,
nitrate and sulfate are examples of such acceptors. The first compound is
of special quantitative importance, its reduction leading to the
formation of methane or in some bacteria to the formation of acetate.

However, a variety of extracellular organic molecules directly derived
from the plant food may serve as electron acceptors as well. First, double
carbon to carbon bounds in unsaturated lipids or in the aliphatic side
chain of aromatic acids (cinnamic, ferulic and caffeic acids) will be
reduced in the rumen. Fig. 1 shows the reduction of caffeic acid as proven
for gut contents of the rat (10).

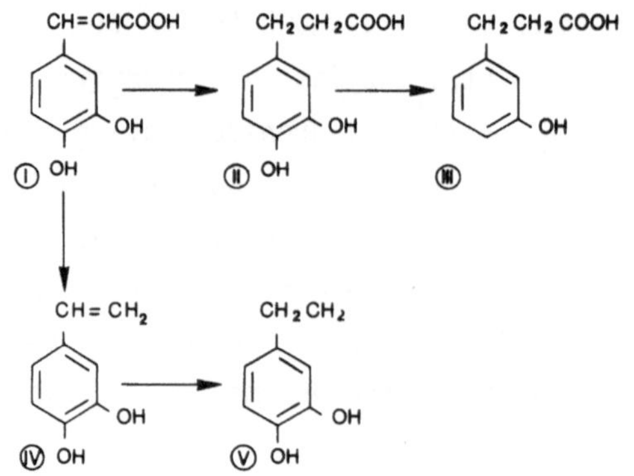

FIGURE 1. Metabolism of caffeic acid. Caffeic acid (I) is reduced to dihydro-caffeic acid (II), which is dehydroxylated to m-hydroxyphenyl-acetic acid (III). In another pathway, caffeic acid can be decarboxylated to yield 4-vinylcatechol (IV) which can be reduced to 4-ethylcatechol (V) (10).

Another example is the reductive fission of pyrrolizidine alkaloids heliotrine and lasiocarpine in the rumen resulting in detoxification (see Fig. 2).

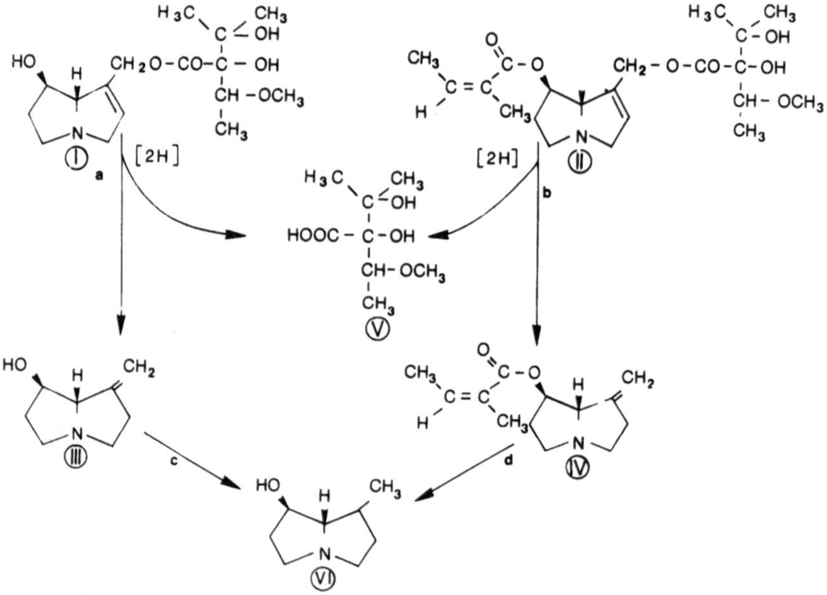

FIGURE 2. Reductive metabolism of the alkaloids heliotrine (I) and lasio-carpine (II) in the rumen. Products are 1-goreensine (III) and heliotric acid (V) (route a) or 7α-angeloxy-1-methylene-8α-pyrrolizidine (IV) and heliotric acid (route b), formed by reductive fission. The detoxification finally leads to the common end product 7α-hydroxy-1α-methyl-8α-pyrroli-zidine (VI) by another reduction step (see review 6).

More recent studies by Shull et al. (11) and Cheeke (12), throw some doubt on the question whether this process occurs in the rumen of animals in the Western US ingesting tansy ragwort (*Senecio jacobaea*). It could be that certain microbes are lacking in these ruminants (see below). Still another example of reduction of carbon to carbon double bonds is the reduction of the alkaloid solanidine to the 5,6-dihydro analogue (13).

Reduction of double nitrogen to nitrogen bonds (azo bonds) in numerous synthetic water-soluble colouring agents (food dyes) has been demonstrated for the gut flora of rats and man. Reduction of 7 azo dyes (amaranth, Ponceau SX, Allura Red, Sunset Yellow, tartrazine, Orange II and methyl orange) by cell suspensions of several important anaerobic intestinal bacteria in pure cultures was studied by Chung et al. (14). The study showed that the reduction of azo compounds -with the production of toxic products- can be accomplished by the major anaerobic bacterial species (*Fusobacterium, Bacteroides* sp.) rather than by facultative species in the gastrointestinal tract.

Reduction of nitro groups in chloramphenicol, parathion, nitrophenols, nitropropanol and other nitro-compounds has been demonstrated for the rumen. With several of the compounds this reduction results in inactivation (detoxification), in other words in a lowering of biological activity. Rumen protozoa are active in nitro group reduction and the protozoal concentration should have a strong influence on the reduction rate.

The reduction of epoxides to olefins in the rumen is a remarkable reaction and a significant detoxification mechanism, because it is the epoxide group which confers biological activity to several alkylating agents, carcinogens and pesticides (15).

II.3. Fission reactions.

A number of lytic reactions are known to occur in rumen or gut during metabolism of foreign compounds and feed constituents. These reactions have arbitrarily been lumped together here as fission reactions and include decarboxylation, dealkylation, dehalogenation, dehydroxylation, deamination and ring fission reactions.

Decarboxylation of amino acids and phenolic acids has been described most often. Decarboxylation of phenolic acids occurs primarily with p-hydroxylated compounds and further substitution in the ring leads to a lowering of the reaction rate, especially with adjacent substituents, e.g.,

p-hydroxyphenylacetic acid but not o-hydroxyphenylacetic acid is
decarboxylated. Phenolic, phenylacetic and cinnamic acids are
decarboxylated but phenylpropanoic acids are not, clearly showing the
influence of the side chain (Fig. 3).

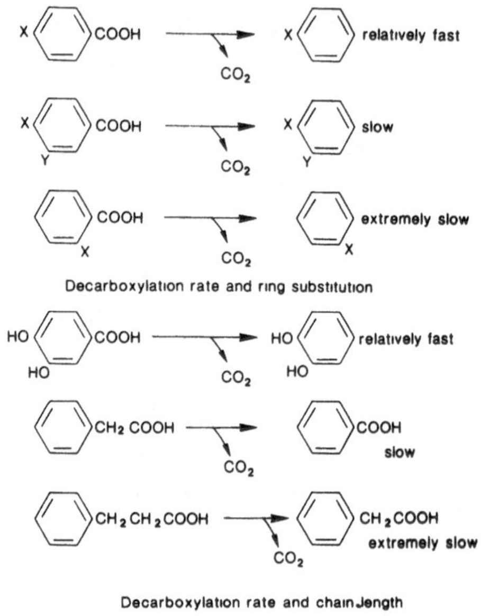

FIGURE 3. Decarboxylation of aromatic acids by mixed gastrointestinal
microorganisms: molecular structure and reaction rate.

O-dealkylation has only been described for methoxyl-compounds and not
for higher homologues. In contrast, N-dealkylation is not restricted to
demethylation and dealkylation of higher homologues is possible. The latter
has been seen e.g. with the herbicide Trifluralin in the rumen or with the
conversion of mimosine to 3,4-DHP (see below).

Dehalogenation in the rumen has been described for organic chlorine
compounds: the conversion of DDT to DDD is a familiar example. Deamination
by deaminases or dehydrogenases are other reactions possible in the rumen.

Rates of C-dehydroxylation of phenolic acids are increased with
compounds having longer side chains, thus following a trend opposite to the
one seen with decarboxylation. E.g. gallic acid or protocatechuic acid are
decarboxylated in the gut, but little dehydroxylation occurs (Fig. 4).

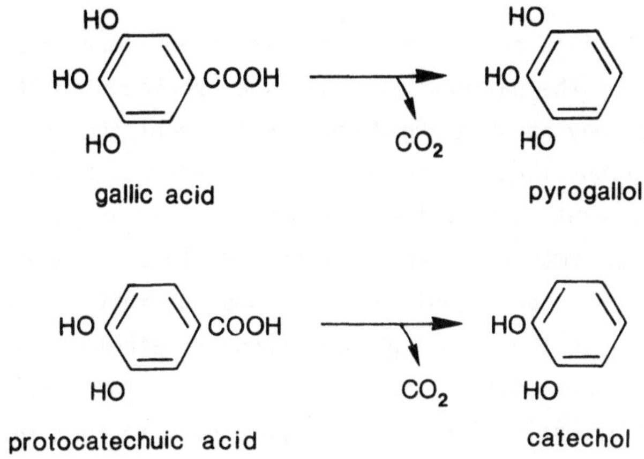

FIGURE 4. Decarboxylation of gallic acid and protocatechuic acid.

Dehydroxylation at the para position of substituted catechols seems rather specific for intestinal microbes and has been described for compounds like L-dopa and caffeic acid.

Heterocyclic ring cleavage in bioflavonoid metabolism and a very slow reductive fission of the benzene nucleus of various compounds may occur in the rumen, although the latter often will not proceed further than reduction of the ring. Coumarins can be cleaved in a reductive process.

Although little work has been devoted to compare reaction rates of metabolic transformations of foreign compounds in the rumen, it can be expected that rates of hydrolysis and reduction are relatively rapid as compared to the reactions we have designated here as fission reactions. Ring fission reactions are notably slow. Perhaps some of these are amenable to adaptation upon prolonged feeding of the compounds under feeding conditions which result in low rumen turnover rates.

III. MAIN CATEGORIES OF FOREIGN COMPOUNDS ENTERING THE RUMEN.

In the following, some discussion will be devoted to the types of compounds that may enter the rumen. A selection of these will be treated thereafter with special reference to their possible fate in the rumen and the consequences of their metabolism.

III.1. Non-intentional (accidental) intake of foreign compounds in ruminants.

III.1.1. Intake of feed contaminants (pesticides).

Numerous chemicals may inadvertantly be present as contaminants in animal feed. Pesticides are among the chemicals of importance in this respect. Studies on the pathways of pesticide breakdown in the rumen are of interest in that they have enlarged our knowledge of the types of biochemical reactions that may occur (6). The evidence available suggests that these contaminants are of little concern as far as their possible negative effect on rumen function is concerned. In some cases, however, as with the reduction of the organic nitro groups in dinitrocresol or dinitrobutylphenol to the 6-aminophenols causing methemoglobinemia and hemoconcentration, metabolism results in increased toxicity. A similar reduction of the aromatic nitro group in parathion to form the less toxic aminoparathion which is excreted by the animal is an example of detoxification. Malathion is inactivated by microbial phosphatase (16).

III.1.2. Toxic principles formed in feeds during storage (mycotoxins).

A number of compounds produced by fungi infecting pasture plants, produced by infected plants or taken in with soil may cause disorders in grazing animals. Examples of such diseases are facial eczema, annual ryegrass toxicity, ryegrass staggers, paspalum staggers and lupinosis. These ailments are discussed by Hegarty (17) and will not be dealt with in detail here, but hepatotoxic mycotoxins are among the compounds involved and include compounds like deoxynivalenol (vomitoxin), chetomin, ochratoxin A, zearalenone, aflatoxin and patulin. Not much is known of their fate in the rumen or their influence on rumen function (18), although it is to be expected that a number of mycotoxins will inhibit microbial activity (reviewed by Allison, 8) as has actually been proven for aflatoxin B1."Ovine-J11-Thrift" in Nova Scotia has been brought in connection with an inhibition of rumen function by toxic fungal products (19). One such product is chetomin, an antibiotic metabolite of the fungus *Chaetomium* sp. This compound was found to act bacteriostatically on a number of rumen bacterial strains, especially on gram-positive species. The minimal inhibitory concentration of chetomin for cellulose hydrolysis by *Ruminococcus albus* strain 7 was 20 μg/ml (20).

A recent study on the fate of six mycotoxins (21) disclosed that ochratoxin A, zearalenone, T-2 toxin and diacetoscirpenol were metabolized by mixed rumen microorganisms or suspensions of rumen bacteria or protozoa in vitro. The protozoa were most active in this respect. The following reactions were shown to take place:

ochratoxin A------------------▶ ochratoxin a + phenylalanine
         peptide hydrolysis

zearalenone------------------▶ a-zearalenol + b-zearalenol
      reduction

diacetoxyscirpenol-------------▶ monoacetoxyscirpenol
        deacylation

T-2 toxin -------------▶ HT-2 toxin
      deacylation

Two of the mycotoxins studied were not changed by incubation with rumen
microorganisms: aflatoxin B1 and deoxynivalenol. The authors discussed the
question whether the conversions found were to be considered a first line
of defense against toxic compounds present in the feed. Except for the
reduction of zearalenone, the processes led to the production of
metabolites with a lowered toxicity as compared with the parent molecules.
According to the authors, microbial metabolism would increase water
solubility of the mycotoxins, thereby lowering the toxicity of these
compounds for the microbes themselves. The increased polarity would also
facilitate excretion by the animal. Also, absorption from the
gastrointestinal tract would be changed.

    This would offset the problem of the increased biological activity of
zearalenol as compared to zearalenone (21).

III.1.3. Naturally formed toxic principles in plants (plant secondary
       compounds).

    Ruminants are able to satisfy their nutritional requirements with only
a limited number of compounds, yet plants contain a very large number of
chemical constituents which often do not seem to have a clear function in
nutrition (22). In fact, an enormous list could be made of plants known to
contain deleterious compounds. This list is still growing as new pasture
plants are found which have negative effects on herbivores.

    Another point to consider is the fact that concentrations of such
deleterious compounds (or "toxins", "poisons") can be extremely high (see
Table 2). Then, there is a great number of other compounds such as
coumarins, cardiac glycosides (digitalis e.g.), dianthrones, mustard oils,
saponins, phenols (gossypol, tannins), polypeptides, toxalbumins,

triterpenes, quinones, resins, resinoids, etc.

TABLE 2.

Maximal concentrations of some plant constituents considered toxic or of limited value for herbivores consuming these plants (from 23).

Compound	Concentration as % of dry matter	Plant name
fluoroacetate	0.1	*Gastrolobium* sp.
isoflavones	5	*Trifolium subterraneum*
mimosine	10	*Leucaena leucocephala*
oxalate	14	*Oxalis pes-caprae*
potassium nitrate	11	*Avena sativa*
sodium chloride	20	*Atriplex vesicaria*

The biological significance of toxic plant constituents, which do not play an important role in the nutrition of the plant, is not always clear, but many of them play a role in the interaction between plant and plant pathogens or between plants and their herbivorous predators. It is believed that a considerable number of the compounds act as feeding deterrents. McDonald (23) cites Culvenor, who postulated the following steps in the evolution:

(1) mutations will occur in plant species leading to the elaboration of a toxic secondary metabolite,

(2) the toxic mutant will experience reduced predation and become fitter for survival,

(3) the toxic mutant replaces the non-toxic form by the process of natural selection,

(4) as a consequence a large number of plant species have become toxic.

Direct losses of domesticated animals grazing poisonous plants in rangelands of the Western United States amount to 3-5% of the livestock and estimates of losses have been similar over the last 20 years (24). An even greater but unknown loss results from decreased production of intoxicated animals and costs of specialized management techniques to avoid poisonous plants. The secondary compounds can roughly be divided in two groups. One (the quantitative group) comprises the tannins, resins, polyphenols and silicates. These chemicals are of low toxicity and have to be present in rather large amounts to have an impact on the animal consuming the plant. The spectrum of action is broad, however, and little or no adaptation seems to be possible. Tannins are known to depress digestion. A highly significant relationship was seen between the in vitro rumen digestibility of West African pasture plants and their tannin content (25). The second (qualitative) group contains the more toxic compounds of specific action, such as the plant alkaloids or cyanogenic compounds. Adaptation and thus a successful defense by the animal is more likely to occur. Additional influences from high levels of copper or selenium in plants containing secondary plant compounds enhance the toxic action of the latter group. This is the case with the combined action of copper and hepatotoxins from *Heliotropium* species.

The circumstances leading to poisoning of domesticated ruminants often are consequences of husbandry procedures, of the loss of feed selection in these breeds or of the lack of suitable alternative feeds. Wild animals have learned to avoid the dangerous species or will use them only to a moderate extent. A very interesting observation was made by Van Hoven (26) during a study of nutritional problems in wild ruminants grazing in game farms. When plants were injured, e.g. by grazing herbivores, some quickly produced chemical defenses. The promptness and the extent with which trees (*Acacia* sp.) increased their condensed tannin contents in reaction to being browsed varied from species to species. *Acacia caffra* (sweet thorn) showed the quickest increase: about 94% in the first fifteen minutes. On average it took 50 - 100 hours to reach normal tannin levels, when plants were left undisturbed after the attack.
The behaviour of kudu antelope in the field - when free to roam about - is such that the animals graze a specific bush or tree for a limited time only before moving on. This has been brought in connection with the reported increase in tannin content. Numerous books (27,28) and reviews (29,30,31,32,33) have been published on the interactions of plant secondary compounds and wild herbivores.

III.1.4. Toxicological consequences of rumen metabolism of toxic principles
          in plants.
Inactivation, detoxification.

Examples of detoxification by the gut microflora of monogastric animals are limited in number (9). As for the rumen, a number of toxic compounds are inactivated by enzymes already present in the rumen microbiota. The hydrolysis of *Clostridum botulinum* toxin C (34), the hydrolysis of the mycotoxin ochratoxin A (35), the assumed hydrolysis of proteinaceous inhibitors of proteases such as present in leguminous seeds, the hydrolysis of mushroom toxins and plant lectins are all examples of inactivation by hydrolysis, probably followed by fermentation of the products of hydrolysis.

Digitalis is inactivated in the rumen of sheep to a varying extent (36). The alkaloids heliotrine and lasiocarpine are metabolized to non-toxic methylene derivatives by ruminal microorganisms of sheep in Australia (reviewed by Carlson and Breeze, 37) (Fig. 2).

Complete fermentation of a compound after slow adaptation of the animal to the toxic principle is another possibility of detoxication, as witnessed by the interesting oxalate story.

The Oxalate Story

This story is an example of the situation where an organism already present in the rumen, is able to increase in number when its favorite energy source is offered with the ration.

A variety of plants contain high levels ($\pm$ 5% of the dry matter) of oxalic acid or oxalate salts. For some of these plants oxalates serve as energy sources. Ingestion of the plants may be harmfull to the animal due to the removal of circulating ionized calcium and/or formation of insoluble calcium oxalate crystals causing tissue damage.

It has been shown that gradual adaptation of ruminants to increasing quantities of oxalate containing plants will allow the animals to survive without signs of toxicity (38). When sheep were changed to a diet of *Halogeton glomeratus* (halogeton) containing 12% (w/w) oxalic acid, a transition of low ($> 0.05 \; \mu mol.ml^{-1}.h^{-1}$) to high ($< 0.2 \; \mu mol.ml^{-1}.h^{-1}$) oxalate degradation rates by sheep rumen fluid was found within 3-4 days. Further tests showed that anaerobic rumen bacteria were responsible for the oxalate breakdown and that methanogenesis was "coupled" to oxalate degradation (39,40). Finally, an obligately anaerobic gram-negative oxalate-degrading bacterium was isolated (41). The organism (OxB) uses only a limited range of substrates and its numbers in the rumen are closely regulated by the oxalate supply.

Numbers of this organism in the rumina of adapted sheep were between 1 and $5 \times 10^5 g^{-1} h^{-1}$, while the oxalate degradation rates were between 0.8 and 3.3

$\mu mol.g^{-1}.h^{-1}$ (see 42 for a review). It is perhaps of interest to note that organisms similar to OxB were found by Allison and his colleagues in human faeces. It was speculated that the loss of this organism could be connected with hyperoxaluria as seen after enteric resections and -disease.

Rates of oxalate breakdown in the gut of various animal species (rabbit, guinea pig, horse, swine) were found to increase with increasing oxalate content of the diet (43). Laboratory rats did not show this phenomenon, but wild rats did harbour gastrointestinal oxalate degraders, which were able to colonize the gut of white laboratory rats (see 42).

Initial toxication followed by detoxification.

In certain cases the metabolites produced by the microflora are more toxic than the parent compound (lethal synthesis). Examples for the monogastric animal are the reduction of the food dye Brown FK to toxic polyamino compounds in the rat, the hydrolysis of the glycoside amygdalin to the cyanogenic benzaldehyde-cyanohydrin and the production of nitrosamine from nitrite and secondary amines, a reaction also occurring in the rumen. Walker (9) stresses that e.g. the hydrolysis of biliary conjugates in the lower gut frequently results in the liberation of more lipophilic (and more toxic) compounds, initiating enterohepatic cycling.

In the rumen, e.g. the breakdown of the isoflavone formononetin results in the formation of the weakly estrogenic equol, cyanides are produced from cyanogenic glycosides and 3-methylindole - the causative agent of acute lung oedema and emphysema - is formed from the amino acid tryptophan (Fig. 5).

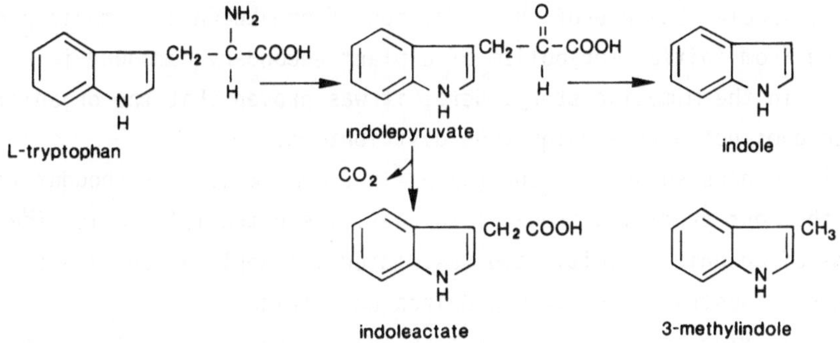

FIGURE 5. Tryptophan fermentation by ruminal bacteria leading to the formation of 3-methylindole and indole (37).

Certain of such toxic initial products can be processed further in the rumen but this often needs a period of adaptation. A microbe may be stimulated by the continuous presence of a new metabolite to use it as an energy source or as an electron acceptor. Research on the fate of miserotoxin in the rumen highlights this latter possiblity.

The Miserotoxin Story

It has been mentioned in the beginning of this review that the compound miserotoxin is the beta-glucoside of 3-nitro-1-propanol and that this compound is present in *Astragalus miser* (timber milk vetch). It is also present in many other species of *Astragalus*. In the rumen this glycoside is hydrolyzed to glucose and 3-nitro-1-propanol (NPOH) is the toxic compound. Severe respiratory distress, pelvic limb weakness, recumbency and death are symptoms commonly associated with NPOH poisoning. Majak and Cheng (44) have shown that nitrotoxins such as NPOH can be degraded by pure or mixed cultures of rumen bacteria. Diet variation can produce a sixfold difference in the in vitro rates of NPOH degradation. In their latest publication, Majak and Cheng (45) have shown that the detoxification of NPOH can be stimulated in the rumen by offering potential inducers of nitro group-reducing activity. Nitroethane supplements stimulated the rate of nitropropanol degradation. The induced activity was transferred between groups of animals in adjacent pens. Allison and Reddy (42) reviewed the rumen microbial adaptation to dietary nitrate.

The Mimosine Story

A very special example of the induction of breakdown of a toxic product resulting from initial metabolism of a plant secondary compound is presented in the mimosine story. Here, it was proven that the organism involved does not have a ubiquitous distribution.

The leguminous shrub leucaena (*Leucaena leucocephala*) is thought to be one of the most promising tropical forages. Its potential use is wide, but problems of chronic toxicity have restricted its application as a feed for ruminants in Australia, Papua New Guinea and Africa.

The unusual amino acid mimosine in both leaves and seeds (3-12% of the dry weight!) of leucaena is behind these problems, since it is converted in the rumen by ruminal microbes or by enzymes present in the leucaena leaves itself to a toxic product: 3-hydroxy-4(1H)-pyridone (3,4-DHP) (46). DHP interferes with the use of iodine by the thyroid gland and induces goitre. There follows a deficiency in thyroxine, the growth regulatory hormone. Low weight gains or weight loss, lack of appetite, esophageal ulcerations, hair loss and profuse salivation are some of the symptoms seen in cattle in northern Australia after prolonged feeding of leucaena.

The attention was drawn to the surprising observation that in other countries leucaena is fed to cattle and goats without signs of poisoning. In fact, ruminants in Hawaii were known to thrive on natural stands of leucaena at levels of about 90% of the total dry matter intake. The lack of toxicity of the leucaena in Hawaii was ascribed to the observation (47) that DHP is degraded rapidly in the rumen of the Hawaiian animals by microbes which were not present in Australian ruminants.

Mixed enrichment cultures of DHP-degrading microbes obtained from the rumen contents of goats in Hawaii were introduced into Australian ruminants and this resulted in a remarkable tolerance of the treated animals against leucaena. The microorganisms responsible for the breakdown of DHP apparently spread easy from animal to animal, once they were introduced into one animal of the herd. Persistence of the DHP-degrading microorganisms in the rumens of two steers that had not been grazing leucaena for 9 months was seen (48,49). Both by the group of Allison in Iowa and the group of Jones in Australia obligately anaerobic gram negative rods fermenting some amino acids but not mimosine or carbohydrates were isolated from the enrichments. Thus the organism ferments the DHP produced in the rumen. This case is unique, since it shows that the detoxication of DHP is carried out by a non-ubiquitous organism with a limited geographical distribution. Certain rumen protozoa are known to be limited in distribution (e.g. *Ophryoscolex* species), but so far no connection with a difference in rumen function has been demonstrated.

III.2. Foreign compounds added to feed or otherwise dosed orally.
III.2.1. Drugs used in the treatment of rumen disorders or microbial
          infections (antibiotics and chemotherapeutics).
Antibiotics

Not all antibiotic compounds act similarly on the rumen microflora. Of 12 antibiotics tested (on 11 strains of rumen bacteria in pure culture) chloramphenicol and penicillin G were most effective, but penicillin G was rapidly inactivated (50,51). Streptomycin did not inhibit the organism *Anaerovibrio lipolytica* (strain 5S). Wright (52) found that this antibiotic

had no effect on lipolytic activity of rumen contents, while penicillin
decreased lipolysis in vitro and in vivo.

Studies on the antibiotic sensitivity of rumen bacteria with no previous
history of contact with antibiotics, indicated that these were susceptible
to: bacitracin, chloramphenicol, erythromycin, novobiocin, oleandomycin,
oxytetracycline, penicillin, tetracycline, tylosin and vancomycin (53,50,
51). Quite a number of species were not inhibited by kanamycin, neomycin,
streptomycin and polymyxin.

The selective action of antibiotics is shown in the work of Cafantaris
(54). Salinomycin, flavomycin and avoparcin stimulated in vitro breakdown
of starch by mixed rumen microorganisms. Effects on breakdown of cellulose
were quite different: salinomycin was inhibitory, flavomycin was
stimulatory, while avoparcin had no effect. Salinomycin decreased acetate
percentage, while flavomycin increased it and avoparcin increased
propionate and butyrate. In vivo results were not studied and these might
be different again.

Several antibiotics which are effective in inhibiting in vitro rumen
cellulolysis (Table 3) can be assumed to damage the rumen ecosystem. These
include penicillin, oxytetracycline, ampicillin, erythromycin, methicillin
and oleandomycin.

TABLE 3

Effect of some antibiotics on in vitro rumen cellulose breakdown (from 55).

Antibiotics	Amount 2) µg/20 ml	Cellulose breakdown 1) %
Colistin	50	100
Kanamycin	5	100
Neomycin	10	100
Streptomycin	10	100
Chloramphenicol	10	91
Cloxacillin	5	67
Fusidicacid	10	83
Novobioxin	5	44
Penicillin G	1.5	35
Oxytetracycline	10	5
Ampicillin	2	0
Erythromycin	10	0
Methicillin	10	0
Oleandomycin	5	0

1) Cellulose digestion as % of the controls.
2) Penicillin G is in "units" per 20 ml.

Treatment of rumen disorders with antibiotics or chemotherapeutics has been advocated from time to time. Penicillin has been suggested for the treatment of bloat. Thiopeptin has been found effective against lactic acidosis (56) as were lasalocid and monensin (57). Monensin and other ionophore antibiotics may be of value in the prevention of amino acid decarboxylation, thus e.g. interfering with the genesis of 3-methyl indole from tryptophan. Such treatments may serve some purpose in cases of acute bloat, rumen lactic acidosis or emphysema, but the digestive upsets and the massive destruction of the rumen microflora result in appetence and a reduced ruminal motility. Animals may be unthrifty for weeks after such a treatment. Diarrhea may follow.

Oral application of penicillin (400.000 IU), streptomycin (0.5-1.0 g daily), chloramphenicol (0.25-0.5 g), terramycin (0.5 g) or aureomycin (0.8 g) severely depressed rumen function in sheep (58).

Time of addition of antibiotics in relation to feeding will influence the outcome. When rumen microorganisms were exposed to antibiotics prior to receiving substrate, inhibition of microbial fermentation is more pronounced then when substrate and antibiotics are added simultaneously (59).

Chemotherapeutics

It was mentioned before that chloramphenicol is reduced in the rumen to the amino derivative as are many compounds containing nitro-groups. This is strongly related to the stage of microbial development of the rumen (60, 61). Chloramphenicol administered orally to adult ruminants is not absorbed (62).

The protozoa are thought to be responsible for the transformation but other organisms already present in the first stages of microbial colonization of the rumen are capable of this reduction too.

Trimethoprim (63) is broken down to less active metabolites in rumen fluid of calves with developing rumina. Products were not studied, but demethylation seems a probable reaction. The breakdown is age-dependent in calves. Sulfamerazine is inactivated in the rumen (64). A glance at the formula of sulfamerazine suggests hydrolysis is a possible rumen reaction followed by reduction of the sulfoxide group. Sulfamerazine was not very active against cellulolytic bacteria in 20-hr in vitro incubations with rumen fluid inocula (55; Table 4).

TABLE 4

Effect of some sulphonamides on in vitro rumen cellulose breakdown
(from 55).

Sulfonamide 1)	Cellulose breakdown 2) %
sulfisomidine	89
sulfisoxazole	89
sulfamerazine	87
sulfamethoxypyridazine	84
sulfadiazine	74
sulfathiazole	41
sulfamethylthiadiazole	21

1) Dosed at 150 µg/20 ml
2) See Table 3.

For the treatment of coccidiosis and gastrointestinal infections the
sulphonamides sulfaguadin and sulfamidin can be administered orally in a
dose of 0.1 kg/kg body weight to fully-grown ruminants for a period of up
to 5 days without endangering rumen function. It must be added, however,
that the test used to prove this were very simple and inadequate (65).

Both antibiotics and sulfonamides can be excreted through the rumen wall
or the salivary glands after being administered intravenously. In addition
to direct analysis this can be demonstrated by the inhibition of the
methylene blue reduction test (66) or the (slight) inhibition of cellulose
breakdown (67). This should be kept in mind when these drugs are injected
(68).

Other compounds

Against ketonaemia certain chemicals are dosed orally to ruminants in
veterinary practice. Among these are chloral hydrate, potassium chlorate
and propylene glycol. Chloral hydrate is decomposed to chloroform, a
structure analogue of methane which is inhibitory to methanogenesis and
increases propionate production on the rumen. Propionate in turn serves as
a glucose precursor and the extra glucose produced restores the balance
between glucose needed for milk production and glucose formed in the body,
at least for some time. This then restores appetite in diseased cattle.

Propylene glycol serves as a direct glucose precursor in the tissues of the ruminant.

Several surface active agents have been tested for the treatment of bloat. These may severely affect the microbes in the rumen (e.g. see 69).

III.2.2. Additives used to improve animal production by manipulating the rumen fermentation (feed additives)

A number of drugs are in use as feed additives in order to increase beef cattle production. Especially some ionophore antibiotics (monensin, lasalocid, narasin) are advocated as suitable agents for an increased retention of feed energy in the animal. In general this is achieved by a manipulation of the fermentation leading to lower rates of methane production and increase rates of propionate production. These compounds will not be discussed here as they are the subject of another presentation in this book.   It   must be mentioned here that microbial adaptation is thought to occur with these drugs when administered over a long time. Earlier attempts to modify the rumen microbial fermentation by halogenated compounds (methane analogues and derivatives) failed, among other reasons because of microbial adaptation (6).

Now, even to ionophores, which specifically transport certain ions across the bacterial cell membrane partial adaptation has been found (70). The underlying adaptation mechanisms are not known.

III.2.3. Drugs in veterinary practice aimed at the treatment of non-rumen disorders.

A limited number of drugs is added orally to ruminants in the treatment of non-rumen disorders. Anthelmintics are the main group to be considered here. Certain anthelmintics were found to be less active when added orally, while other anthelmintics were found to need rumen metabolism for activation.

III.2.4. Nutritional and pharmacological consequences of drug-microbe interactions in the rumen.

Our knowledge of the pharmacological consequences of oral dosing of drugs to ruminants is limited. The need for a more systematic approach in this field was stressed by Dunlop (71) and Koritz (72). Only in a handful of experiments have the main factors been studied which determine the final

outcome of the oral or intraruminal administration of drugs. Most often
speculations are offered in the discussion portion of scientific papers
which deal with the possibility of rumen bypass or microbial degradation
of a drug. Even worse is the situation with respect to diseased ruminants.
Very few studies on the effectiveness of orally dosed drugs in ruminants
have dealt with diseased animals, although it is known that these may
display strongly altered rumen characteristics.

The main considerations regarding the consequences of oral drug
administration can be grouped in two categories. The first group comprises
the effects of the forestomachs on the drug and its bioavailability. This
would include the role of the rumen as a slow mixing reservoir, diluting
the drug and retarding its passage along the gastrointestinal tract. Also
would be included the microbial drug transformation processes in the rumen.
A second group of considerations involves the effects of the drug or its
rumen metabolites on the functioning of the rumen itself, whether this
occurs by influencing the microbes or by affecting processes such as feed
intake, rumen motility, etc.

The rumen as a slow mixing reservoir

The form in which a drug is administered is of great importance. When
given in liquid form, a disproportionate amount of the drug may pass
through the reticulo-omasal orifice before retention in the reticulo-rumen
can occur. Dilution in the rumen, delay in transport of the drug down the
alimentary tract and microbial influences are largely prevented in such a
case. When closure of the oesophageal groove can be induced, this bypass
will be maximized. This may not always be desirable. For instance, if
anthelmintics are passed rapidly through the gut, worms are exposed for a
shorter time to the therapeutic compounds.

Drugs added in solid form can be lodged in the ventral regions of reticulum
or rumen when the density of the material (pellet, bolus) is high enough.
Slow-release intraruminal devices have been developed for all sorts of
applications.

A point to remember is the possibility of a depressed rumen motility in
diseased animals. Dunlop (71) stresses the need to verify that no
irritation of the static reticulo-rumen wall occurs upon drug
administration in solid form.

The physico-chemical nature of the drug is of importance. Lipophilic drugs will be absorbed directly from the rumen to a large extent. With ionized compounds the rate of absorption is a function of the concentration of the unionized form of the compound. The latter is influenced by the concentration of the drug, the pKa of the drug and the pH of the rumen fluid.Hydrophilic compounds, especially when these are weak bases, may be absorbed to a small extent only. Rumen pH values in intensively fed cattle fluctuate over a range of 2 pH-units, which would cause a 100-fold variation in the degree of ionization of the compounds and therefore feeding practice and time of application in relation to feeding time are very important in determining bioavailability. Dobson (73) has formulated the principles underlying the partitioning of acidic and basic drugs between plasma, rumen and saliva (see also 71). Turnover rates of rumen contents are influenced by feeding practice (feed intake parameters: quality and quantity of the ration, time of feeding, frequency) and motility of the rumen. Outflow rates differ between ruminant species as a result of considerations of energetics and body size. In cattle fed high rations, fractional outflow rates of liquid may be as high as 0.25 h-1, indicating a 4 h - turnover time. Solids outflow rates are much lower, turnover times may range from 12-24 h or more. In diseased ruminants outflow rates may be extremely low. Microbial drug transformation rates will be influenced by rumen microbial species composition and the degree of adaptation to the compound as well as by the chemical nature of the drug. Species composition is a function again of animal and feed characteristics. The main metabolic transformations were discussed in the preceeding pages of this chapter.

Effects of the drug on the rumen functions

Drugs may have an effect on feed intake, mostly in a negative sense by depressing motility or by inhibiting microbial species. A direct effect on rumen motility is another possibility. All of these processes will influence a number of the factors discussed earlier. In this way interactions between host animal, microbes and drugs become extremely complicated and difficult to predict. As we have concluded before, it is time that a systematic knowledge is built up with regard to the factors that determine bioavailability of drugs in ruminants after oral application. Marker studies, in vitro rumen experiments and sampling of body and gut compartments should accompany in vivo evaluations of oral drug bioavailability in ruminants.

REFERENCES

1. Baldwin, R.L. and Allison, M.J.: J. Anim. Sci. 57 (Suppl 2): 461-477
   (1983).
2. Hungate, R.E.: The rumen and its microbes. Academic Press, New York
   and London, 533 pp. (1966).
3. Hungate, R.E.: Indian J. Vet. Med. 1: 1-20 (1981).
4. Scheline, R.R.: Pharmacol. Rev. 25: 451-523 (1973).
5. Drasar, R.S. and Hill, M.J.: Human intestinal flora. Academic Press,
   London, New York and San Francisco, 263 pp. (1974).
6. Prins, R.A.: In: Nutrition and Drug interrelations. J.N. Hatcock and
   J.M. Coon (eds.), pp. 189-251 (1977).
7. Scheline, R.R.: Acta Pharmacol. Toxicol. 26: 189-205 (1968).
8. Allison, M.J.: In: Effects of poisonous plants on livestock. R.F.
   Keeler, K.R. van Kampen and L.F. James (eds.), Academic Press, Inc.
   New York, San Fransisco and London, pp. 101-118 (1978).
9. Walker, R.: Proc. Nutr. Soc. 32: 73-78 (1973).
10. Goldman, P., Peppercorn, M.A. and Goldin, B.R.: Amer. J. Clin. Nutr.
    278: 1348-1355 (1974).
11. Shull, L.R., Buckmaster, G.W. and Cheeke, P.R.: J. Anim. Sci. 43:
    1247-1253 (1976).
12. Cheeke, P.R.: Can. J. Anim. Sci. 64: 201-202 (1984).
13. King, R.R. and McQueen, R.E.: J. Agr. Food Chem. 29: 1101-1103 (1981).
14. Chung, K.T., Fulk, G.E. and Egan, M.: Appl. Environm. Microbiol. 35:
    558-562 (1978).
15. Ivie, G.W.: Science 191: 959-961 (1976).
16. O'Brien, R.D., Dauterman, W.C. and Niedermeier, R.P.: J. Agr. Food
    Chem. 9: 39-42 (1961).
17. Hegarty, M.P.: In: Nutritional limits to animal production from
    pastures. J.B. Hacker (ed.), Commonwealth Agricultural Bureaux,
    Farnham House, U.K., pp. 133-150 (1982).
18. Mertens, D.R.: In: Interactions of mycotoxins in animal production.
    Proc. Symp. Michigan State Univ., Nat. Acad. of Sciences, Washington,
    pp. 118-136 (1979).
19. Brewer, D., Duncan, J.M., Jerram, W.A., Leach, C.K., Safe, S., Taylor,
    A., Vincing, L.C., Archibald, R.M., Stevenson, R.G., Mirocha, C.J. and
    Christensen, M.: Can. J. Micribiol. 18: 1129-1137 (1972).

20. Jen, W.C. and Jones, G.A.: Can. J. Microbiol. 29: 1399-1404 (1983).
21. Kiessling, K.H., Petterson, H., Sandholm, K. and Olsen, M.: Appl. Environm. Microbiol. 47: 1070-1073 (1984).
22. Butler, G.W. and Bailey, R.Q.: Chemistry and Biochemistry of Herbage. Academic Press, London, San Fransisco, New York (1973).
23. McDonald, I.W.: In: Grazing Animals, F.H.W. Morley (ed.), World Animals Science B1. Ch. 19: 349-360 (1981).
24. James, L.F., Keeler, R.F., Johnson, A.E., Williams, M.C., Cronin, E.H. and Olsen, J.D.: USDA, Agr. Inf. Bull. 415, 90 pp. USDA, SEA, Poisonous Plant Research La. Logan, Utah (1980).
25. Diagagayete, M. and Huss, W.: Anim. Res. Development 16: 79-90 (1982).
26. Hoven, W. van: Custos 13: 11-16 (1984).
27. Rosenthal, G.A. and Janzen, D.H.: Herbivores: their Interaction with Secondary Plant Metabolites. Academic Press, Inc., New York, San Francisco and London, p. 718 (1979).
28. Crawley, M.J.: Herbivory: the Dynamics of Animal-Plant Interactions. Blackwell Sci. Publ., London, 448 pp. (1983).
29. Bryant, J.P. and Kuropat, P.J.: Ann. Rev. Ecol. Syst. 11: 261-265 (1980).
30. Labov, J.B.: Comp. Biochem. Physiol. 57A: 3-9 (1977).
31. Levin, D.A.: Ann. Rev. Ecol. Syst. 7: 121-159 (1976).
32. Janzen, D.H.: In: The Ecology of Arboreal Foliovores. G.G. Montgomery (ed.), Smithsonian Institution Press, Washington, D.C. (1978).
33. Freeland, W.J. and Janzen, D.H.: Am. Naturalist 108: 269-299 (1974).
34. Allison, M.J., Maloy, S.E. and Matson, R.R.: Appl. Environm. Microbiol. 32: 685-688 (1976).
35. Galtier, P. and Alvinerie, M.: Ann. Rech. Vet. 7: 91-98 (1976).
36. Westermarck, H.: Acta Vet. Scand. 1: 67-72 (1959).
37. Carlson, J.R. and Breeze, R.G.: J. Animal Sci. 58: 1040-1049 (1984).
38. Allison, M.J., Littledike, E.T. and James, L.F.: J. Animal Sci. 45: 1173-1179 (1977).
39. Allison, M.J., Cook, H.M. and Dawson, K.A.: J. Animal Sci. 53: 810-816 (1981).
40. Dawson, K.A., Allison, M.J. and Hartman, P.A.: Appl. Environm. Microbiol. 40: 840-846 (1980).
41. Dawson, K.A., Allison, M.J. and Hartman, P.A.: Appl. Environm. Microbiol. 40: 833-846 (1980).

42. Allison, M.J. and Reddy, C.A.: In: Current Perspectives in Microbial Ecology, M.J. Klug and C.A. Reddy (eds.), Proc. 3rd Int. Symp. Microbial Ecol., pp. 248-256 (1984).
43. Allison, M.J. and Cook, H.M.: Science 212: 675-676 (1981).
44. Majak, W. and Cheng, K.J.: Can. J. Microbiol. 27: 646-650 (1981).
45. Majak, W. and Cheng, K.J.: Can. J. Animal Sci. 64: 33-34 (1984).
46. Hegarty, M.P., Lee, C.P., Christie, G.S., Court, R.D. and Haydock, K.P.: Austr. J. Biol. Sci. 32: 27-40 (1979).
47. Jones, R.J.: Austr. Vet. J. 57: 55-56 (1981).
48. Jones, R.J. and Lowry, J.B.: Experientia 4: (in press) (1984).
49. Ralph, W.: Rural Res. 123 (1984).
50. El-Akkad, I. and Hobson, P.N.: Nature 209: 1044-1047 (1968).
51. El-Akkad, I. and Hobson, P.N.: Zentralbl. Vet. Med. A 13: 700-708 (1966).
52. Wright, D.E.: New Zeal. J. Agr. Res. 4: 216-233 (1961).
53. Fulghum, R.S., Baldwin, B.B. and Williams, P.P.: Appl. Microbiol. 16: 301-307 (1968).
54. Cafantaris, B.: Ph.D. Thesis, Universitaet Hohenheim, Stuttgart, 141 pp. (1981).
55. Prins, R.A.: Brit. Vet. J. 125: xviii-xx (1969).
56. Muir, L.A., Duquette, P.F., Rickes, E.L. and Smith, G.E.: J. Animal Sci. 51: 1182-1188 (1980).
57. Nagaraja, T.G., Avery, T.B., Bartley, E.E., Roof, S.K. and Dayton, A.D.: J. Animal Sci. 54: 649-658 (1982).
58. Nesic, P. and Ibrovic, M.: Veterinaria 12: 39-44 (1963).
59. Klopfenstein, T.J., Purser, D.B. and Tyznik, W.J.: J. Animal Sci. 23: 126-131 (1964).
60. De Backer, P. and Debackere, M.: J. Vet. Pharmacol. Therap. 2: 195-202 (1979).
61. De Backer, P., Debackere, M. and De Corte-Baeten, K.: J. Vet. Pharmacol. Therap. 1: 135-140 (1978).
62. De Corte-Baeten, K.: J. Vet. Pharmacol. Therap. 1: 129-134 (1978).
63. Nielsen, P., Romvary, A. and Rasmussen, F.: J. Vet. Pharmacol. Therap. 1: 37-46 (1978).
64. De Backer, P., Belpaire, F.M., Bogaert, M.G. and Debackere, M.: Amer. J. Vet. Res. 43: 1744-1751 (1982).
65. Nesic, P. and Ibrovic: Berl. Muench. Tieraerztl. Wochschr. 73: 403-407 (1962).

66. Behravesh, S., Wolstrup, J. and Dirch Poulsen, J.S.: Proc. XIIth World Congr. Diseases of Cattle 2: 1118-1121 (1982).

67. Atef, M., Salem, A.A., Al-Samarrae, S.A. and Zafer, S.E.: Zentralbl. Vet. Med. A28: 113-121 (1981).

68. Jenkins, W.L., Davis, L.E. and Boulos, B.M.: Amer. J. Vet. Res. 36: 1771-1776 (1975).

69. Burggraaf, W. and Leng, R.A.: New Zeal. J. Agr. Res. 23: 287-291 (1980).

70. Mackie, R.I., Bahrs, P.G. and Therion, J.J.: Can. J. Animal Sci. 64: 351-353 (1984).

71. Dunlop, R.H.: In: Veterinary Pharmacology and Toxicology. Y. Ruckebusch, P.L. Toutain and G.D. Koritz (eds.), MTP-Press, Lancaster, United Kingdom, pp. 165-181 (1983).

72. Koritz, G.D.: In: Veterinary Pharmacology and Toxicology. Y. Ruckebusch, P.L. Toutain and G.D. Koritz (eds.), pp. 151-163 (1983).

73. Dobson, A.: Fed. Proc. 26: 994-1000 (1967).

9. CHEMICAL MANIPULATION OF RUMEN METABOLISM.

D.I. DEMEYER AND C.J. van NEVEL

I. INTRODUCTION

Ruminant feed is exposed to fermentative digestion by the rumen microbial population before hydrolytic digestion by animal enzymes can occur. Total digestion may be optimized by adjusting the proportion of feed fermented in the rumen to that escaping fermentation and hydrolyzed by animal enzymes. Essentially, feed components that can be hydrolyzed in the animal (true protein, starch) should be protected from rumen fermentation whereas components not available to animal enzymes (plant cell walls and non-protein N) should be brought into an optimal fermentation.It should be realized however that optimal fermentation of the latter components may require fermentation of the former for provision of energy (e.g. starch with urea) or growth factors (e.g. branched chain fatty acids with crude fibre).

Fermentation by mixed rumen microbes can be described as an anaerobic oxydation of mainly carbohydrate, protein and glycerol to acetate, CO_2 and NH_3 involving electron transfer in methane, propionate and butyrate as reduced end products. Energy (ATP) generated during oxydation is mainly

228

derived from substrate linked phosphorylation (SLP) but also from anaerobic electron- and proton transport (ETP). ATP generation is coupled to synthesis of microbial matter to a variable extent when supply of N or other growth factors is not limiting. Energy yield is reflected in microbial growth yield (E) measured e.g. as g of microbial N formed per kg of organic matter fermented (apparently digested) in the rumen (E = g Ni/kg OM_f). Maximal energy yield may be with maximal SLP, involving interspecies hydrogen transfer and methanogenesis (75). At higher rates of fermentation however electron transfer is shifted from methane to propionate without apparent lowering of E (1,2).

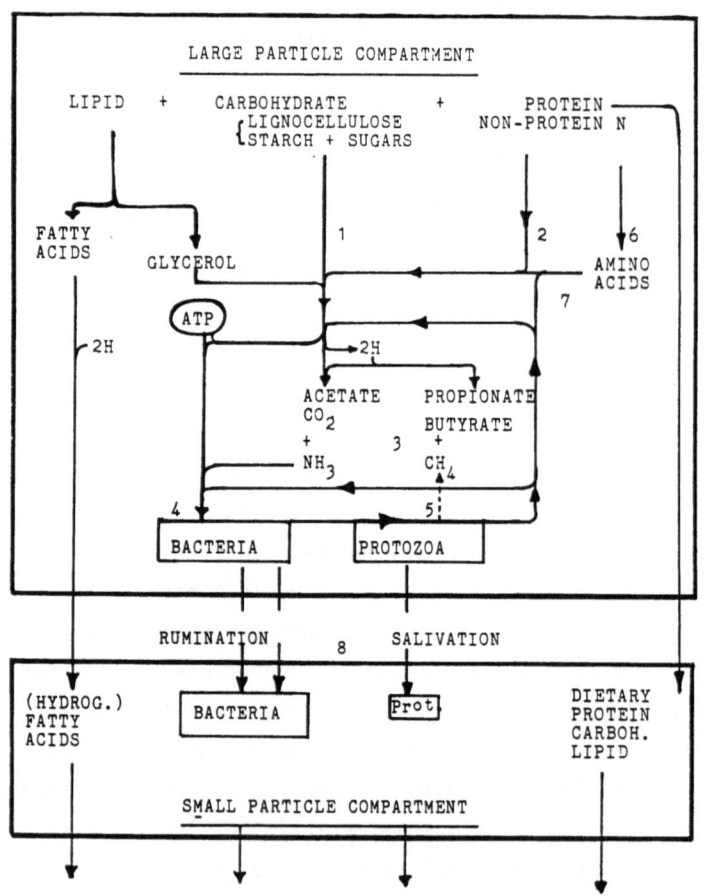

FIGURE 1. Fermentation, predation and compartmentation in the rumen microbial system. Figures indicate possible sites for manipulation.

The relative proportions of reduced end products (fermentation pattern) and E characterize fermentation but are not only related to pathways of hydrogen transfer and energy yield in fermentation. Indeed, recently the importance of compartmentation and differential rumen particle outflow (3) and of protozoal retention and predation (4) for E has been recognized. Figure 1 summarizes some aspects and interactions in the rumen microbial system of fermentation, predation and compartmentation. Some sites for possible manipulation (optimisation, modulation) are indicated.

II. SITES FOR OPTIMISATION OF FERMENTATION.

1. Feed carbohydrates can be treated to increase rate and extent of rumen degradation. Alkali treatment of low quality roughage (5) and processing of grain (6) are good examples of dietary interventions.
2. Regulation of ammonia release from non protein N sources to synchronize release with carbohydrate fermentation. The introduction of glycosylureides (7) and inhibition of urease activity (8) belong to this category.
3. Optimisation of fermentation by alteration of fermentation pattern. Up to 10% of dietary gross energy may be lost as methane and considerable efforts have been directed towards inhibition of methanogenesis (1,9). It was soon observed that such inhibition shifts electron transfer to propionate as alternative electron sink in fermentation (10) providing more energy, and carbon in the volatile fatty acids available to the animal (11). The use of buffers may prevent excessive acidulation and lactate production and shift fermentation to acetate (12).
4. Yield of microbial protein (E) may be increased by addition of limiting microbial nutrients to the diet. Use of nicotinic acid, branched chain fatty acids and protein (13) can be cited as examples here.
5. Yield of microbial protein (E) may be increased by defaunation omitting recycling of microbial N due to protozoal retention and/or predation (14,15).

III. SITES FOR PROTECTION AGAINST FERMENTATION

1. Hydrolysis of feed proteins to amino acids (proteolysis) may be inhibited, protecting amino acids from further fermentation. Treatment of feed proteins by heat, aldehyde and tannins, encapsulation of proteins and amino acids and the use of amino acid analogues can be

cited here (16,17) as well as the potential use of metal ions and chemicals inhibiting rumen proteases (18,19).

2. Inhibition of amino acid deamination and fermentation by chemicals such as diaryliodonium compounds (20), hydrazine, sodium arsenite and thymol (21) can be considered.

TABLE 1.

Chemical agents that adjust fermentative digestion (ref.22)

Ionophores	Herbicides and Insecticides
Monensin	Cotoran
Lasalocid	Dalapon
Salinomycin	2,4-D
ICI 139603	M_{15}
Laidlomycin	DDT
Narasin	Ronnel
Polyether A	Others
Halogen-containing	Nonylphenol ethoxylate
Methane analogues	Buquinolate
Alcohols	Hydroxamates
Aldehydes	$Na^+, K^+, Co^+, Zn^+, Fe^{2+}, Cu^{2+}$
Acids	Long-chain fatty acids
Esters	Reducing dyes
Amicloral	Fumarate
Benzol-1,3 dioxins	Sulphate, Sulphite
Antibiotics	Nitrate, Nitrite
Avoparcin	Antipain
Thiopeptin	Leupeptin
Actaplanin	Pepstatin
Capreomycin disulphate	Chymostatin
Oxamycin	Merthiolate
Diaryliodonium	Iodoacetate
Diphenyliodonium chloride	p-Chloromercuric benzoate
Diphenyliodonium bromide	PMSF
4,4'-dimethyldiphenyliodonium chloride	Dithiothreitol
4,4'-difluorodiphenyliodonium chloride	Trypsin inhibitors
	Orotic acid

Many of the examples cited above involve the use of chemicals (drugs, antibiotics, etc.) as single repeated doses or, more often, sustained at relatively low concentrations (ppm) in the diet. In an excellent review, Chalupa (22) has listed most of the compounds used to manipulate rumen fermentation (Table 1) whereas some of them have also been discussed by Prins (23), Durand (24), Demeyer & van Nevel (1) and van Nevel & Demeyer (25).

IV. POSSIBLE EFFECTS OF CHEMICALS ON INTERACTIONS IN RUMEN METABOLISM.

Most of the compounds listed in table 1 were studied initially in short-time incubations of rumen contents *in vitro* obtained from adapted or unadapted animals and the effects observed may only partly relate to long-term effects observed *in vivo*. Such discrepancies may be due to differences in rumen microbial resistance to the compounds but also to disturbances of the balance between the many interacting and integrated processes in the rumen ecosystem. Some of these interactions can be observed *in vitro*, others can only be apparent *in vivo*.
Our earlier work on chemical manipulation of rumen metabolism (1,14,26-29) made us realize the nature and importance of such interactions. They can be predicted from present knowledge of rumen microbial metabolism and it seems appropriate to list them here as a check list for possible effects of chemicals on rumen metabolism:

Interactions in vitro:
1. Extents of protein and carbohydrate fermentation.
   Rumen protein degradation varies with diet and is enhanced by roughage feeding (30) whereas proteolytic rumen micro-organisms ferment carbo-hydrate (16,31). It can therefore be expected that inhibition of protein degradation will affect lignocellulose and/or carbohydrate fermentation.
2. Methanogenesis and extent of fibre and protein fermentation.
   Compounds shifting hydrogen transfer from methane to propionate (methane analogues,ionophores) may be expected to lower lignocellulose fermentation because of the removal of methanogenesis as supporting process for optimal fibre degradation by maximal ATP yield. As fibre degradation is linked to protein degradation, the latter may also be affected.
3. Methanogenesis and yield of microbial N.

Inhibition of methanogenesis may lower E because of lowered SLP in fermentation.

4. The presence of protozoa, methanogenesis, microbial N yield and extent of fermentation.

It is known that methane bacteria may be associated with protozoa (32,33; dotted line in Fig.1) whereas the presence of protozoa lowers microbial N yield (14). Removal of protozoa may therefore lower methanogenesis and vice versa with opposite effects of both actions on microbial N yield. As protozoa may be involved in physical plant cell wall degradation, their removal as well as inhibition of methanogenesis may impaire fibre and protein degradation (4).

Interactions in vivo.

Besides interactions measurable *in vitro,* effects observed *in vivo* may reflect changes in compartmentation and differential fractional rumen outflow. Decreases in extent of fermentation (apparent digestion in the rumen) may decrease intake and increase rumen retention. The use of buffers may increase fractional rumen liquid outflow rate and thus affect microbial N yield. Removal of protozoa may affect particle retention. Also, it is evident that interactions of compounds with animal physiology beyond the rumen are to be considered. According to Owens et al (34) e.g. as much as 50% of ionophores may be absorbed from the gastro-intestinal tract and rapidly re-excreted via the bile, exposing liver cellular mineral metabolism to ionophores. Significant changes in rumen and serum mineral concentrations have been observed after dosing with monensin (35).

The interactions discussed suggest that many chemical compounds may have similar effects on rumen metabolism, as indeed summarized by Chalupa (22; Table 2) although the relative magnitude of the effects is often different. The further discussion will be confined to three groups of compounds our laboratory has gained some experience with over the past years: halogenated compounds, antibiotics including ionophores and higher fatty acids. In a final paragraph, effects of some compounds on animal performance will be summarized.

TABLE 2

Effects of types of chemical agents on rumen digestion and fermentation in vitro (ref. 22).

	Ionophores	Halogen-containing	Chemical type Diaryl iodonium	Avoparcin
Fermentation				
Methane	-	-	-	-
Hydrogen	0	+	0	0
Acetate	-	-	-	-
Propionate	+	+	+	+
Butyrate	-	+	+	0
Lactate	-	?	?	?
Digestion				
Organic matter	-	0	?	?
Protein	-	?	?	?
Amino acids	-	-	-	-
Cellulose	-	?	?	?
Starch	0	?	?	?
Micro-organisms				
Total yield	-	0	?	?
Growth efficiency	-	0	?	?

V. EFFECTS OF HALOGENATED COMPOUNDS

The inverse relationship between methanogenesis and propionate production in the rumen (10) suggested methane inhibitory properties of chloral hydrate, a propionate enhancing therapeutic against ketosis. Such inhibition was soon confirmed (27) and is probably related to formation in the rumen of the active compound $CHCl_3$ (25). It was shown that halogenated compounds are directly toxic for methane bacteria (36) probably acting through interference with co-enzymes active in methyl transfer (37,38). Related compounds such as a hemiacetal of chloral and starch (amichloral or HCS) (25) and, more recently, trichloroethyl adipate (39,40) and halogenated-1,3-dioxins (41,42) were developed. All compounds shift methane to propionate production in the rumen with concomittant production of H_2. In line with the expected effects on metabolic interactions, extents of carbohydrate and amino acid utilisation in vitro were often depressed

(26,43,44). Inhibition of substrate utilisation was more outspoken with a low than with a high concentrate diet using HCS (43), whereas ICI 111075 did not inhibit utilisation of a mixed diet *in vitro* (Table 3) in contrast to monensin (41).

TABLE 3

Percent change in fermentation end products by addition of methane analogues to incubations of rumen contents.

Reference[1]	(1)	(2)	(3)	(4)	(5)
Inhibitor	HCS[2]	ICI 111075	$CHCl_3$	HCS	CH[2]
Substrate	Sugars	hay + conc.	A.acids	hay+conc. (A.acids)	Sugars
Substrate fermented[3]	- 5	+ 31	- 5	- 10(-40)[6]	+ 18
End products					
Acetate	- 2	- 13	- 17	- 36	- 3
Propionate	+ 3	+ 66	+ 37	+ 25	+ 13
Butyrate	- 11	- 20	+ 14	+ 27	- 13
Methane	- 100	- 86	- 98	- 81	- 62
Microbial N yield[5]					
Total	-	-	-	-	- 12
Net	-	- 10	-	-	- 15

References (1) Marty & Demeyer (26) (2) Stanier & Davies (41)
(3) Russell & Martin (44) (4) Chalupa et al. (43) (5) Van Nevel & Demeyer (29).

[2]HCS = amicloral, CH = chloralhydrate

[3]Calculated from volatile fatty acids produced Marty & Demeyer (26).

[4]Per unit substrate fermented

[5]g N_i / kg OM_f

[6]( ) = = % inhibition of A. Acid utilisation

Microbial N yield was decreased *in vitro* (Table 3) possibly because of an impairment of SLP. Chloralhydrate lowered total microbial N yield *in vitro* (29) in contrast to linseed oil hydrolysate. The lack of effect of the latter methane inhibitor was probably related to its toxicity for protozoa, resulting in less turn-over of microbial N as indicated by a similar inhibitory action of both compounds in the absence of protozoa (29). In line with these findings Mathers & Miller (45) in a model experiment *in vivo* found no change in total duodenal N flow but suggest an increase in dietary N flow and a decrease in microbial N flow following chloralhydrate addition. Total and rumen O.M digestibility were little affected by the additive. Effects of these additives on rumen fractional outflow rates and protozoa have not been investigated. Animal performance tests with non-volatile halogenated compounds have shown lack of response possibly by flora adaptation to the compounds (46,47). Table 4 shows some recent data on animal performance, illustrating that favourable effects can only be expected with high roughage diets, normally associated with significant methane production, although dietary protein protection may be involved, whereas past of the energy gain from methane inhibition may be lost as hydrogen. A positive response on high roughage diets, in contrast to monensin (Table 6) indicates that rumen fibre degradation may not be significantly impaired.

TABLE 4

Effect of halogenated methane analogues on cattle performance.

Reference	Inhibitor	Dose	Period (days)	Diet	Intake[4]	Gain (kg/d)	FCR[5]
(1)	-	-	84	80% conc.	12.3	1.40	8.84
	Amicloral	0.2[1]	84	75% lucern	4.2	1.35	8.31
		0.1-0.3[2]	84		10.4	1.10	9.86
(2)	-	-	112	60% barley	9.50	1.31	9.50
	Amicloral	0.15[1]	112	36% lucern	8.84	1.34	8.84
(3)	-	-	196	2.5 kg conc.	7.27	0.89	8.19
	ICI 13409	3[3]	196	hay ad. lib.	7.25	0.93	7.77
		6[3]	196		6.88*	0.96*	7.17*

References (1) Cole & McCroskey (50)   (2) Horton (51)   (3) Davies et al. (42)

[1]% of diet   [2] % of diet, increasing with 28 day intervals
[3]mg/kg body wt.   [4] kg/day   [5] Feed conversion ratio (kg feed/kg gain)
*Significantly different from control p < 0.05 at least.

VI. EFFECTS OF ANTIBIOTICS, INCLUDING IONOPHORES
VI.1. Ionophores

Since the original publication of the effects of monensin (Eli Lilly) on rumen fermentation and cattle performance in 1976, more than 150 articles on such effects have been published. A complete survey of this work is not intended here as recent specialized reviews are available (48,22). We will try to summarize known effects briefly and refer to own work and some representative papers only. Monensin is a carboxylic polyether antibiotic and an ionophore, meaning that it carries cations through lipoprotein membranes. There are at least 76 known polyether ionophores (22) but besides monensin, only lasalocid and salinomycin have been tested in ruminants to some extent (24). Monensin increases propionate production (not always) in the rumen from carbohydrate both *in vitro* and *in vivo* with a concomittant decrease in methanogenesis and acetate and/or butyrate production. No direct effect on methane bacteria is involved, in contrast to halogenated methane analogues (28). A toxic effect on ruminococci - like H_2 producing bacteria (or hydrogenases) with a selection towards succinate producing and utilizing bacteria in the mixed flora seems to be the main mechanism of action (49).

TABLE 5

Effect of monensin on rumen OM digestibility, duodenal N flow and rumen microbial N yield.

Refe-rence	Monensin	Diet	ADOMR[2]	Duodenal N flow(g/d) NAN[3]	Microb. N	Feed N	gNi/kgOM$_f$
(1)	0	90% whole	0.36	75	45	30	16.1
	33ppm(31)[1]	shelled corn	0.29	73	39*	34	14.7
(2)	0	ground corn	0.58	140	70	71	19.1
	200mg/d(10)	cobs + grain	0.52	144	47*	97*	14.4*
	0	sorghum	0.60	124	84	40	22.3
	200mg/d(10)		0.63	117	56*	61*	14.1*
(3)	0	Coastal	0.49	80	55	12	22.7
	133mg/d(20)	Bermuda	0.54	90	49	29*	18.9
	0	grass	0.49	106	53	41	16.0
	133mg/d(20)		0.47	104	48	44	20.6

Reference (1) Muntifering et al. (66)   (2) Poos et al. (67)
(3) Moore et al. (68)

[1] ( ) adaptation period   [2] OM apparently digested in the rumen
[3] Non ammonia N

*Significantly different from control with $p < 0.05$ at least

Recently these findings were confirmed (52) although an inhibition of Ni uptake in a methanogen has been observed (53). As monensin specifically inhibits cellulolytic organisms (54), a depression in rumen fibre degradation can be expected and has been demonstrated (55) even after adaptation (56). No effect has been observed however using cotton fibre strips in the rumen (57). Fecal digestibilities of fibre may be decreased (58) as well as increased (59) but may be affected by a shift in site of digestion from rumen to hindgut. Experiments *in vivo* using cannulated animals indicate no unequivocal effect of monensin on rumen digestibility (Table 5).

A consistent effect however is a decrease in microbial non-ammonia N (NAN) flow to the duodenum, concomittant with an increase in feed NAN flow, the result being no change in total NAN flow (Table 5). A decrease in microbial NAN flow may be due to a lowered microbial N yield (g Ni/kg OMf), or, in adapted animals, to a lowered extent of fermentation in the rumen (Table 5). The latter effect is in line with expected effects on metabolic interactions and with the consistent depression of rumen feed protein degradation (Table 5), confirming earlier work *in vitro* (28,60,61). Inhibition of protein degradation *in vitro* was accompanied by an accumulation of peptides and amino acids, indicating that deamination was more inhibited than proteolysis. Negative results on animal performance using monensin were obtained with animals fed low quality diets and non-protein N (Table 6)

TABLE 6

Effect of monensin on steer growth using low quality roughage diets with urea.

Reference	Basal ration	Supplement	Monensin	Intake[3] (kg/d)	Weight gain (kg/d)
(1)	Cotton	80 urea	0	8.44	0.71
	seed	20 SMB[1]	500 ppm[2]	6.94	0.42*
	hulls	80 urea	0	8.33	0.58
		20 F-SBM[1]	500 ppm[2]	6.78	0.31*
(2)	Pelleted wheat	urea	0	6.23	0.33
	straw		30 ppm	4.48*	0.03*
	Alkali treat.	urea	0	8.34	0.73
	and pelleted				
	wheat straw		30 ppm	6.68*	0.57
(3)	Corn silage +	urea	0	6.91	0.52
	NaOH treated	(10.5% CP)	200 mg/d	6.94	0.51
	husklage 60/40	urea	0	6.94	0.58
		(12.5% CP)	200 mg/d	6.94	0.53

[1] SBM = soybean meal, SBM-F = formaldehyd-treatment SBM
[2] in Supplement   [3] roughage only
References: (1) Oltjen et al. (62)   (2) Coombe et al. (63)
          (3) Hanson & Klopfenstein (69)
* Significant difference from control p < 0.05.

Such results may be related to depressions of rumen microbial N yields and/or rumen fibre digestion. The latter effect is suggested by lowered concentration of rumen total volatile fatty acid concentrations (62,63). Inhibition of rumen urease activity, lowering microbial N supply may be an additional factor. Such effect was suggested by Van Nevel & Demeyer (64) and Bartley et al. (65), may be related to an impaired Ni transport into ureolytic bacteria and was recently clearly confirmed by Starnes et al. (35).

Rumen wall associated bacteria (70) may be involved, as no effect was observed *in vitro* by Wallace et al. (55). Although counts of rumen protozoa do not always show an effect of monensin (64,71,72), unequivocal evidence of an inhibitory effect of monensin on rumen protozoa with a shift in metabolism to lactate was obtained by Hino (73). Selective toxicity to large ciliates may be involved (74) and such effect may lower microbial N recycling in the rumen and thus contribute to the overall effect on animal performance. Lowered protozoal activity may also be involved in lowered rumen fibre digestion as it was shown that the presence of protozoa contributes to rumen fibre degradation (75). Negative effects on fibre digestion may however be balanced by a longer retention time of particles and fluid as is evident from most published experiments although statistical significance is rarely obtained.

TABLE 7

Effect of monensin on rumen fractional liquid (k_l) and particle (k_p) outflow rates (h^{-1}) (ref. 48).

Monensin dose[1]	Liquid outflow (k_l) Control	Monensin	Particle outflow (k_p) Control	Monensin	Reference
33 ppm	0.103	0.090	-	-	(1)
33 ppm	0.106	0.098	-	-	(2)
33 ppm	0.051	0.046	0.046	0.039	(3)
170 ppm	0.074	0.056	0.059	0.044	(4)
200 mg	0.065	0.045*	0.027	0.015*	(5)
20 mg	0.053	0.048	-	-	
100 mg	0.053	0.048	-	-	
200 mg	0.053	0.042*			

[1] ppm in ration DM or mg/steer/day
* Significant difference from control at least $p < 0.05$

References: (1) Adams et al. (76) (2) Rogers & Davis (78)
(3) Ricke et al. (57) (4) Bull et al. (79)
(5) Lemenager et al. (77)

A decrease in rumen fractional outflow rate will also affect microbial N
yield, fermentation pattern and feed protein degradation. The reasons for
such effect of monensin on the interaction between rumen outflow rate and
metabolism are not known, but demand further research in view of their
possible importance (48).
According to Wedegaertner and Johnson (80) 1/3 of the improved energy
utilization in animals fed the drug is due to reduced methanogenesis. From
our discussion it is clear that additional effects may involve (Fig. 1):
- an increase in post ruminal digestion of feed OM (protein, starch
  and fibre)
- changes in rumen fibre digestion by inhibition of protozoa and
  muralytic bacteria and increases in retention time.
- changes in microbial N yield by inhibition of bacteria and protozoa,
  N supply to microbes and increases in retention time.
Additional effects may involve reduction of parasite loads in the lower
gut, prevention of pulmonary emphysema, reduction of feed intake, changes
in energy expenditure by the sodium pump system, changes in rumen
osmolality and inhibition of lactate production in the rumen (34,48). All
effects are of course subject to variation with diet and level of intake.
Results from 35 experiments conducted in nine European countries showed
that monensin decreased feed intake by 4%, gain was increased by 5% and
feed:gain ratio improved by 9%. In 12 pasture studies in Europe monensin
increased daily gain by 14% (22). Responses were greater in diets
containing marginal rather than adequate levels of protein, whereas the
additive was not effective when diets contained 40% of the crude protein
as urea.
Other ionophores recently introduced are lasalocid (Hoffman-Laroche),
salinomycin (Hoechst), laidlomycin (Syntex Research), narasin and
ICI 139603 (ICI). Most experimental evidence was obtaind with lasalocid,
that was found to have properties similar to monensin on rumen fermentation
in vitro: a shift from methanogenesis to propionate production, inhibition
of protein degradation and lowered microbial N yield (65,81). The antibiotic inhibited lactate producing bacteria and resistant organisms were
succinate producers or lactate fermenters (82) whereas ciliate protozoa
are affected (83). Thivend and Jouany carried out a model experiment using
sheep with cannuleae in rumen, duodenum and ileum fed sugar beet pulp
supplemented with up to 64 ppm lasalocid after a 4 week adaptation period

(83).

Table 8 summarizes their data:

- a shift from rumen methane to propionate
- a lowered protozoal count
- a shift from rumen to large intestine digestion
- a lowered microbial N flow
- an increased dietary N flow.

Similar effects were reported by Thonney et al. (84), Gutierrez et al. (85), Patersen et al. (86) and Spears and Harvey (87), whereas Starnes et al. (35) also reported inhibition of urease activity.

Other ionophores may show similar effects (88-90), which really reflect a rather non-specific over-all depression in rumen microbial activity. Such effects cannot completely explain the growth promoting activity of iono- phores and effects in the hindgut and at the tissue level are probably involved (34).

TABLE 8

Effect of lasolocid on rumen digestion (ref. 83).

	Lasalocid sodium (ppm)		
Rumen	0	21	64
Total VFA (mmol/l)	74.2	73.6	70.4*
mmol/mol			
Acetic	60.6	59.0	55.7*
Propionic	23.2	26.6	32.5*
Butyric	11.3	10.0	8.6*
CO_2/CH_4	2.23	2.75*	2.55
Entodinia $(10^3/ml)$	103.7	105.1	5.2*
Cellulolysis (%)	24.8	27.8*	27.7*
OM flow (g/day)			
Intake	823	824	785*
Apparent Digestion (%)			
In rumen	59.5	52.4*	50.8*
In rumen + S.I[1]	81.6	75.9	72.3*
Total	82.8	82.8	78.5*
N flow (g/day)			
Intake	20.7	21.2	20.2
Duodenal flow:			
NAN[2]	20.1	19.7	20.8
Bact. N	14.2	12.3*	11.9*
Diet N[3]	5.9	7.4*	8.6*
gNi/kgOMF	29.0	28.5	29.8

[1] S.I. = small intestine   [2] NAN = non ammonia N
[3] includes protozoal and endogenous N

* Significant difference from control at least $p < 0.05$.

VI.2. Other antibiotics

The glycopeptide antibiotic avoparcin (Cyanamid) shows growth promoting activities for cattle and increases rumen propionate (58,91) but does not seem to induce significant changes in rumen protein degradation or microbial cellulolytic activity (92,93). One study reported an increase in rumen organic matter digestion following avoparcin use (94) although reductions in rumen volatile fatty acid concentrations following avoparcin use (95) indicate an opposite effect. This compound deserves further research, also because its effect on small intestinal protein absorption has been demonstrated (94,96). Virginiamycin (Smith-Kline) is a growth promoting antibiotic for fattening pigs (97) acting at least partly through effects on bacterial carbohydrate metabolism in the lower intestinal tract (98). Growth promoting effects with steers have been reported (99) and we have recently investigated the effect of this antibiotic on rumen carbohydrate metabolism *in vitro* (100). Results indicate similar effects as with other antibiotics with most outspoken effects on net microbial N yields, suggesting extensive microbial lysis induced by the antibiotic (Table 9).

TABLE 9

Effect of virginiamycin on rumen metabolism *in vitro*.

	Virginiamycin added (ppm)		
	0	1	5
Hexose fermented (μmoles)[1]	696	667	651*
End products (mmol/mol C_6)			
Acetate	1022	964*	941*
Propionate	568	605*	613*
Butyrate	203	210	218*
Methane	342	298*	303*
Hydrogen recovery (%)[1]	84	84	86
g Ni/kg OMf			
Total[2]	72	75	74
Net	16	4*	-1

[1] Calculated from end products from incubations of rumen contents *in vitro* with cellobiose and maltose (100).

[2] From $^{32}PO_4^{3-}$-incorporation (101)
Values may be overestimated due to acid solubilization of insoluble inorganic P.

VII. EFFECT OF UNSATURATED FATTY ACIDS AND DEFAUNATION

Unsaturated fatty acids were originally investigated as methane inhibitors (103), but are also toxic to rumen protozoa (review in 75). Chemical defaunation of the rumen has resulted in increased microbial N yields in the rumen *in vitro* and *in vivo* (14,104,105) and may thus be expected to promote animal production when limited by rumen microbial production.

A growth promoting effect of defaunation using a detergent was indeed observed in lamb growth trials (102), but effects were least outspoken with straw diets (Table 10).

TABLE 10
Effect of defaunation of the rumen on lamb growth using different diets (102).

Diet	Period	Growth (g/day)	Feed intake (g/day)
Sugar beet pulp	Faun. Defaun.	181 213*	871 857*
Alkali treat. straw	Faun. Defaun.	102 140*	878 964
Alkali treat. straw + starch	Faun. Defaun.	239 192	1766 1895
Molasses	Faun. Defaun. Faun. + Fishmeal	135 208* 228*	1127 1530* 1428*

* Significant difference with control for $p < 0.05$ at least.

Growth promoting effects from defaunation can be due to higher microbial N yields (gNi/kgOMf) in the rumen as well as to decreased energy losses in CH_4 (106) and decreases in feed protein degradation (107). Such effects may be balanced however by decreases in extent of OM and fibre fermentation in the rumen, lowering the total amount of bacterial N flowing to the duodenum (4). A decrease in fibre degradation in sacco was observed following defaunation but effects of defaunation on particle retention may also be involved (108).

As chemical defaunating agents are often toxic to the animals (109) we recently tried to use free higher fatty acids as defaunating agent to study the effect of defaunation on particle retention (110).

TABLE 11

Effect of defaunation of the rumen on fractional outflow rate of fluid (k_1) and particles (k_p) (h^{-1}).

| Period | Fractional outflow rates k (h^{-1})[3] | | | |
| | Expt. 1[1] | | Expt. 2[2] | |
	kl	kp	kl	kp
Faunated	.078	.036	--	--
Defaunated	.085	.071*	.068	.014*
Refaunated	.076	.049	.075	.011

[1] Kayouli et al. (108)   [2] Demeyer & Dendooven (110)

[3] PEG was used for determination of kl and Cr mordanted soya bean meal (expt. 1) or Cr mordanted hay particles (expt. 2) for k_p.

* Significant difference from either faunated or refaunated period.

Table 11 shows that defaunation significantly increases fractional outflow of Cr mordanted hay or soya bean meal particles, an effect certainly contributing to the decrease in rumen fibre digestion after defaunation. Higher fatty acids are different from other chemicals in manipulation of rumen fermentation, because of their nature and the amounts used. They are mentioned here however because they provide a very good example of the intricacies involved in the interpretation of effects of a compound on rumen digestion.

So far, evidence has been found for the following interrelated effects of higher fatty acids on rumen digestion:

- They kill protozoa and as such are defaunating agents.
- They lower extent of rumen fibre digestion not by a coating effect on the fibres but by a direct effect on the microbial rumen population (111,112). Such effect may be related to the removal of protozoa and toxicity to bacteria (113).
- They increase fractional particle outflow rate from the rumen, an effect contributing to changes in rumen protein and fibre degradation and microbial N yield.

It is obvious that all compounds that influence rumen digestion will have similar interrelated effects, varying in relative importance with diet, level of feeding, etc.... Manipulation of digestion by a chemical will have to be based on careful study of these effects, as adapted to a particular feeding situation.

VIII. COMPARATIVE EFFECTS ON ANIMAL PERFORMANCE

Comparative beef production trials have been carried out in the U.S.A. under feedlot conditions and results have been summarized by Chalupa (27) and Owens et al. (34). Their data have been summarized in Table 12 and indicate that the newer ionophores might depress feed intake less than monensin and lasalocid. Feed conversion is similar, resulting in slightly better gain. Avoparcin shows a similar effect whereas results using halogenated compounds are more erratic. Feed intake is depressed and gain and feed conversion less improved than by ionophores. A promising compound may be ICI 13049 showing considerable improvement in both gain and feed conversion in one experiment.

TABLE 12

Comparative effects of chemicals on beef cattle performance mainly under feedlot conditions (% of control values; ref. 22,34 and 42).

	Feed intake (kg/d)	Gain (kg/d)	Feed:gain
Monensin	94-98	99-104	92-95
Lasalocid	95-97	103-107	90-94
Salinomycin	99	106	90-93
Narasin	99	106	93
Avoparcin	99	106	93
Halogen Compounds			
HCS	88-98	101-103	87-96
ICI 11075	96	101	96
ICI13409[1]	95	108	88

IX. CONCLUSION

Most chemicals introduced as such or with feed to manipulate rumen fermentation show an array of interrelated effects of varying relative importance: methane inhibition, propionate stimulation, decreased extent of rumen degradation of dietary organic matter (fibre and protein), lowered microbial N yield and changes in protozoal activity and rumen liquid and particle retention. Such changes are often indicative of an overall depression of rumen microbial activity and may result in shifts of digestion from the rumen to further in the intestinal tract. Effects on animal production may be beneficial depending on feeding conditions as evident in the use of ionophores. Animal response to ionophores and antibiotics however is almost certainly due to additional effects other than on rumen digestion, in the lower intestinal tract and at the tissue level. It can be predicted that other chemicals not discussed here will have similar interrelated effects on rumen digestion as described for example for diaryliodonium compounds (20), recently also shown to have neural toxicity (114). Development of new chemicals to manipulate rumen digestion will require careful study of the relative quantitative importance of their interrelated effects, also beyond the rumen. Animal response may then be evident under defined feeding conditions as was illustrated for defaunating compounds.

Acknowledgement
Own work reported in this review was supported by the I.W.O.N.L. (Brussels).

REFERENCES

1. Demeyer, D.I. and Van Nevel, C.J.: In: Digestion and Metabolism in the ruminant. Proceedings of the 4th Physiology. I.W. McDonald and I.J.C. Warner (eds.), The univ. of New England publ. unit, pp. 366-382 (1975).
2. Demeyer, D.I. and Van Nevel, C.J.: Reprod. Nutrit. Develop. 26: 161-179 (1986).
3. Owens, F.N. and Goetsch, A.L.: In: Control of Digestion and Metabolism in Ruminants. L.I. Milligan, W.L. Grovum and A. Dobson (eds.), Proc. 6th Int. Symp. Ruminant Physiol., A. Reston Book, Prentice Hall, Englewood Cliffs, New Jersey, pp. 196-223 (1986).
4. Demeyer, D.I. and Vervaeke, I.: Proc. OECD Workshop on Improved utilisation of ligno-cellulosic materials with special reference to animal feed, Braunschweig (1984).
5. Capper, B.S., Morgan, D.J. and Parr, W.H.: Tropical Sci. 19: 73-88 (1977).
6. Orskov, E.R.: Livestock Proc. Sci. 6: 335-347 (1979).

7. Merry, R.J., Smith, R.H. and McAllan, A.B.: Brit. J. Nutr. 48: 305-318 (1983).

8. Voigt, J., Piatkowski, B. and Bock, J.: Arch. Tierernahr. 30: 811-823 (1980).

9. Czerkawski, J.W.: World. Rev. Nutr. Diet. 11: 240-282 (1969).

10. Hungate, R.E.: The Rumen and its microbes, Academic Press, New York (1966).

11. Chalupa, W.: J. Anim. Sci. 46: 585-599 (1977).

12. Tamminga, S.: Proc. Symp. on observations on the practical use of new sources of protein in relation to energy supply for high production of milk and meat. FAO - UNO - Geneva (1981).

13. Schaetzel, W.P. and Johnson, D.E.: J. Anim. Sci. 53: 1104-1108 (1981).

14. Demeyer, D.I. and Van Nevel, C.J.: Brit. J. Nutr. 42: 515-524 (1979).

15. Bird, S.H., Hill, M.K. and Leng, R.A.: Brit. J. Nutr. 42: 81-87 (1979).

16. Chalupa, W.: J. Dairy Sci. 58: 1198-1218 (1975).

17. Hobson, P.N. and Wallace, R.J.: Microbial ecology and activities in the rumen part II, CRC-Crit. Revs. Microb. 9: 264 (1982).

18. Brock, F.M., Forsberg, C.W. and Buchanan-Smith, J.G.: Appl. Env. Microbiol. 44: 561-569 (1982).

19. Wallace, R.J.: In: Protein Metabolism and Nutrition, R. Pion, M. Arnal and D. Bodin (eds.), INRA, nr. 16, vol. II, p. 219-222 (1983).

20. Chalupa, W., Patterson, J.A., Parish, R.C. and Chow, A.W.: J. Anim. Sci. 57: 186-194 (1983).

21. Broderick, G.A. and Balthrop Jr., J.E.: J. Anim. Sci. 49: 1101-1111 (1979).

22. Chalupa, W.: In: Recent Advances in Animal Nutrition, W. Haresign and D.J.A. Cole (eds.), Butterworths, London, pp. 143-160 (1984).

23. Prins, R.A.: cited in Chalupa (1984) (22) (1978).

24. Durand, M.: Ann. Zoot. 31: 47-76 (1982).

25. Van Nevel, C.J. and Demeyer, D.I.: Landbouwtijdschrift 29: 431-451 (1976).

26. Marty, R.J. and Demeyer, D.I.: Br. J. Nutr. 30: 369-376 (1973).

27. Van Nevel, C.J., Henderickx, H.K., Demeyer, D.I. and Martin, J.: Appl. Microbiol. 17: 695-700 (1969).

28. Van Nevel, C.J. and Demeyer, D.I.: Appl. Env. Microbiol. 34: 251-257 (1977).

29. Van Nevel, C.J. and Demeyer, D.I.: Arch. Tierernahr. 31: 141-151 (1981).

30. Ganev, G., Orskov, E.R. and Smart, R.: J. Agric. Sci. Camb. 93: 651-656 (1979).

31. Forsberg, C.W., Lovelock, L.K.A., Krumholz, L. and Buchanan-Smith, J.G.: Appl. Env. Microbiol. 47: 101-110 (1984).

32. Vogels, G.D., Hoppe, W.F. and Stumm, C.K.: Appl. Env. Microbiol. 40: 608-612 (1980).

33. Stumm, C.K., Gijsen, H.J. and Vogels, G.D.: Br. J. Nutr. 47: 95-99 (1982).

34. Owens, F.N., Weakly, D.C. and Goetsch, A.L.: In: Herbivore Nutrition in the Tropics and Subtropics. F.M.C. Gilchrist and R.I. Mackie (eds.), The Science Press, Johannesburg, pp. 435-454 (1983).

35. Starnes, S.R., Spears, J.W., Froetschel, M.A. and Croom Jr., W.J.: J. Nutr. 114: 518-525 (1984).

36. Prins, R.A., Van Nevel, C.J. and Demeyer, D.I.: Ant. Leeuwenhoek J. Microb. Serol. 38: 281-287 (1972).

37. Wood, J.M., Kenney, F.S. and Wolfe, R.S.: Biochemistry 7: 1707-1713 (1968).

38. Wolfe, R.S.: Experientia 38: 198-200 (1982).

39. Czerkawski, J.W. and Breckenridge, G.: Brit. J. Nutr. 34: 429-446 (1975).

40. Czerkawski, J.W. and Breckenridge, G.: Brit. J. Nutr. 34: 447-457 (1975).

41. Stanier, G. and Davies, A.: Brit.J.Nutr. 45: 567-578 (1981).

42. Davies, A., Nwaonu, H.N., Stanier, G. and Boyle, F.T.: Brit. J. Nutr. 47: 565-576 (1982).

43. Chalupa, W., Corbett, W. and Brethour, J.R.: J. Anim. Sci. 51: 170-179 (1980).

44. Russell, J.B. and Martin, S.A.: J. Anim. Sci. 59: 1329-1338 (1984).

45. Mathers, J.C. and Miller, E.L.: J. Agric. Sci. 99: 215-224 (1982).

46. Trei, J.E., Parish, R.C. and Scott, G.C.: J. Anim. Sci. 33: 1171 (1971).

47. Clapperton, J.L.: Anim. Prod. 24: 169-181 (1977).

48. Schelling, G.T.: J. Anim. Sci. 58: 1518-1527 (1984).

49. Chen, M. and Wolin, M.J.: Appl. Env. Microbiol. 38: 72-77 (1979).

50. Cole, N.A. and McCroskey, J.E.: J. Anim. Sci. 41: 1735-1741 (1975).

51. Horton, G.M.J.: J. Anim. Sci. 50: 1160-1164 (1980).

52. Dellinger, C.A. and Ferry, J.G.: Appl. Env. Microbiol. 48: 680-682

(1984).

53. Jarrell, K.F. and Sprott, G.D.: J. Bact. 151: 1195-1203 (1982).

54. Henderson, C., Stewart, C.S. and Nekrep, F.V.: J. Appl. Bact. 51: 159-169 (1981).

55. Wallace, R.J., Czerkawski, J.W and Breckenridge, G.: Brit. J. Nutr. 46: 131-148 (1981).

56. De Jong, A. and Berchauer, F.: S. Afr. J. Anim. Sci. 13: 67-70 (1983).

57. Ricke, S.C., Berger, L.L., Van Der Aar, P.J. and Faney Jr., G.C.: J. Anim. Sci. 58: 194-202 (1984).

58. Cottyn, B.G., Fiems, L.O., Boucque, V.C., Aerts, J.V. and Buysse, F.X.: Zeitschr. Tierphys. Tierernahr. Futtermittelde. 49: 277-286 (1983).

59. Horton, G.M.J. and Nickolson, H.H: Can. J. Anim. Sci. 60: 919-924 (1980).

60. Whetstone, H.D., Davis, C.L. and Bryant, M.P.: J. Anim. Sci. 53: 803-809 (1981).

61. Russell, J.B., Bottje, W.G. and Cotta, M.A.: J. Anim. Sci. 53: 242-252 (1981).

62. Oltjen, R.R., Dinius, D.A. and Goering, M.K.: J. Anim. Sci. 45: 1442-1451 (1977).

63. Coombe, J.B., Dinius, D.A., Goering, H.K. and Oltjen, R.R.: J. Anim. Sci. 48: 1223-1233 (1979).

64. Van Nevel, C.J. and Demeyer, D.I.: Ann. Rech. Vet. 10: 338-340 (1979).

65. Bartley, E.E., Herod, E.L., Bechtle, R.M., Sapienza, D.A. and Brent, E.: J. Anim. Sci. 49: 1066-1075 (1979).

66. Muntifering, R.B., Theurer, B. and Noon, T.H.: J. Anim. Sci. 53: 1565-1573 (1981).

67. Poos, M.I., Manson, T.L. and Klopfenstein, T.J.: J. Anim. Sci. 48: 1516-1524 (1979).

68. Moore, C.K., Amos, H.E., Evans, J.J., Lowrey, R.S. and Burdick, D.: J. Anim. Sci. 50: 1145-1159 (1980).

69. Hanson, T.L. and Klopfenstein, T.: J. Anim. Sci. 48: 474-479 (1979).

70. Cheng, K.J. and Costerton, I.W.: In: Digestive Physiology and Metabolism in Ruminants. Y. Ruckebusch and P. Thivend (eds.), MTP Press Ltd., Lancaster, Proceedings of the 5th International Symposium on Ruminant Physiology, pp. 227-250 (1979).

71. Jouany, J.P. and Senaud, J.: Ann. Zoot. 27: 61-74 (1978).

72. Dinius, D.A., Simpson, M.E. and Marsh, P.B.: J. Anim. Sci. 42: 229-234 (1976).

73. Hino, T.: Jap. J. Zoot. Sci. 52: 171-179 (1981).

74. Stevenson, G.T. and Nolan, J.V.: Anim. Prod. Austral. 15: 752 (1984).

75. Demeyer, D.I.: Agric. Env. 6: 295-337 (1981).

76. Adams, D.C., Galyean, M.L., Kiesling, H.E., Wallace, J.D. and Finkner, M.D.: J. Anim. Sci. 53: 780-789 (1981).

77. Lemenager, R.P., Owens, F.N., Shokey, B.J., Lusby, K.S. and Totusek, R.: J. Anim. Sci. 47: 255-261 (1978).

78. Rogers, J.A. and Davis, C.L.: J. Dairy Sci. 65: 944-952 (1982).

79. Bull, L.S., Rumpler, W.V., Sweeney, T.F. and Zinn, R.A.: Fed. Proc. 38: 2713-2719 (1979).

80. Wedegaertner, T.C. and Johnson, D.E.: J. Anim. Sci. 57: 168-177 (1983).

81. Fuller, J.R. and Johnson, D.E.: J. Anim. Sci. 53: 1574-1580 (1981).

82. Dennis, S.M., Nagaraja, T.G. and Bartley, E.E.: J. Dairy Sci. 64: 2350-2356 (1981).

83. Thivend, P. and Jouany, J.P.: Reprod. Nutr. Develop. 23: 817-828 (1983).

84. Thonney, M.L., Heide, E.K., Duhaime, D.J., Hand, R.J. and Perosio, D.J.: J. Anim. Sci. 52: 427-433 (1981).

85. Gutierrez, G.G., Schake, L.M. and Byers, F.M.: J. Anim. Sci. 54: 863-868 (1982).

86. Paterson, J.A., Anderson, B.M., Bowman, D.K., Morrison, R.L. and Williams, J.E.: J. Anim. Sci. 57: 1537-1544 (1983).

87. Spears, J.W. and Harvey, R.W.: J. Anim. Sci. 58: 460-464 (1984).

88. Nakashima, T., Masuno, T., Sakauchi, R. and Hoshino, S.: Jap. J. Zoot. Sci. 53: 541-546 (1982).

89. Spires, H.R. and Algeo, J.W.: J. Anim. Sci. 57: 1533-1560 (1983).

90. Rowe, J.B., Davies, A. and Brooms, A.W.: In: Protein Metabolism and Nutrition, R. Pion, M. Arnal and D. Bonum (eds.), INRA, Paris, pp. 259-262 (1983).

91. Johnson, R.J., Herlugson, M.L., Bola-Ojikutu, L., Corvova, G., Dyer, I.A., Zimmer, P. and Delay, R.: J. Anim. Sci. 48: 1338-1342 (1979).

92. MacGregor, R.C. and Armstrong, D.G.: Proc. Nutr. Soc. 43: 21A (1983).

93. Stewart, C.S., Crossley, M.V. and Garrow, S.H.: Eur. J. Appl. Microbiol. Biotechn. 17: 292-297 (1983).

94. MacGregor, R.C. and Armstrong, D.G.: Anim. Prod. 34: 55A (1982).

95. Froetschel, N.A., Croom Jr., W.J., Res Gaskins, H., Leonard, E.S. and Whitacre, M.D.: J. Nutr. 113: 1355-1362 (1983).

96. Parker, D.S., MacGregor, R.C., Finlayson, H.J., Stockill, P. and Balios, J.: Can. J. Anim. Sci. 64(suppl): 136-137 (1984).
97. Casteels, M., Bekaert, H., Eeckhout, W. and Buysse, F.X.: Recent observations with some new antibiotics as feed additives for swine, 28th Ann. Meet. E.E.A.P.
98. Vervaeke, I.J., Decuypere, J.A., Dierick, N.A. and Henderickx, H.K.: J. Anim. Sci. 49: 846-856 (1979).
99. Parigini-Bini, R.: In: Performance in Animal Production. G. Piana and G. Piva (eds.), Minerva Medica, Torino, pp. 59-72 (1979).
100. Van Nevel, C.J., Demeyer, D.I. and Henderickx, H.K.: Archiv Tierernahr. 34: 149-155 (1984).
101. Van Nevel, C.J. and Demeyer, D.I.: Brit. J. Nutr. 38: 101-114 (1977).
102. Demeyer, D.I., Van Nevel, C.J. and Van De Voorde, G.: Archiv Tierernahr. 32: 595-604 (1982).
103. Demeyer, D.I. and Henderickx, H.K.: Biochim. Biophys. Acta 137: 484-497 (1967).
104. Sutton, J.D., Knight, R., McAllan, A.B. and Smith, R.H.: Brit. J. Nutr. 49: 419-432 (1983).
105. Demeyer, D.I., Van Nevel, C.J. and Aerts, J.: In: Proc. OECD/COST Workshop on Improved utilization of lignocellulosic materials for animal feed. Kh. Domsch, M.P. Ferranti and O. Theander (eds.), pp. 69-71 (1981).
106. Whitelaw, F.G., Eadie, M., Bruce, L.A. and Shand, W.J.: Brit. J. Nutr. 52: 261-275 (1984).
107. Kayouli, C., Van Nevel, C.J., Demeyer, D.I.: 4th Int. Symp. Protein Metabolism and Nutrition, Clermont-Ferrand vol. II, INRA ed., pp. 251-259 (1983).
108. Kayouli, C., Demeyer, D.I., Van Nevel, C.J. and Dendooven, R.: Anim. Feed Sci. Technol. 10: 165-172 (1983/84).
109. Lovelock, K.A., Buchanan-Smith, J.G. and Forsberg, C.W.: Can. J. Anim. Sci. 62: 299-303 (1982).
110. Demeyer, D.I. and Dendooven, R.: Defaunering van de pens door onverzadigde vetzuren en het effect op uitvloeisnelheid in de pens. 10de Studiedag Nederlandstal. Voedingsonderz., Louvain-La-Neuve, 2 pp. (1985).
111. Orskov, E.R., Hine, R.S. and Grub, D.A.: Anim. Prod. 27: 241-245 (1978).

112. McAllan, A.B., Knight, R. and Sutton, J.D.: Brit. J. Nutr. $\underline{49}$: 433-440 (1983).

113. Henderson, C.: J. Agric. Sci., Camb. $\underline{81}$: 107-112 (1973).

114. Hedde, R.D.: Personal communication (1983).

10. THE RUMEN AS A PHARMACOKINETIC COMPARTMENT

J.A. BOGAN AND S.E. MARRINER

I INTRODUCTION

It is surprising that so little work has been done on the effects of
the reticulo-rumen on the pharmacokinetics and pharmacodynamics of drugs
given to ruminant animals. Considering the large effort and expense that
has been made evaluating drugs, especially antibacterials and anthelmintics, in clinical trials, much of this effort could have been saved by an
initial understanding of the fate of the drug.

The potential of the rumen to affect drug action is great. The rumen contents with a pH 5.5 - 6.5 occupying up to 20% of the animal's volume (13), at equilibrium, should contain about 80% of a weakly basic drug - and the majority of drugs are weakly basic - whether the dose is administered orally or parenterally thus minimising the systemic effect of basic drugs. Conversely, for an acid which should not distribute well into the rumen there is the potential for an 20% overdosage if dosage is based on a body-weight basis.

There are many possible influences on drug kinetics in the ruminant and many of these will be discussed later but the essential question is whether drugs readily transfer into and out of the rumen through the ruminal epithelium.

II ABSORPTION THROUGH THE RETICULO-RUMEN EPITHELIUM

For most body compartments, distribution of drugs is by passive diffusion of the unionized fraction of the drug. Passage will proceed until there is an equilibrium on either side of the tissue barrier.

Distribution of an acid (pka=4.4) between rumen and plasma

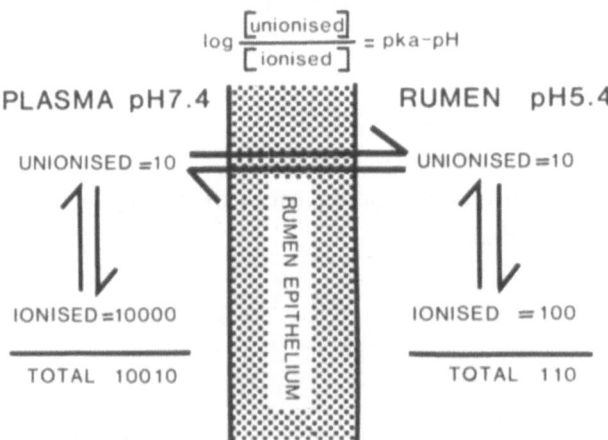

FIGURE 1. Theoretical distribution of an acid (pKa 4.4) between ruminal fluid and plasma.

The *extent* of distribution, i.e. the total amount of drug on either side of a barrier, will be affected by the degree of ionization which is dictated by the pH on either side of the barrier. For example, for the rumen epithelium for a weak acid of pKa = 4.4 the distribution equilibrium is as shown in Fig. 1. The distribution between rumen and plasma for acids and bases is theoretically as shown in Fig. 2.

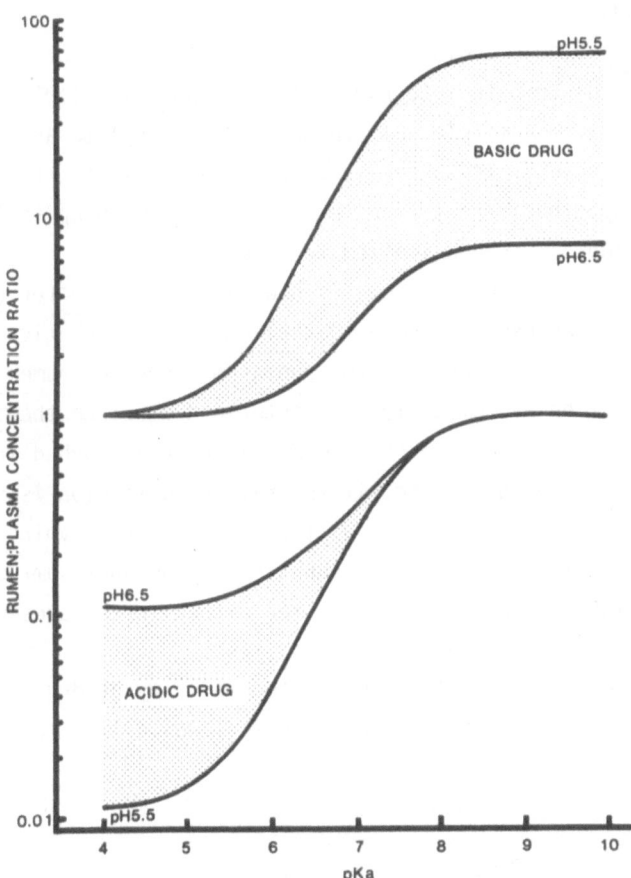

FIGURE 2. The theoretical rumen: plasma ratio for acidic and basic drugs of different pKa.

What is the evidence that drugs passively diffuse through the reticulo-rumen epithelium?

The earliest experiments were those of Trautman (35) who demonstrated effects on the eye of atropine and pilocarpine after these had been added to a tied-off rumen and Rankin (31) showed that cyanide and strychnine could also be absorbed in sufficient quantity from a tied-off rumen to kill sheep.

Since then, there has been a considerable amount of data to demonstrate that for many drugs passive diffusion occurs in the ruminal epithelium. This has been satisfactorily demonstrated for sulfonamides (2), salicylate, pentobarbitone, quinine (15) and thiabendazole (24), using tied-off rumens in *in vivo* situations.

Also, after systemic administration, the following drugs have been demonstrated to distribute into rumen fluid - ephedrine (10), amphetamine (5), quinine (15), levamisole (8) (bases) and salicylate and pento-barbitone (15) (acids). In these experiments, adjustments of the rumen pH confirmed the hypothesis that transfer across the rumen epithelium is by passive diffusion of the non-ionized fraction.

The important question, however, is how fast does transfer occur? If the rate of diffusion across the rumen epithelium is slow relative to the onward passage of gut contents to the abomasum, then the rumen will have negligible effect on systemically administered drug since the small amounts of drug diffusing into the rumen will be re-absorbed in the more distal portions of the gut. Also, if the rate of diffusion is slow, for orally administered drug the rumen will serve as a "reservoir" of drug, drug becoming available for rapid absorption in the abomasum/duodenum at the rate at which contents leave the rumen either in the aqueous phase if dissolved or in the solid phase if undissolved.

This we believe is the situation for the majority of drugs and before describing the consequences of such a result I would like to describe the evidence.

II.1. Weak bases

Weak bases, such as quinine and levamisole, should concentrate in rumen fluid after systemic administration. Jenkins, Davis and Boulos (15) measured the rate of transfer of quinine (pKa 8.4) to the tied-off rumen of goats from plasma (Fig. 3). Although their experiment demonstrates well the diffusion hypothesis, the rate of equilibration is slow. Additionally this experiment provides, if anything, an over-estimate of the transfer rate. The rumen contents had been removed and the rumen fluid was replaced with Krebs-Ringer phosphate solution which was well-stirred (circulated at

1 1/min), thus presenting drug to the epithelium at an optimum rate.

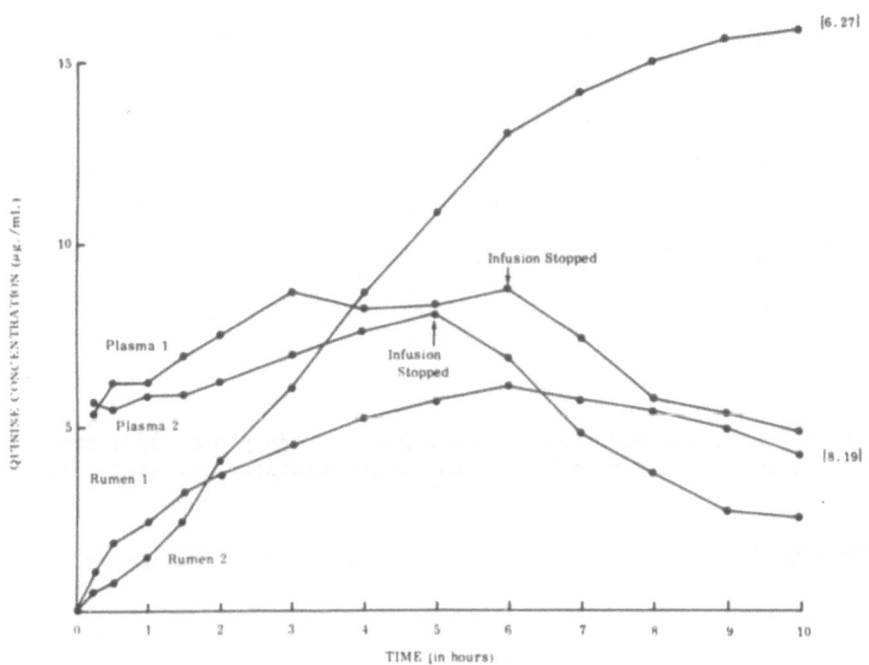

FIGURE 3. The concentration of quinine in the plasma and rumen of goats
after constant intravenous infusion of quinine (ref. 15).

Similar experiments in sheep with levamisole (8), a base of similar pKa
(pKa 8.0) of high lipid and water solubility showed that rumen
concentrations were relatively much lower. In these sheep, with ruminal
fluid sampled through rumen cannulae, the rumen was not tied-off (Fig. 4).

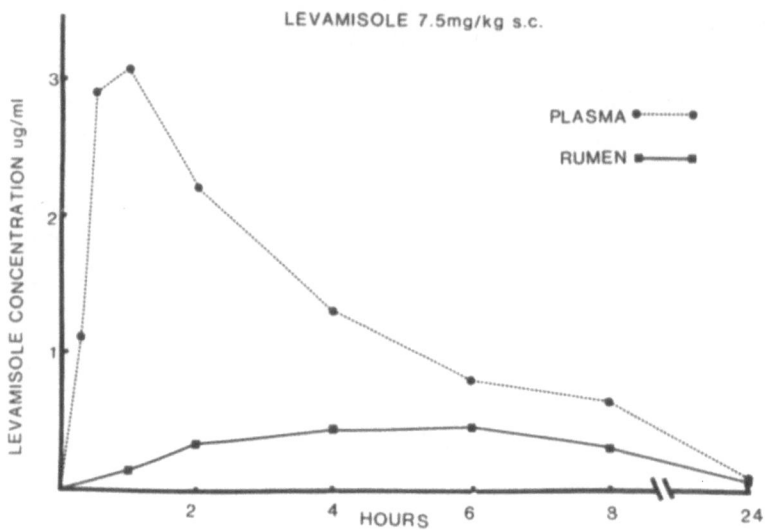

FIGURE 4. The mean concentration of levamisole in the plasma and rumen of sheep (n = 6) after levamisole administration s.c. (ref. 8).

II.2. Weak acids

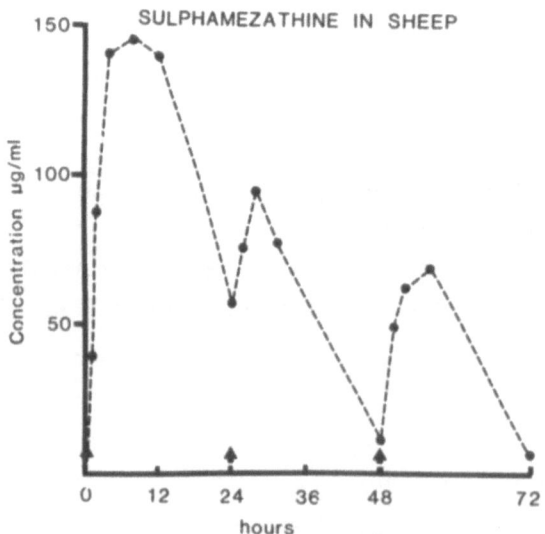

FIGURE 5. The mean concentration of sulphamezathine in the plasma of sheep (n = 12) given sulphamezathine tablets orally (200 mg/kg initially and 100 mg/kg at 24 and 48 h).

Weak acids, such as the sulfonamides, whose pKa and lipid solubility should favour rapid absorption from the rumen do not reach maximum concentrations in plasma for 6-8 h after oral dosage (36) (Fig. 5).

II.3. Stronger acids

Stronger acids also take some time to reach maximum concentrations in plasma of ruminants; 8 h for phenylbutazone (3) (pKa 4.5) in cattle and 4-8 h for salicylic acid (12) (pKa 3.8) given orally to goats and 5-6 h for meclofenamic acid (pKa 3.8) given intraruminally to sheep (19) (Fig. 6).

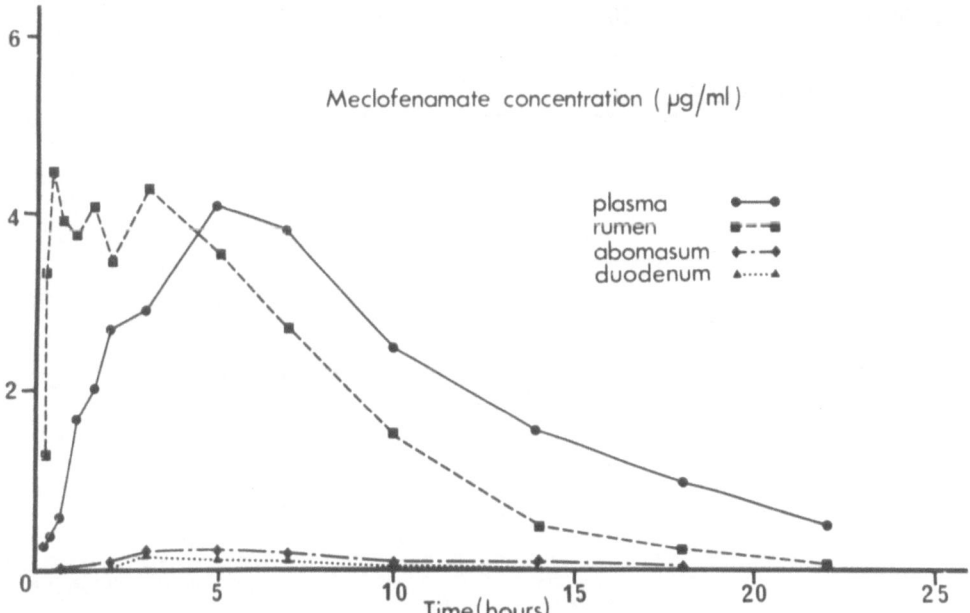

FIGURE 6. Mean plasma, rumen, abomasum and duodenum concentration of meclofenamic acid after intra-ruminal administration of meclofenamic acid (20 mg/kg) to 3 sheep (ref. 19).

Meclofenamic acid was not absorbed to any measurable extent from a tied-off rumen whereas in the same sheep maximum plasma concentrations were obtained 30 min after intra-abomasal administration (18). The time to maximum plasma concentration after intra-ruminal administration correlates well with the appearance of maximal abomasal concentrations. For example, this occurs for levamisole, meclofenamic acid, oxfendazole and albendazole (Table 1).

TABLE 1. The time to maximum concentrations of meclofenamic acid, oxfendazole, levamisole and albendazole sulfoxide (after albendazole) in plasma and abomasal fluid after oral administration in sheep.

Drug	ORAL ADMINISTRATION IN SHEEP	
	Time to maximum plasma concentration (hours)	Time to maximum abomasal concentration (hours)
Meclofenamic acid	5	5
Oxfendazole	20-24	16-24
Levamisole	4- 6	4- 6
Albendazole (Sulfoxide)	16	16

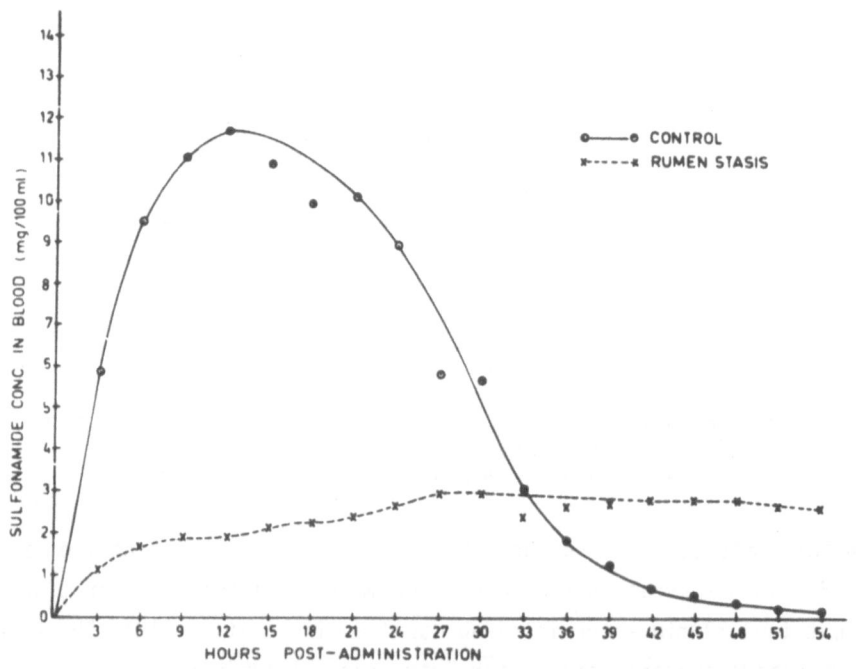

FIGURE 7. The mean concentration of sulfamethazine in plasma from normal and atropine treated sheep (n = 4) given 214 mg/kg orally (ref. 6).

Bischop et al. (6) showed that abolition of rumen-reticulum motility by atropine dramatically slowed absorption of sulfamethazine such that therapeutic concentrations (> 50 μg/ml) were maintained for 30 h in the normal sheep but were never attained in the atropinised animals (Fig. 7).

III   REASONS FOR SLOW RATE OF DIFFUSION ACROSS THE R-R EPITHELIUM

There are a number of reasons for the slow rate of diffusion out of the rumen compared with other parts of the gastro-intestinal tract.

III.1. Poor mixing of the aqueous phase in the rumen

The rumen epithelium is not presented with a continuous even concentration. From the rate of appearance of drug in the abomasum it would appear that the aqueous phase moves forward to produce maximal concentrations in the abomasum around 6 h in sheep after intra-ruminal administration. Observations of the time to maximal plasma concentrations of the same drugs suggest that in cattle and goats the rate of progress of the aqueous phase is similar. For example, oral administration of meclofenamic acid takes a similar time to reach maximum plasma concentrations in cattle (1) and sheep (19).

Additionally the concentration gradient of unionized drug between rumen and plasma is never great (Fig. 2) (much less than for abomasum-plasma) and therefore, especially with poorly stirred contents, the equilibrium pressure is low.

III.2. Relatively low surface area to volume ratio

In monogastric animals, it is known that for acids, although gastric pH is more favourable for absorption than duodenal pH, the much greater absorptive surface of the small intestine leads to a more extensive and rapid absorption (27) (Fig. 8). It is probable that the relatively low surface area/volume ratio of the rumen compared with the abomasum/duodenum could markedly reduce absorption.

Although the various involutions and papillae of the forestomachs increase surface area (estimated about seven times for cattle and goats) increase in useful absorptive capacity may not be as great because many papillae are of heavily keratinised epithelium (14). The increase in absorptive capacity of the small intestine caused by villi and surface microvilli is much greater.

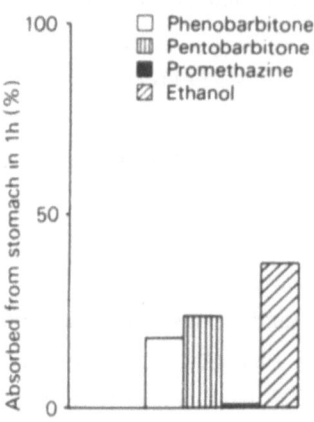
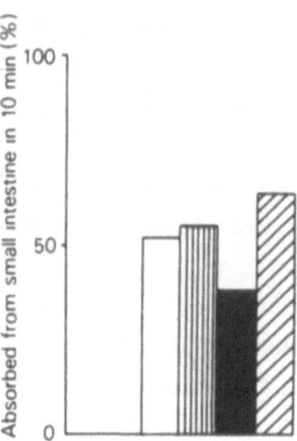

FIGURE 8. Comparison of the rate of absorption of drugs from the stomach
and small intestine in rats (ref. 27 using data from Magnussen,
ref. 17).

III.3. Blood flow

The rate of removal of absorbed drug in the bloodstream is important in
maintaining the concentration gradient. For its size, the rumino-reticulum
receives a relatively low blood supply - about 20% of the portal blood
before feeding and about 40% after feeding. In the goat stomach, blood flow
was highest to the fundic abomasal mucosa (28).

III.4. Adsorption to rumen contents

Feeding can affect drug availability. Cellulose has a high capacity for
drug binding. In the horse, for example, feeding reduces the plasma
bio-availability of trimethoprim and phenylbutazone (7). It is probable
that drug binding occurs in the rumen and although the drug may be
released on cellulose digestion, this will also serve to delay the
absorptive process.

IV ABSORPTION IN OTHER AREAS OF THE GASTRO-INTESTINAL TRACT OF RUMINANTS

Absorption from the abomasum and more distal areas of the gastrointestinal tract of the ruminant is similar to that from the stomach and

distal portions of the G.I.T. of simple-stomached species; viz. rapid
passive diffusion of non-ionized drug with acids being absorbed to some
extent in the abomasum, but both acids and bases being absorbed more
rapidly and more extensively in the upper small intestine due to its larger
surface area/volume. The only difference between the ruminant animal and
the simple-stomached species appears to be that the pH of the duodenal
contents remains lower for longer.

V EFFECT OF CLOSURE OF THE OESOPHAGEAL RETICULAR GROOVE

Since absorption from the abomasum and duodenum is relatively much
faster than from the rumen, rumen by-pass could have significant effects on
drug absorption. This reflex occurs commonly in younger ruminant animals
and is mainly a psychological reflex. We have observed it to occur
frequently in adult ruminants (cattle and sheep) after oral administration
of solutions and suspensions and is responsible for the early appearance
of plasma concentrations (Fig. 9).

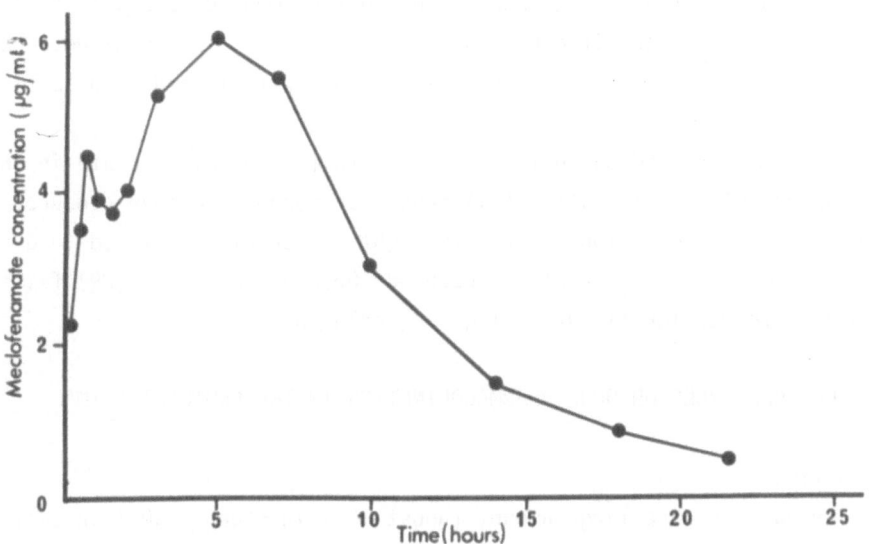

FIGURE 9. Mean concentration of meclofenamate (µg/ml) in plasma of sheep
(n = 3) after oral administration of meclofenamic acid (20 mg/kg)
as a drench.

Only liquids or suspensions can by-pass the rumen and oral tabletted
formulations, e.g. sulphamethazine boluses, (Fig. 5) do not result in early
concentrations. It has been proposed that ruminal by-pass may account for
the occasional failure of activity of benzimidazole anthelmintics
especially against inhibited larval species (16). Although by-pass appears
to occur to some extent in most adult animals with oral drenches it has
probably been over-rated as a cause of anthelmintic failure. Even if the
groove closed, with small volume drenches, especially suspensions, it is
probable that the majority of drug is still spread along the oesophageal
groove and omasum rather than arriving in the abomasum as a discrete slug
of drug. For the benzimidazole anthelmintics, albendazole (19), fenbendazole
(21) and oxfendazole (20), their overall plasma and abomasal kinetics were
not altered markedly in these animals where groove closure could be shown
to have occurred (by the appearance of drug in the abomasum within 20 min
of oral administration). Oxfendazole, given intra-ruminally or orally, to
cattle in a cross-over experiment, gave rise to areas under the plasma
concentration/time curve which were not significantly different (26) and
albendazole had similar kinetics in sheep given as a paste or as a drench
suspension (23).

It is surprising how few studies show a biphasic pattern of drug
absorption; one of the consequences of presenting meaned values is that
this initial peak, since it can occur at varied times, is minimised, and
most pharmacokinetic computer models cannot cope with it and also abolish
it.

Early work which indicated that metal salts (sodium bicarbonate in sheep
(37), copper sulphate in cattle (9)) caused oesophageal groove closure,
and which led to suggestions that this might be usefully utilised in drug
administration has been largely discounted. Orskov and Benzie (29) failed
to demonstrate regular closure using such solutions.

VI OTHER INFLUENCES ON DRUG PHARMACOKINETICS IN THE RUMINANT ANIMAL

VI.1. Saliva

The production of a large amount (about 10 l in sheep; 140 l in cattle)
of alkaline saliva (pH 8.2) (13) can be a source of drug to the rumen.
Drugs diffuse into saliva rapidly by diffusion and as predicted the
highest concentrations are obtained with acidic drugs (barbiturates/sulfo-

namides) with maximal concentrations up to 3.8 times the free (non-protein bound) drug in plasma (32). Salivary production, which is one to two times the extracellular volume daily, could therefore have some major influence in prolonging drug kinetics for drugs not metabolized in the rumen, or as a route of drug excretion for systemically administered drugs destroyed by the rumen flora.

VI.2. Protein-bound drug

TABLE 2. The protein binding of various drugs at the same concentration in plasma of different species.

PROTEIN (%) BINDING OF DRUGS IN DIFFERENT SPECIES

	Salicylic Acid	Amphetamine	Quinine	Chloramphenicol
Goat	62	41	72	30
Pony	54	25	69	30
Dog	60	27	75	40
Cat	59	26	85	38
Swine	68	40	85	35
Human	69	--	82	46

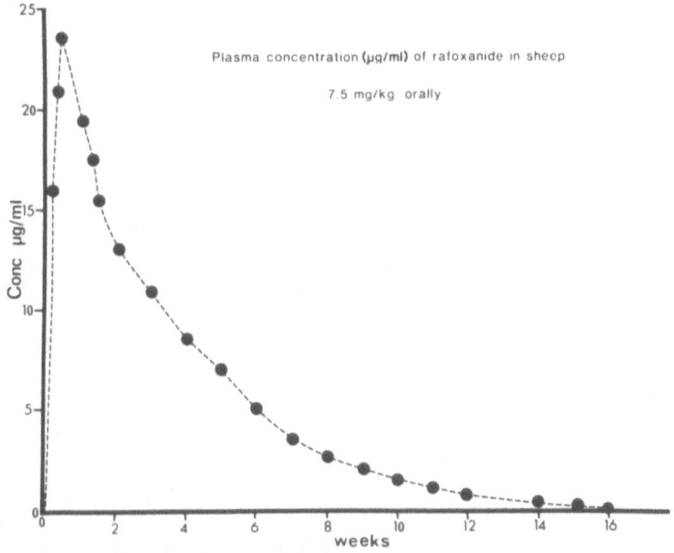

Plasma concentration (µg/ml) of rafoxanide in sheep

7.5 mg/kg orally

FIGURE 10. The mean concentration of rafoxanide in the plasma of sheep (n = 6) after oral administration of 7.5 mg/kg.

266

As in all other species, many drugs are extensively bound to plasma
proteins (principally albumin) in ruminant animals. Bound drug is unavailable for distribution/metabolism or excretion. No obvious pattern of
differences in protein binding exists between ruminants and monogastric
animals (11) (Table 2). For some drugs, for example, the salicylanilide
flukicides, strong extensive protein binding produces exceptionally long
half lives (Fig. 10).

VI.3. Drug metabolism - liver
Ruminants and other herbivorous animals have a much greater capacity for
metabolism by conjugation mechanisms (Phase II metabolism) than carnivores
or omnivores. Thus drugs such as chloramphenicol (25) and salicylic acid
(conjugated as glucuronide) have a relatively short half-life in sheep,
goats, cattle and horses (11). However, Phase I metabolic reactions (principally oxidative reactions) are more unpredictable between species. It is
our observation that cattle have a greater capacity for oxidative reactions
than sheep (goats similar to cattle) especially for the benzimidazole
anthelmintics resulting in higher dosage rates being necessary for cattle.

VI.4. Drug metabolism - rumen

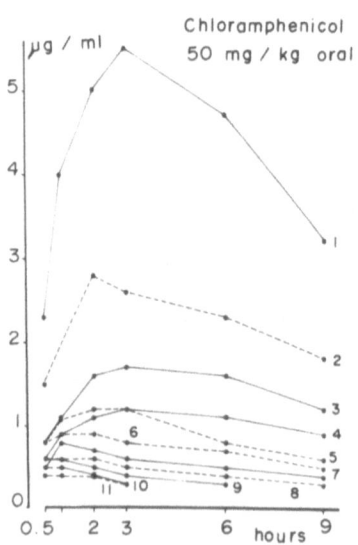

FIGURE 11. Plasma concentrations
of chloramphenicol after oral
administration (50 mg/kg) to a
calf at weeks 1-11 after birth
(ref. 4).

Metabolism by the rumen flora (see chapter 8 in this book) is principally by reduction and rapid destruction of chloramphenicol (34) and trimethoprim occurs. As the rumen develops in the young animal so the rate of destruction increases (4) (Fig. 11). Oxfendazole and albendazole sulfoxide are reduced to the respective sulfides by ruminal flora and ivermectin also appears to be rapidly destroyed by ruminal contents (30).

VII CONCLUSIONS AND PRACTICAL CONSEQUENCES OF THE RETICULO-RUMEN AS A PHARMACOKINETIC COMPARTMENT

1. For solubilised or readily dissolving drugs, the rumen serves to delay the onset of action. Whether the drug is a weak acid, strong acid or weak base, since absorption from the abomasum/duodenum is relatively rapid, time to maximum concentration is similar - 4-8 h in sheep, similar in goats/cattle - and is due to the arrival of the aqueous phase of the rumen contents in the abomasum.

If the drug has a short plasma half life (as determined by intravenous administration), then useful systemic concentration will not be achieved except at excessive dosages e.g., salicylate, xanthines, chloramphenicol and trimethoprim.

Strong bases, such as neomycin and apramycin, will remain essentially ionized at all gut pHs and will not be extensively absorbed. For example, only 11% of apramycin is absorbed after oral administration (38).

2. For drugs which are poorly soluble in rumen contents, the time to maximum concentration will be longer due to slower passage of solid forms from the rumen. Drugs in this category are the more insoluble benzimidazoles, albendazole, fenbendazole, oxfendazole and the flukicide, rafoxanide. This has been of value in extending their plasma-kinetics. For the benzimidazoles this makes them much more effective than earlier benzimidazoles at a single dose in the ruminant animal. For such drugs micronisation of drug particles will assist ultimate dissolution and will aid the extent of absorption as has been shown for oxfendazole (33). Drugs too insoluble in rumen or abomasal contents may be relatively unavailable, some of the drug being excreted undissolved in faeces. This may be the case with fenbendazole (22) where the relative bioavailability compared with an equivalent dose of oxfendazole (21) is reduced.

3. The view of the reticulo-rumen as a relatively inert reservoir allows its use for slow-release drug forms when the rumen boluses are

made of sufficient size and density to be retained there. This has been
used with morantel ("Paratect" bolus, Pfizer) with about 1 mg/kg/day
being released through a semi-permeable membrane. The technique will
become widely used in steady-release and pulse-release rumen boluses for
endo and ecto parasiticides.

REFERENCES

1. Aitken, M.M. and Sanford, J.: Res. Vet. Sci. 19, 241-244 (1975)

2. Austin, F.H.: Fed. Proc. 26, 1001-1005 (1967)

3. De Backer, P., Braeckman, R., Belpaire, F. and Debackere, J.: J. Vet.
   Pharmacol. Therap. 3, 29-33 (1980)

4. De Backer, P., Debackere, M. and De Corte-Baeten, K.: J. Vet.
   Pharmacol. Therap. 2, 195-202 (1979)

5. Baggot, J.D., Davis, L.E. and Reuning, R.H.: Arch. Int. Pharmacodyn.
   Therap. 202, 17-23 (1973)

6. Bischop, C.R., Janzen, R.E., Landals, D.C. et al.: Can. Vet. J.
   14, 269-271 (1973)

7. Bogan, J.A., Galbraith, E.A., Baxter, P., Ali, N.M. and Marriner, S.E.:
   Vet. Rec. 115, 599-600 (1984)

8. Bogan, J.A., Marriner, S.E. and Galbraith, E.A.: Res. Vet. Sci. 32,
   124-126 (1982)

9. Clunies, Ross, I.: Austr. Vet. J. 10, 11 (1934)

10. Corker, E.: M.S. Thesis, Univ. of Minnesota (1966)

11. Davis, L.E., Davis, C.N. and Baggot, J.D.: In: Research Animals in
    Medicine. Harrison, L.T. (ed), Washington, D.C., U.S. Dept. of Health
    Education and Welfare Publ. No. (NH) 72-33, pp. 715-732 (1973)

12. Davis, L.E. and Westfall, B.A.: Am. J. Vet. Res. 33, 1253-1262 (1972)

13. Dobson, A.: Fed. Proc. 26, 994-1000 (1967)

14. Hofmann, R.R.: In: The Ruminant Stomach. East African Literature
    Bureau, Nairobi, p. 27 (1973)

15. Jenkins, W.L., Davis, L.E. and Boulos, B.M.: Am. J. Vet. Res. 36,
    1771-1776 (1975)

16. Kelly, J.D., Hall, C.A., Whitlock, H.V., Thompson, H.G., Campbell, N.J.
    and Martin, I.C.A.: Res. Vet. Sci. 22, 161-168 (1977)

17. Magnussen, M.P.: Acta Pharmacol. Toxicol, 26, 130-144 (1968)

18. Marriner, S.E.: Ph.D. Thesis, University of Glasgow (1981)

19. Marriner, S.E. and Bogan, J.A.: J. Vet. Pharmacol. Therap. 2, 109-115

(1979)

20. Marriner, S.E. and Bogan, J.A.: Am. J. Vet. Res. 41, 1126-1129 (1980)

21. Marriner, S.E. and Bogan, J.A.: Am. J. Vet. Res. 42, 1143-1145 (1981)

22. Marriner, S.E. and Bogan, J.A.: Am. J. Vet. Res. 42, 1146-1148 (1981)

23. Marriner, S.E., Bogan, J.A. and Vandaele, W.: Zbl. Vet. Med. B, 28, 19-26 (1981)

24. McManus, E.C., Washko, F.V. and Tocco, D.J.: Am. J. Vet. Res. 27, 849-855 (1966)

25. Neff, C.A., Davis, L.E., Baggot, J.D. and Powers, T.E.: Am. J. Vet. Res. 33, 2259-2266 (1972)

26. Ngomuo, A.J., Marriner, S.E. and Bogan, J.A.: Vet. Res. Commun. 8, 187-193 (1984)

27. Nimmo, W.S.: In: Drug Absorption. Prescott, L.F. and Nimmo, W.S. (eds), M.T.P. Press, Lancaster, p. 12 (1981)

28. Olowookorun, M.O.: Res. Vet. Sci. 28, 254-255 (1980)

29. Ørskov, E.R. and Benzie, D.: Brit. J. Nutr. 23, 788 (1970)

30. Prichard, R.K., Steel, J.W., Lacey, E. and Hennessy, D.R.: J. Vet. Pharmacol. Therap. 8, 88-94 (1985)

31. Rankin, A.D.: Fed. Proc. 1, 70 (1942)

32. Rasmussen, F.: Acta Pharmacol. Toxicol. 21, 11-19 (1969)

33. Shastri, S., Mroszezak, E., Prichard, R.K., Parekh, P., Nguyen, T.H., Hennessy, D.R. and Schlitz, R.: Am. J. Vet. Res. 41, 2095-2101 (1980)

34. Theodorides, V.J., Di Cuollo, C.J., Guarini, J.R. and Pagano, J.F.: Am. J. Vet. Res. 29, 643-645 (1968)

35. Trautman, A.: Arch. Tierernähr. Tierzucht 9, 178 (1933)

36. Tunnicliff, E.A. and Swingle, K.F.: Am. J. Vet. Res. 26, 920-927 (1965)

37. Wester, J.: In: Die Physiologie und Pathologie der Vormagen beim Rinde. Schoetz, R. (ed), Berlin, p. 34 (1926)

38. Ziv, G., Bar, A., Soback, S., Elad, D. and Nouws, J.F.M.: J. Vet. Pharmacol. Therap. 8, 95-104 (1985)

11. DRUG-INDUCED EFFECTS ON RETICULAR GROOVE REFLEX, ERUCTATION AND RUMINATION

L.A.A. OOMS , A.D. DEGRYSE , A. WEYNS , S. BOUISSET AND Y. RUCKEBUSCH

I   INTRODUCTION

The alimentary canal function of ruminants in terms of rumen volume, passage of digesta and particle size is a topic worthwhile being investigated. Extensive studies on the manipulation of its function, using chemical as well as mechanical stimuli have been performed over the years.

For example the closure of the reticular groove could be prevented by dosing via a tube in the thoracic oesophagus (1) and by the use of anticholinergic drugs which are known to suppress its closure during sucking (2). Its activation could be obtained by antidopaminergic agents. It could be beneficial in early phases of growth to bypass the rumen or to increase rumen emptying by relaxation of the reticulo-omasal orifice (3).

Feeding increases the frequency and amplitude of primary rumen contractions but also stimulates salivation with release of osmotically active ingredients in the rumen (4). The diversion of saliva, entering the rumen, elevate the volatile fatty acids (VFA) concentration, resulting in pH decrease which in turn reduces rumen motility (5,6). In steers, saliva secretion during eating was increased more than four times when fed hay instead of concentrates; in dairy cows, saliva flow (about 200 liter per day) was reduced by 40 to 50% when ground hay replaced long hay diets (7).

Local blood flow could also be involved in the neutralization of the acid pH after intake of concentrates. In conscious sheep, total forestomach capillary blood flow (7.5 ml/min/kg) was about 7% of the cardiac output. Although 95% of the flow was in the mucosa and only 5% in the muscle layers no studies have been done about the relation between blood flow and control of rumen pH. Blood flow in the rumen was 6 times higher than in the reticulum and 4.4 times higher than in the omasum. Mucosal capillary flow per unit area of mucosal epithelium in the omasum (disregarding the increment in area due to papillae) was only one-third of that in the ventral rumen (long papillae), notwithstanding the fact that there is a considerable uptake of ions and fluid in the omasum. Flow in the dorsal rumen (short papillae) was about half the flow in the ventral rumen (8).

Dairy cows suffering from water deprivation during dry weather in summer, during freezing weather in winter and during transport can lose 100 kg body-weight in 72 h, a value about twice that observed in steers deprived of water for three days, the difference being due to cumulative losses of water in milk (9). In such cases, anorexia with a very low rate of reticulo-rumen contractions is observed.

When cows are given hay directly into the rumen, the amount of time spent ruminating is increased: 630 min (44% of 24 h) versus 430 min (30%). The beneficial effects of an increased time spent chewing the cut is an

increased salivary secretion rate, hence the carbonate-phosphate buffering
of the rumen contents by saliva flow. The activity of the ascending
reticular formation is at a low level during rumination, hence a drowsy
state which is facilitated by neuroleptic drugs. The increased afferent
nerve discharge subsequent to activation of the reticulum by adrenaline (6)
is enhanced by interaction with the opioid inhibitory system (10,11).

The purpose of this work is to present recent trials in manipulating
rumen bypass, in enhancement of rumination and alleviation of free-gas
bloat and in enhancement of rumen motility and manipulation of rumen
metabolism.

II SMOOTH MUSCLES

Smooth muscle membrane permeability changes usually affect membrane
potential by allowing one or more ions to pass through the membrane more
freely. Since none of the ions in smooth muscle cells is in equilibrium at
a membrane potential of - 50 to - 60 mV, there will be a net flow of ions
into and out of the cells, tending to move the membrane potential closer
to equilibrium. Membrane depolarization usually results in a contraction,
although membrane potential is not a prerequisite for induction of
contraction in all smooth muscle cells (12). Two pathways exist for
transmembrane influx of Ca^{2+} : activation by changes in membrane potential
and a receptor-linked Ca^{2+} channel, activated by binding of agonists to
their receptors. Contraction of smooth muscles can be initiated by changes
in membrane permeability either after binding of agonists to their
receptors or after exposure to high K^+ concentrations (13,14). In either
instance, electrical or chemical cell membrane signals indirectly activate
contractile elements by releasing membrane-bound Ca^{2+}, or increasing Ca^{2+}
influx, or both. Three sources of Ca can be distinguished: the free Ca in
the extracellular fluid, the Ca bound to the surface membrane and the
intracellular Ca in endoplasmic reticulum and mitochondria. Ca influx
during receptor activation seems to be different from Ca influx induced by
membrane depolarization (15). Two pathways of transmembrane flux of Ca^{2+}
exist: a voltage-dependent Ca^{2+} channel, activated by changes in membrane
permeability, and a receptor-linked channel, activated by binding of
agonists to their receptors (Fig. 1). The plasma membrane of vascular,
intestinal and myometrical smooth muscle seems to be equipped with the

274

exchange system to regulate intracellular Ca^{2+} concentration (16).

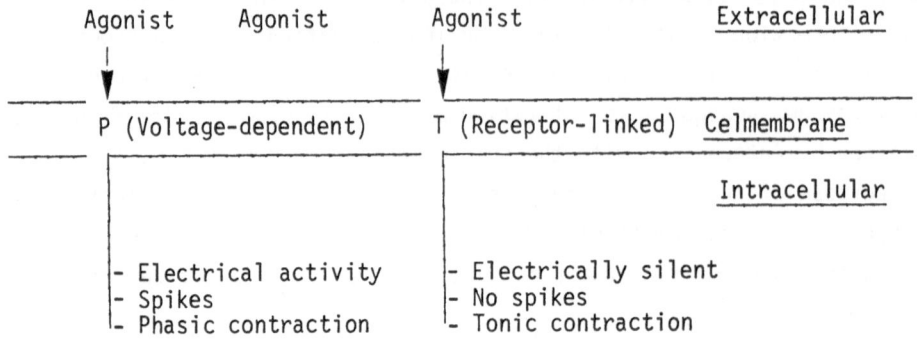

FIGURE 1. Scheme of the differences between activation of the voltage-dependent and receptor-linked channel.

A $(Ca^{2+}-Mg^{2+})$-ATPase was demonstrated in pig stomach muscle, which could be purified on a calmodulin affinity column and is calmodulin-dependent (17,18). This protein is able, when incorporated into lipid vesicles, to transport Ca^{2+} in an uphill fashion if ATP is present in the medium (19).

Receptor agonists induce contraction without changing membrane potential in smooth muscles that do not generate action potentials or in depolarized smooth muscles (13). All eukaryotic cells contain inositol lipids. Phospholipase C catalyses the breakdown of phosphatidylinositol 4,5-biphosphate, a multiple-charged anion that has a very high affinity for Ca^{2+} (higher than that of EDTA) and exhibits a rapid turnover in vivo. Its hydrophilic/hydrophobic solubility partition coefficient is markedly altered when Ca^{2+} replaces monovalent phosphate counterions (20,21). The receptor-mediated breakdown of phospholipids is not mediated by an increase in cytosol Ca^{2+} but closely coupled to receptor occupation. Inositol triphosphate (IP_3) and also the lipid soluble product of phosphatidyl-inositol 4,5-biphosphate breakdown, 1,2 diacylglycerol (DAG), act as second messengers in the cells (22). The phosphoryl groups, covalently attached to PI_3, turn over extremely rapidly. The rise in IP_3 may be the means by which the intracellular (nonmitochondrial) pools of calcium are mobilized (23). The less Ca^{2+} bound to inositol 1,4,5-triphosphate, the stronger the attraction of Ca^{2+}. Diacylglycerol acts on its own right and activates a specific, calcium-activated, phospholipid-dependent protein kinase, C-kinase, which catalyzes the phosphorylation of a specific group of protein substrates. Diacylglycerol is one of the sources of arachidonic acid (liberated by phospholipase A_2) which serves as the substrate for prostaglandin, leukotrine and/or thromboxane synthesis (24,25).

A group of organic Ca^{2+} antagonists or Ca^{2+} channel blockers (including verapamil, methoxyverapamil (D600), nifedipine, diltiazem and flunarizine) are specific inhibitors of Ca^{2+} influx through voltage-dependent Ca^{2+} channels (26,27,28). Nitrocompounds, especially sodium nitro-prusside, are selective inhibitors of the receptor-linked Ca^{2+} channel (29). Tetraethyl-ammonium (TEA) increases spike activity of many spike-generating smooth muscles and induces spike potentials in spontaneously inactive guinea-pig fundic muscles (30,31). No effect was observed on the spontaneously inactive ruminal preparations by micromolar TEA. Acetylcholine (10^{-6} g/ml) applied to TEA (3×10^{-3} to 10^{-2} M) pretreated ruminal preparations produced no spike-free tonic contraction but spike activity and phasic contractions (32).

On mucosa-free circular smooth muscle strips of the dorsal ruminal sac of sheep, acetylcholine (10^{-9} - 10^{-6} g/ml) induces dose-dependent spike-free tonic contractions. These contractions are verapamil and methoxyverapamil (D600) resistant and are suppressed by sodium nitro-prusside (10^{-6} M). In Ca^{++}-free EGTA-containing solutions, no tonic activity was observed. EGTA not only inactivates extracellular Ca^{2+}, but also the membrane-bound Ca^{2+}. Ba^{2+} or Sr^{2+} applied in normal Krebs solution led to the appearance of spike activity, determining phasic contractions in the spontaneously inactive ruminal muscle, and clear-cut membrane depolarization and the appearance of spike potentials. The electrical activity was accompanied by an increase in muscle tone and the occurrence of phasic contractions. Verapamil or D600 completely eliminated the Ba^{2+}- or Sr^{2+}-induced spike potentials and the related phasic muscle contractions.

The organic Ca^{2+} antagonists or Ca^{2+} channel blockers (verapamil and methoxyverapamil) are specific inhibitors of Ca^{2+} influx through voltage-dependent Ca^{2+} channels and inhibit both the increase in Ca^{2+} influx and the contraction. In spontaneous inactive ruminal preparations incubated in nutrient solution in which Ca^{2+} was substituted by Ba^{2+}, the application of Ach did not lead to an increase in the spike-free tone as was observed in normal Krebs solution, but induced spikes and phasic contractions (32). These experiments clearly demonstrate that a voltage-

linked and also a receptor-linked contraction is present in the smooth
muscle of the sheep dorsal ruminal sac.

Many hormones and neurotransmitters (e.g. glucagon and adrenaline
acting through its beta receptor) trigger the activation of adenylate
cyclase (AC). Stimulation of AC (Fig. 2) results in an elevation of the
intracellular concentration of cAMP, which transmits the hormonal signal
by activating cyclic AMP dependent protein kinase (PK).

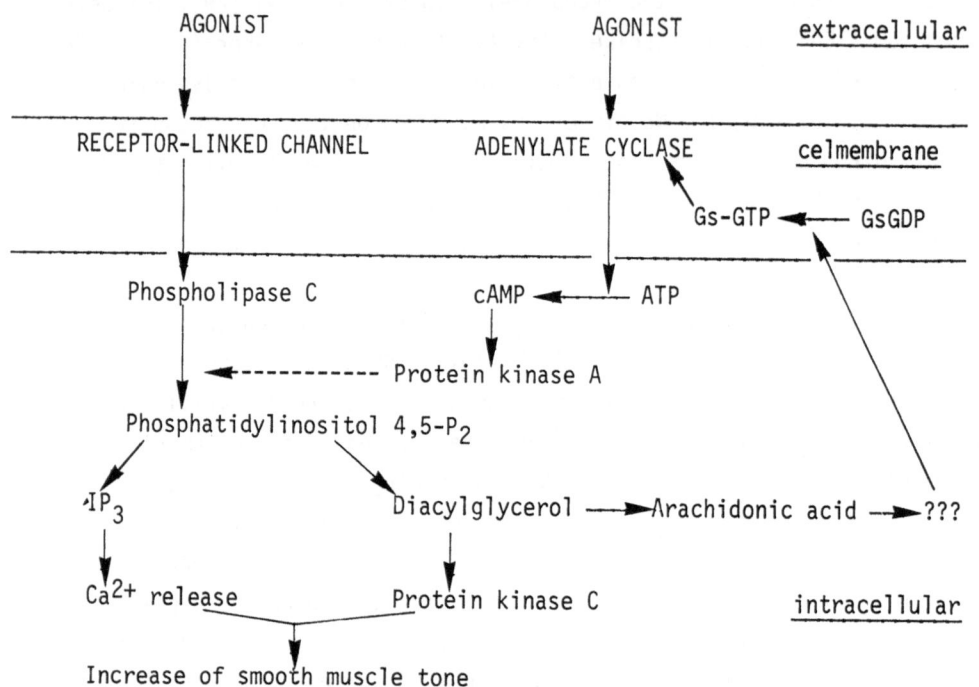

FIGURE 2. Possible mechanism of action of adenylate cyclase in the control
of smooth muscle tone (receptor-linked channel).

This enzyme phosphorylates a variety of intracellular proteins and thereby
regulates their activities (e.g. serine (and occasionally threonine)
residues C-terminal to pairs of adjacent basic amino acids: ARG-ARG-X-SER
and LYS-ARG-X-Y-SER- (33). Some hormones inhibit adenylate cyclase
(including enkephalins and adrenaline (acting through its alpha 2
receptor)) and activate the GTPase activity of a guanine nucleotide binding
protein converting it from a GTP-liganded form (Gs-GTP) that stimulates

adenylate cyclase to an inactive GDP-liganded form (Gs-GDP). Hormones that activate adenylate cyclase exert their effect by promoting the conversion of Gs-GDP to Gs-GTP (34). Indeed, adenylate cyclase consists of a recognition component (a stimulatory receptor unit and an inhibitory receptor unit) and a catalytic unit. Mg^{2+} stimulates activity to levels approaching that observed with hormones. Ca^{2+} at physiological concentrations can stimulate as well as inhibit smooth muscle adenylate cyclase activity. The stimulation of adenylate cyclase activity is mediated by calmodulin. The level of calmodulin associated with smooth muscle adenylate cyclase may modulate the response (both stimulatory and inhibitory) of the enzyme to Ca^{2+} (35). Forskolin, a steroid-like compound, stimulates the activity of all animal cell cyclase systems, but acts on a component distinct from the 45,000 or 55,000 dalton unit through which GTP acts (36). Sodium nitroprusside, nitroglycerin and related smooth muscle relaxants were reported to increase smooth muscle levels of cGMP (37). Nitroprusside is unstable in aqueous solutions and releases nitric oxide. Nitric oxide is a potent activator of guanylate cyclase. cGMP stimulates the activity of the sarcolemmal Ca^{2+} extrusion ATPase in a concentration dependent manner. In this way cGMP seems to be involved in the relaxing effect of AC stimulation.

Especially the smooth muscles of the sphincter regions and also of the stomach (reservoir function) are equiped with both voltage- and receptor-linked channels. The first regulates the phasic contractions while the second is involved in the tonic contractions.

The results of in vitro studies on mucosa-free strips of the smooth muscles of the different compartments of the forestomach of cattle with sodium nitroprusside (10^{-10} - 10^{-5} M; specific blocker of the receptor-linked channel) and verapamil (10^{-10} - 10^{-5} M; blocker of the voltage-dependent channel) are shown in figs. 3-6 (38).

The results of these studies show that a tonic component (inhibition by sodium nitroprusside) is present in LES, RET, RDS, RVS and FUN of the longitudinal muscles and in the LES, RET, RDS, RVS and FUN of the circular muscles. In the OMA, a reduction of the longitudinal muscle tone was found only at a dose level of 10^{-5} M. Verapamil reduced dose-dependent the muscle tone of the RET longitudinal muscles. The action on the longitudinal and circular muscles of the RDS and VDS was variable. OMA smooth muscles nearly responded.

278

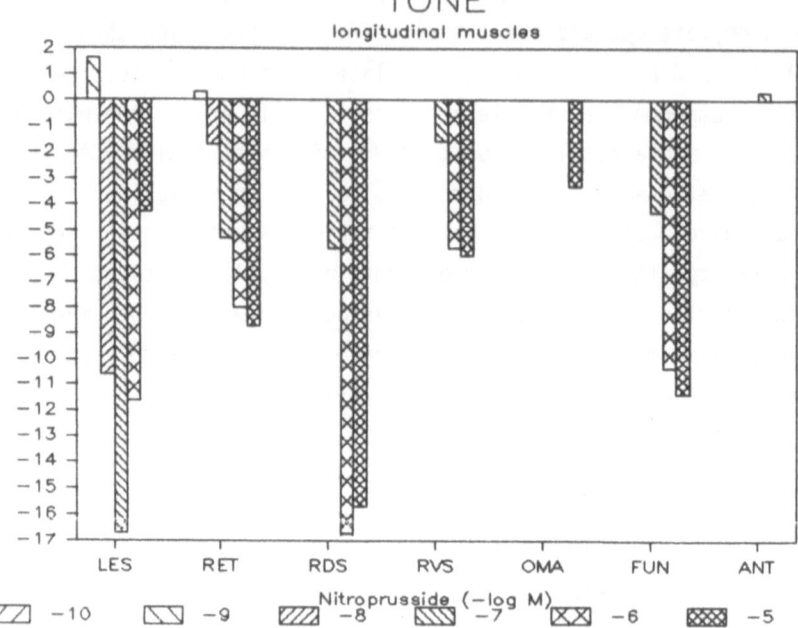

FIGURE 3. Dosis-titration of sodium nitroprusside on the longitudinal smooth
muscle tone. LES = lower oesophageal sphincter; RET = reticulum;
RDS = rumen dorsal sac; RVS = rumen ventral sac; OMA = omasum;
FUN = fundus; ANT = antrum; PYL = pylorus.
1 unit at the vertical axis means 0.2 gram tension

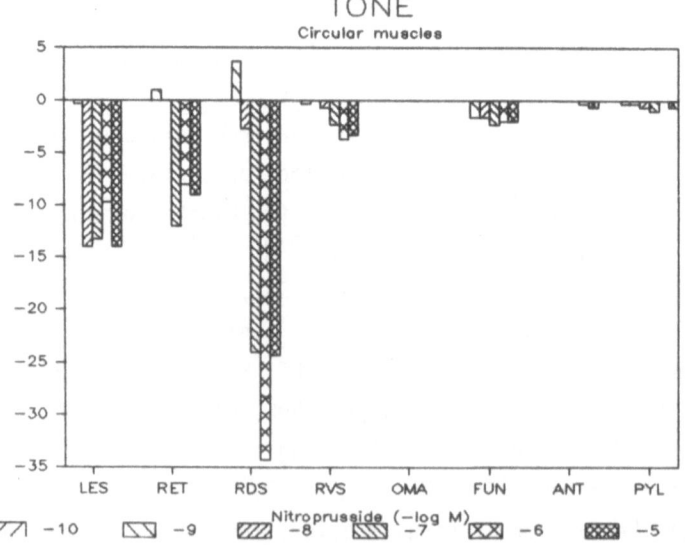

FIGURE 4. Dosis-titration of sodium nitroprusside on the circular smooth
muscle tone. Legends see Fig. 3.

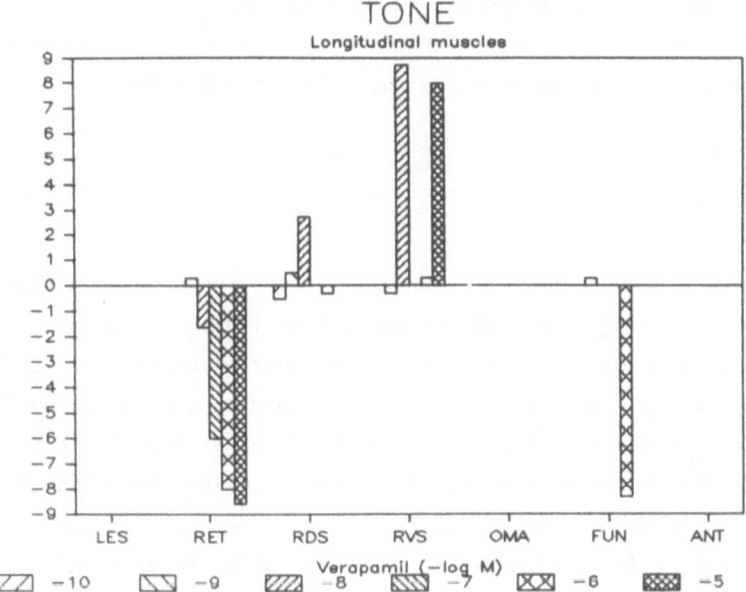

FIGURE 5. Dosis-titration of verapamil on the longitudinal smooth muscle tone. Legends see Fig. 3.

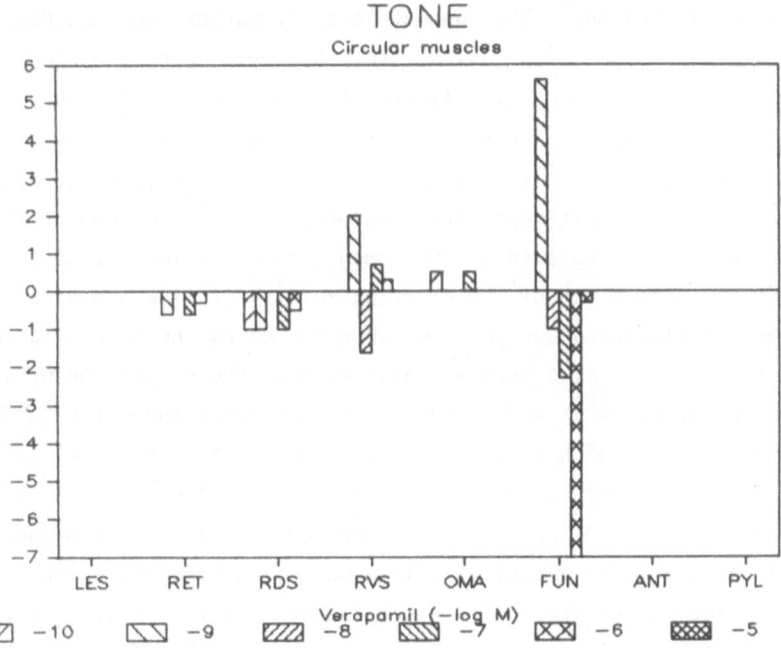

FIGURE 6. Dosis-titration of verapamil on the circular smooth muscle tone. Legends see Fig. 3.

On the FUN circular smooth muscles, a reduction of tone was observed; the FUN longitudinal muscles responded only at 10^{-6} M.

These data indirectly suggest that muscle tone may be of importance for the adaptation to changing intraluminal volume and for the control of digesta flow.

III RUMEN BYPASS

The reticular groove reflex is an all or none response in bottle-fed lambs or calves allowing the direct passage of liquids into the abomasum. The oesophageal groove contracts in two distinct movements. First, by shortening the right and left lips become firmly opposed allowing direct passage of 30 to 40% of the volume of liquid towards the abomasum. Then, the closure can be complete if the lips invert, mainly the right lip. In this case, 75 to 90% of the liquid ingested is recovered in the abomasum.

The closure reflex, activated in adult ruminants (copper salt in sheep, sodium salts in weaned calves) was studied in animals fitted with rumen fistules by measuring the proportion of ingested liquid feed found in the rumen, using polyethylene glycol (PEG 4000) as a marker at a low concentration in the meal. The concentration of markers such as PEG, xylose (39,40) or a drug like sodium salicylates (5% w/v) can be measured directly in the blood or in the content delivered in the abomasum of calves fitted with a reentrant cannula placed immediately distal to the pylorus. Less than 20% of the milk given to calves until the age of 1 year is recovered in the rumen and for milk-replacers, the proportion of soybean or fish protein concentrate recovered in the rumen (10%) is lower than for whey protein (45%). Alteration of the clotting ability of milk proteins or their replacement by alkanes grown yeats or whey increases the rate of abomasal emptying (41). It has also been established that the proportion of water recovered in the rumen is much higher in calves receiving water *ad libitum* (60%) than in those which did not receive water during the night (30%). Finally, young ruminants given milk to appetite, will eat little solid food. Conversely, solid food will be eaten earlier, if the allowance of milk is restricted. The amount of solid food eaten (chopped dried grass) is not affected by the dry-matter concentration (10 versus 20%) of the milk substitute, but is decreased by the amount of milk consumed (12 versus 20% of body weight). Large amounts of milk in the first month of life, then followed by restriction of milk, should help to ensure rapid and early growth. However, this practice is accompanied by a higher risk of digestive disorders, e.g. gastric paresis resulting in abnormal abomasal emptying (42,43).

III.1. Manipulation of the reticular groove reflex

The two reasons for manipulating this closure reflex in ruminants are: (i) to avoid activation of the reflex from oropharyngeal origin in mature ruminants during oral dosing; (ii) to activate the reflex in calves thus avoiding the escape of milk into the rumen, e.g. when pharyngitis or oropharyngeal abcesses prevent the afferent arc of the reflex to be operative.

III.1.1. Intraruminal drug delivery

In adult sheep, to ascertain that the drug remains into the reticulorumen for a local action, three possibilities are at hand to prevent the activation of the reflex: injection of atropine, application of local anaesthetics to the oral cavity and drug delivery into the thoracic oesophagus via a gastric tube. The latter procedure is to be recommended for its simplicity and effectiveness. As shown by the peaks of blood concentration of meclofenamic acid, a single peak occurs at 2.5 h after oesophageal dosing, instead of two peaks after oral dosing: the first due to the rumen bypass and the second due to ruminal release (Fig. 7).

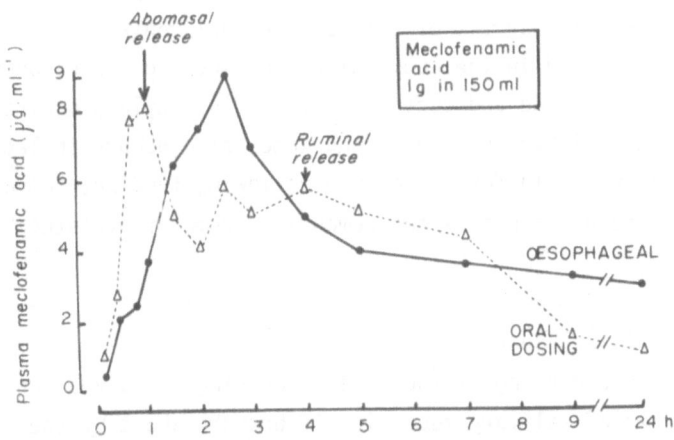

FIGURE 7. Plasma concentrations after oral dosing in 150 ml of water (drenching bottle) or via a tube of soft PVC passed through the centre of a small wooden gag to reach the midthoracic region in mature sheep (from 1).

III.1.2. Teat versus bucket feeding

The xylose absorption test is applied to evaluate the degree of groove closure in sheep after cupric ions administration (10 ml of 10% $CuSO_4$). A detectable rise in xylose concentration occurs after D-xylose (0.5 g/kg BW) administered via an oesophageal tube but not via a rumen cannula (44). In calves, at the time of weaning, no rise in xylosemia is detectable when bucket fed, even after a 24-h fast (food and water). Teat feeding always results in a marked increase of xylosemia within 60 min.

pH measurement of the chyme in the duodenum of calves showed a marked increase by 2 to 3 units due to saliva swallowed during teat feeding, suggesting a closure of the oesophageal groove, while there was only a tendency of increase in pH after bucket feeding. An almost complete closure must occur for teat feeding since duodenal pH values were very similar to those seen after a direct abomasal administration according to the procedure used by Pearson & Aldwin (45).

A major component of the oesophageal groove reflex is evidenced by Orskov et al. (46) showing its closure while seeing teat-bottle. When, in a lamb sodium salicylate containing milk (5% w/v) is administered into the lower oesophagus, the volume collected through an abomasal fistula constitutes 20% and contains 16.6% salicylate derivatives. In a trained subject, the increased excitability provoked by showing the teat-bottle is sufficient to double or triple the volume of liquid collected at the abomasal fistula after administration into the lower oesophagus.

In adult sheep, showing arrest of reticulo-ruminal contractions, the volume of liquid collected in the abomasum during sucking corresponds to 86.4% of the ingested volume and contains 73.3% of salicylate derivatives.

A significant ruminal bypass of drinking water also occurs in lactating cows. When water is withheld for 4.5 or 9 h following feeding, 18% of drinking water was found to bypass the rumen in 8 rumen-fistulated Holstein cows (47).

III.1.3. Role of salivary secretion

Among the changes occurring at the time of weaning in calves, an increase in the rate of salivary secretion is brought about by the roughage intake (Fig. 8), reaching a rate of 0.5 ml/kg.min^{-1} by 10-12 weeks of age (48). The concomitant changes in gastric secretions and motor functions are only partially known, except that the acid secretion

becomes continuous in relation with the permanent delivery of reticulo-
ruminal contents. Accordingly, when a small amount of milk is suckled, a
relatively large quantity of saliva simultaneously passes into the ventral
regions of the abomasum (49). This amount of bicarbonate is sufficient to
transiently increase the pH (1.5-2 units) of the chyme for 60 min. This
rise in pH is enhanced by secretagogues and further increased when the acid
secretion is partially blocked by an antihistaminic drug (histamine 2
antagonist).

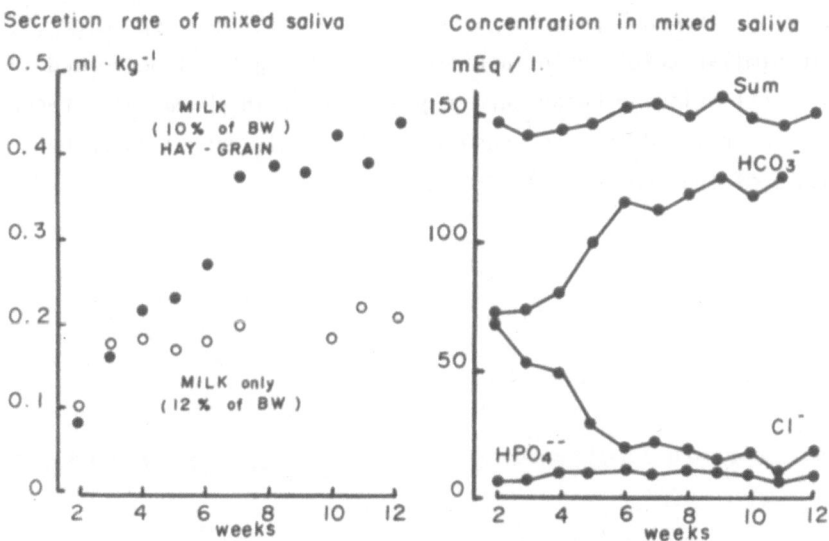

FIGURE 8. Development of the rate of salivary secretion and concentration
of anions in mixed saliva of calves receiving hay in addition to a maximum
milk intake of 6 kg hay and in 3 calves receiving only milk at 12.5% of
body weight (48).

III.1.4. Activation of the reticular groove reflex and rumen motility

The closure of the groove is accompanied by an inhibition of rumino-
reticular contractions as reported by Schalk and Amadon (50) in an adult
cow when licking salt. In a 12 month-old bull fitted with a rumen cannula,
this also occurs when sucking 1 l of milk from a watering can (51). The
inhibition in the rate and amplitude of reticulorumen contractions was
mimiked by L-DOPA (1 mg/kg) and suppressed by metoclopramide (0.2 mg/kg)
pretreatment (52). Metoclopramide is a dopamine antagonist and also acts
via the cholinergic system (53). A similar effect on reticulorumen
contractions was found with domperidone which does not penetrate the CNS to
the same extent as metoclopramide. It is possible that exepanol-HCl (which

is proven to enhance the canine LES pressure) as well as cisapride
(R 51619) behave as metoclopramide or domperidone in improving the
oesophageal groove closure (54,55).

   3 weeks after weaning, young steers (6-month old) were fitted with a
reentrant cannula distal to the pylorus. pH was measured continuously during
oral administration by drenching bottle of 2 l-milk and 30 g $NaHCO_3$. A
complete rumen bypass following domperidone (0.5 mg/kg i.m. or 0.25 mg/kg
i.v.) was found. In such cases the pH values remain at a very high level
for about 2 h. A rumen bypass was also recorded with metoclopramide (0.5
mg/kg). In similar trials using angiotensin II (1 $\mu g.kg^{-1}$) performed in
order to elicit drinking behaviour, a gradual rise in pH was also recorded,
but seem to be related to a decrease in gastric acid secretion rather than
to a closure of the groove reflex (Fig. 9).

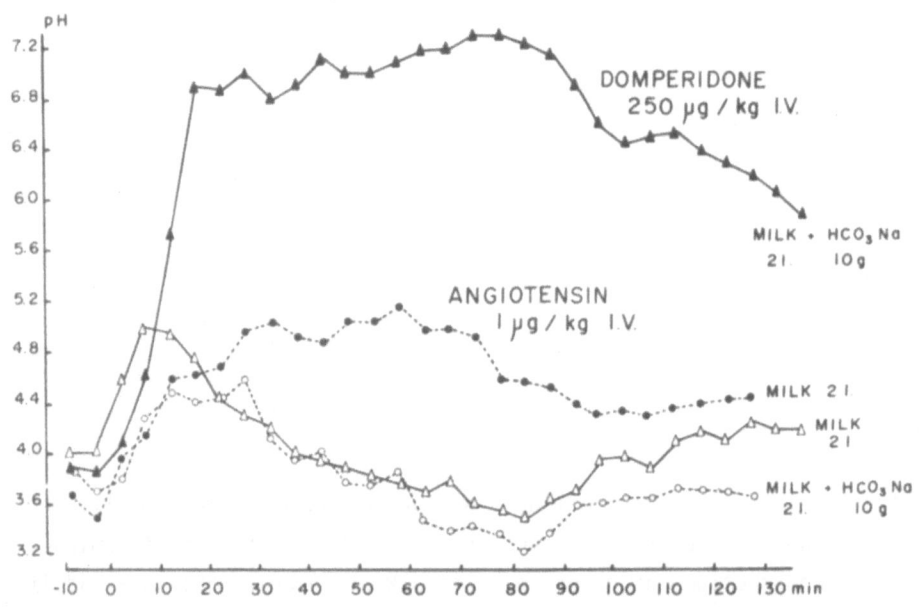

FIGURE 9. pH values of the chyme leaving the abomasum of a young steer
receiving 2 l of milk after angiotensin versus saline (dark spot)
pretreatment or 2 l of milk and sodium bicarbonate (triangle) after
domperidone versus saline.

These results, obtained within 3 weeks after weaning, became progressively
less evident suggesting that the vagally-controlled opposite effects
(closure of the groove and reticulo-ruminal inhibition) could not be
brought about with age. The reticulo-ruminal inhibition is reminiscent to

the vagally-mediated relaxation which is observed in the canine stomach during sham-feeding in experiments in dogs with Pavlov and Heidenhain pouches (56).

III.2. Gastric emptying

The basic pattern of gastric emptying in calves is exponential in form, irrespective of the volume of the meal. The half time of emptying of different volumes (about 20 min) is controlled by receptors in the duodenal bulb (57,58). Isotonic solutions of NaCl and $NaHCO_3$ activate abomasal emptying by positive feedback from the duodenum.

Acid solutions as well as many hypertonic solutions, inhibit gastric emptying by a negative feedback. The inhibitory effect of infusion of acid (60 mM HCl) in the duodenum is not modified by vagotomy but is associated with the endogenous production of somatostatin. All three gastric functions (motility, acid and pepsinogen secretions) are enhanced by duodenal infusions of isotonic $NaHCO_3$ and abolished by transthoracic vagotomy, suggesting a neural-mediated mechanism (59,60).

IV RUMINATION

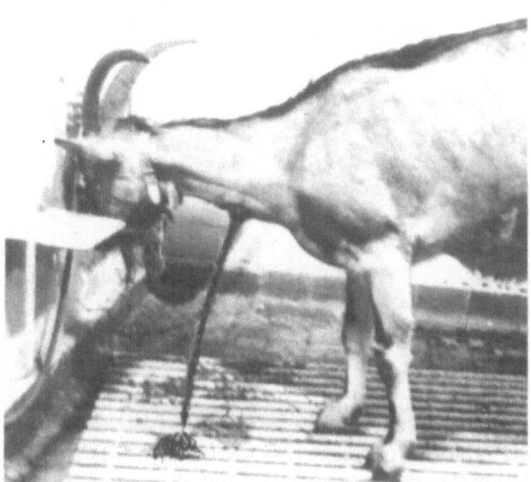

FIGURE 10. Regurgitation of reticulo-ruminal contents propelled at a velocity of 50 cm/sec from the cardia towards the oral cavity in the goat. The oesophageal cannula was opened at the end of the 3rd merycic cycle. The absence of chewing movements initiates a premature extra-reticular contraction.

An increase in the fibre content of roughage decreases the rate of feed
ingestion (expressed in gram of ingested dry matter/hour), and the number
of daily meals, but the time spent ruminating is increased up to 10 hr per
day. Since the rumen is not actively involved in rumination, this act is a
misnomer: the bolus is rejected from the reticulum and then actively carried
past the zone where oesophageal distension evokes a secondary peristaltic
wave. Speed (50 cm/sec) and force (40 mm Hg) of the contraction in the
distal half of the oesophagus during regurgitation may be sufficient to
propel the bolus into the pharynx, without further active contraction in
the proximal oesophagus (Fig. 10). The oesophageal pressure dynamics during
rumination suggest that initially reticulo-oesophageal reflux is
facilitated by the pressure gradient in the LES pressure, as has been
shown by Winship et al. (61) (Fig. 11).

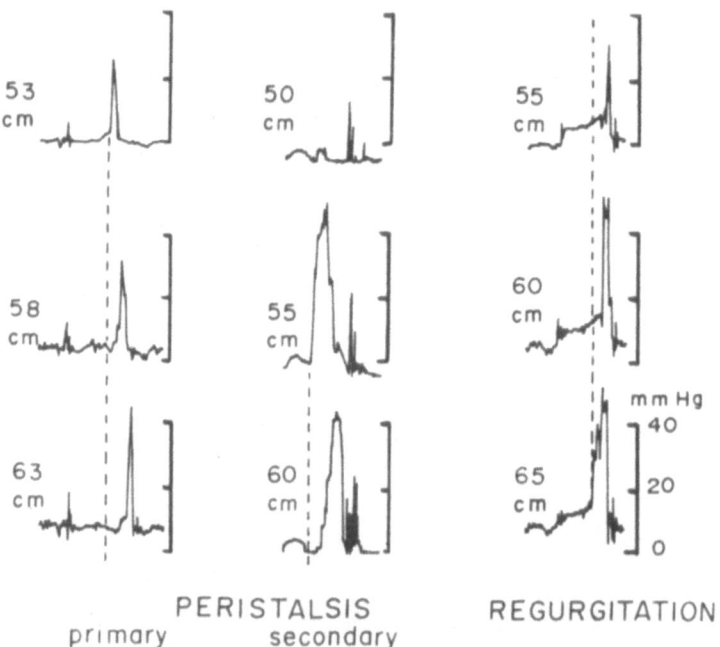

FIGURE 11. A. Primary peristalsis. The wave of positive pressure representing oesophageal muscular contraction moves down the oesophagus following
deglutition (S). B. Secondary peristalsis. Peristaltic response to
intraluminal balloon distension occurring in the distal oesophagus and
distal to the balloon. C. Rumination. An initial plateau of positive
pressure occurs simultaneously in all three leads without coincident
respiratory change and terminates in a rapid retrograde peristaltic wave.
Paper speed 10 mm/sec. The speed of retrograde waves was 42.5-53.8 cm/sec
in two sheep vs. 23 cm/sec for primary peristaltic waves and 112.5 cm/sec
vs. 30 cm/sec in a calf (61).

Tickling the LES area, the reticulo-omasal orifice as well as the reticulo-ruminal folds and the cranial pillar induces attempts to regurgitate within a few minutes, and when successful a series of merycic cycles. Accordingly, the latency between the end of a long silage meal and rumination is increased compared to a short chopped silage meal because a longer time is taken by long silage to move from the rumen into the reflexogenic area (62). Other digestive reflexogenic areas able to induce rumination are: contraction of the reticulum by adrenaline, omasal contractions elicited by pentagastrin, and spasm of the duodenal bulb evoked by several spasmogenic substances like 5-HT, tolazoline... In contrast, omaso-abomasal distension has an opposite effect, i.e. an inhibition via a neural or hormonal pathway.

Several attempts to explain the mechanisms involved in ruminating behaviour have been made. The role of supraspinal influences is based on the attainment of a regurgitation as a conditioned reflex and on the occurrence of rumination as a sequence of stereotyped motor events involving an extracontraction of the reticulum, opening of the cardia, retropulsion and chewing the cud. The replacement of rumination by pseudorumination corresponds to an inherent "drive to ruminate" and occurs where there is lack of peripheral stimulation or when there is no possibility for regurgitation, e.g. when plastic fibres are introduced into an empty rumen. Species specific differences also exist between sheep, goats and cattle, e.g. in the latency between the end of a meal and the occurrence of a period of rumination. This may vary from 10 min in cattle to 20 and 40 min in sheep and goats, respectively for hay.

Finally, the relative importance of peripheral versus central control is unclear. The inherent drive for rumination occurs as early as 5 days after birth in camels, and is present in preruminant lambs maintained on a milk diet. Pseudorumination, which can reach very high levels, is an alternative to rumination in milk-fed calves.

IV.1. Peripheral versus central control of rumination

In calves with complete separation of the rumen from the reticulum, and thus limited possibilities of rumination, the amount of time spent in pseudorumination is nearly doubled by mechanical stimulation of the rumen wall (Fig. 12). Volatile fatty acids (VFA) infusion have opposite effects on ruminating behaviour (63). During the VFA infusion, the animals become

288

restless; this is associated with vasodilation of the digestive tract and
to a large extent a peripheral effect.

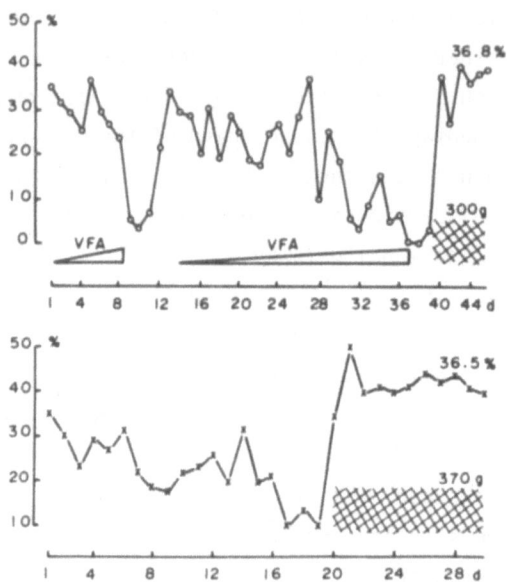

FIGURE 12. Opposite effects of volatile fatty acids and mechanical
stimulation of the isolated rumen on "pseudorumination"
(p. cent per 24 h) in two calves (63).

Central effects resembling those of GABA, a cerebral vasodilator (64),
which facilitates drowsiness and rumination (unpublished results), are
also observed with several substances which modify the metabolism of
serotonin.

It has been suggested that insulin hypoglycaemia may be a triggering
factor for the rumination centre, although the ruminant differs from other
mammals in that little glucose is absorbed from the digestive tract; the
most important source of glucose being the hepatic gluconeogenesis from
aminoacids and propionic acid. In fact, ruminant plasma glucose
concentration normally is only about one-half that of non-ruminants and
the ruminant central nervous system is unusualy resistant to the
deleterious effects of severe hypoglycaemia caused by insulin injection.
Furthermore, it is now well established that the role of insulin in the

short-term control of feeding and/or rumination, if any, depends on the
nutritional status (65). For example, the initiation of rumination in a
few minutes following i.v. insulin injection was not ascertained (66,67).
In addition, factors involved in the decrease of immunoreactive serum
insulin, like clonidine in cattle (68), or able to depress central nervous
system by their alpha2-adrenergic receptor agonistic properties, like
xylazine (69,70), have no major effect on rumination.

IV.2. Indirect enhancement of rumination

In sheep fitted with a reentrant cannula in the duodenum, the physical
stimulation may have been involved in the excess of rumination. For
example, in sheep of 43-44 kg, the time spent ruminating was 369-496 min
per 24 h 3 weeks after surgery instead of 278-343 min/24 h before (71).
This increase by 30-40% could be due to the resistance of the flow of
digesta as well as to the increased antroduodenal motility. Factors which
induce satiety like gastrin-like peptides, when administered centrally or
peripherally may enhance the occurrence of rumination. For example, the
carboxy-terminal octapeptide (CCK-OP) of cholecystokinin (CCK) which has
been identified in sheep brain as a satiety factor, may enhance arrest of
eating which is followed by rumination. The fact that several effects of
CCK-like peptides are antagonized by enkephalins, in a way which suggests
physiological antagonism by occupation of two different but opposite
receptors, is theoretically consistent with the involvement of a neuropeptidergic system in the initiation of feeding and with a role of an
enkaphalinergic pathway in the initiation of rumination. Direct evidence
of such control systems in rumination is still lacking because there seems
to be a direct relationship between the amount of dry matter intake and the
time spent ruminating. However, when growth in lambs is stimulated by
somatostatin immunization (72), both the dry matter intake and rumination
were increased.

IV.3. Role of an inhibitory opioid system

The effects of opiates on ruminant feed-intake are different from those
seen in other species (73). Morphine and apomorphine, administered at low
doses at the level of the IIIrd ventricle, induced compulsive chewing
movements (74) and reduced time spent ruminating (75). In contrast, the
area postrema which lines the margins of the IVth ventricle and is rich in

biogenic amines (76), does not operate as a metabolic sensor that regulates the periodicity of rumination. Its chronic ablation did not alter either the spontaneous feeding or ruminating behaviour in sheep (77). In a pre- liminary study in sheep, drugs able to decrease the time spent ruminating for 100 g of hay (68 ± 8 min), the systemic administration of cardiac glu- cosides was found more potent than monoaminooxydase inhibitors. The time spent ruminating was 32 min after i.v. digitaline (10 µg/kg) versus 49 and 55 min for i.m. iproniazide (20 mg/kg) and s.c. imipramine (1 mg/kg), res- pectively (78). Since the reduction of rumination without anorexia, which occurs as a side-effect of digitalis in sheep, disappears after postrumen- ectomy (77) it is suggested that the reduced time spent ruminating might be an indicator of a nauseant effect of drugs but not of a central control.

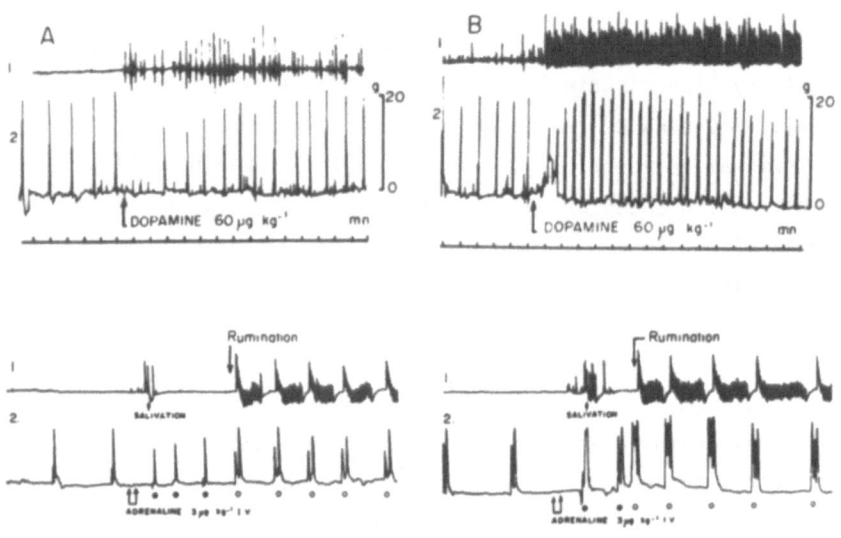

FIGURE 13. Effects of the intravenous administration (bolus) of dopamine before (A) and within 10 min after naloxone (B) on jaw movements (1) and reticular contractions (2) in sheep. The injection of dopamine induced a transient inhibition of reticular extrinsic contractions and increased the salivary flow resulting in frequent swallowing movements. Rumination caused by dopamine after naloxone pretreatment occurred at a high rate. Rumination caused by adrenaline in sheep is accompanied by an increased salivary flow, supplementary contractions of the reticulum and extra- contractions associated to the regurgitation of digestive contents and masticatory movements. The latter effects are enhanced by the previous administration of naloxone.

In contrast, the additional contraction of the reticulum, which occurs at the time of regurgitation, before the normal biphasic contraction can be facilitated by the central administration of opiate antagonists. In sheep, the intravenous (i.v.) and intracerebroventricular (ICV) administration of naloxone (0.1 mg/kg and 10 μg/kg, respectively), enhances the occurrence of rumination caused by adrenaline (Fig. 13). Rumination induced by systemic catecholamines injection occurs in sheep under naloxone, even when the coarseness of the diet is low and even during eating. In contrast, morphine and ICV Leu-enkephalin, but not ethylketazocine, delay the onset of rumination, suggesting the involvement of an inhibitory-opioid system pathway in the occurrence of rumination (79). The fact that kappa opioid agonists do not mimick mu opioid agonists, lend support for a role of multiple opioid receptors in the control of rumination.

V FREE GAS BLOAT

Free-gas bloat is commonly associated with stasis of the ovine ruminant stomach (81). Comparison of the effects of rumen digestion on the rate of eructation in sheep and cattle showed major species differences; e.g. an increased ruminal pressure enhances the secondary contractions in sheep (82,83) but not in cattle (84). On the other hand, eructation is closely linked to the presence of secondary contractions in cattle as evidenced by the use of xylazine (Fig. 14). This phenomenon is paralleled by a relatively more important peripheral action of drugs in cattle than in sheep. The consequence of such differences is that the relief of gas accumulation will be more easily obtained by central acting drugs in sheep than in cattle (Table I). In both species, relief of free-gas bloat by passing a nasogastric tube through the lower oesophageal sphincter (LES), incriminates this structure as a factor involved in the elimination of ruminal gas (85). The effects of exogenous neurotransmitters suggest the presence of adrenergic, cholinergic, serotonergic and possibly substance P receptors at the LES (86). The specific role of the LES tone is assessed by the absence of any improvement in bloating when the frequency and amplitude of reticulo-rumen contractions are stimulated by cholinergic agents like carbachol, bethanechol or pilocarpine in cattle. Conversely, during hypomotility induced by hypocalcaemia in sheep, the volume of gas expelled can be increased by treatment with a serotonin 2 antagonist, without major changes in the magnitude of contractions (87).

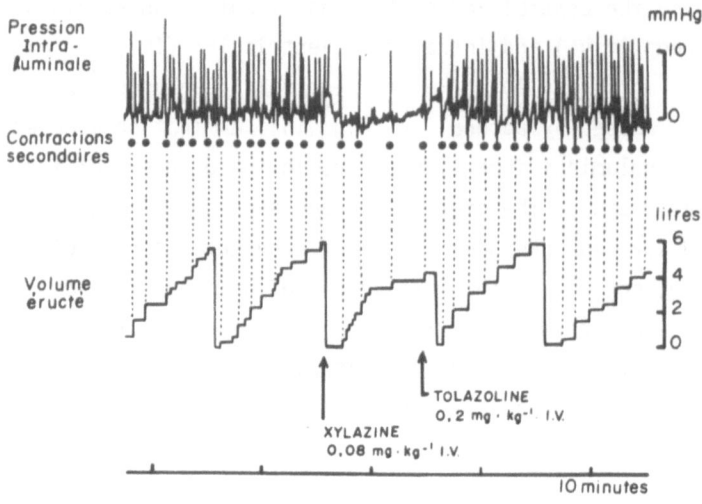

FIGURE 14. Relationship between the eructated volume of gas (in litres per 10 min) and the secondary contractions of the rumen which persist at a lower rate after injection of xylazine in a 3-year old heifer. Note the antagonism by tolazoline which was not found with 4-aminopyridine (80).

TABLE I. Central versus peripheral mechanisms of eructation in sheep versus cattle.

A Belching is restricted to the secondary contractions (the lower their frequency, the lower the volume eructated) in cattle. In sheep, belching also occurs during primary cycles of contractions, hence a higher volume during rumination.

B The enhancement by increased intraruminal pressure concerns both primary and secondary cycles without changes in the ratio. In sheep, ruminal distension evokes an increase in its own frequency with a ratio of 1:2 towards 1:3.

C Peripheral inhibition is a major factor of bloating (suppression of primary cycles of contractions by opiates without causing bloating) and methylnaloxone is as efficient as naloxone in the alleviation of bloat.
In sheep, central inhibition is also involved, hence bloating after treatment with opiates (including s.c. loperamide) or xylazine which blocked primary cycles. Accordingly, naloxone > methylnaloxone in alleviation of bloat.

V.1. Role of smooth muscle tone

Contraction of smooth muscles can be initiated by changes in membrane permeability after binding of agonists to their receptors, or after exposure to high K^+ concentrations (88). In other cases, receptor agonists induce contraction without changing membrane potential. This happens especially in smooth muscles that do not generate action potentials, or in depolarized smooth muscles (89). In both cases electrical or chemical cell membrane signals activate contractile elements by releasing membrane-bound Ca^{2+} or by increasing Ca^{2+} influx, or both.

In ruminal mucosa-free strips of cattle and calves, serotonin increased the muscle tone. This was inhibited by sodium nitroprusside but also by serotonin 2 antagonists as ritanserin. Both substances inhibited the spontaneous contractions. The effect of ritanserin was long lasting (90). This results from the high affinity receptor binding capacities of ritanserin on serotonin 2 receptors.

In sheep, the basal smooth muscle tone of the rumen the posterior dorsal rumen and the ventral sac are selectively increased in response to rumen distension. The increase in muscle tone during bloating, as can be assessed by calculating the pressure reached in the rumen and the time required to return to the basal level after a rapid insufflation of the rumen, seem to be an adverse effect. This part is mimicked following an i.v. injection of serotonin (5-HT) and can be reduced by 5-HT antagonists like methysergide (10 μg/kg and R 50970 (40-100 μg/kg) (Table II, Fig. 15). The pressure changes induced in sheep by 5-HT, comprise an increased muscle tone well-patterned on the ventral sac of the rumen. This was reduced by R 50970 (a $5-HT_2$ antagonist) which facilitates movement of large volume of gas towards the LES area, even for contractions of low magnitude. In cattle too bloating may persist, despite an increase in intraruminal pressure, if the whole reticulo-rumen capacity is reduced by an increased muscle tone. Beyond a threshold level of pressure, e.g. after carbachol, the contractions cease and the only way to facilitate the eructation is the increase in the reticulo-rumen capacity by a local decrease in tone. Such a reduction in smooth muscle tone seems to be involved in the relief of postprandial bloating by $5-HT_2$ antagonists (87).

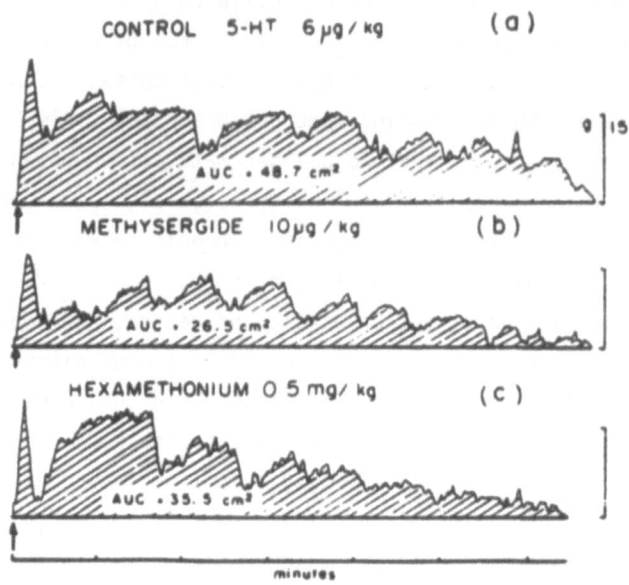

CONTROL 5-HT 6 μg/kg (a)

METHYSERGIDE 10μg/kg (b)

HEXAMETHONIUM 0 5 mg/kg (c)

FIGURE 15. Selective inhibition by a 5-HT antagonist of the increased muscle tone of the rumen ventral sac following the injection of 5-HT (arrow). (a) The area under the curve (AUC) resulting from the shift of the recording pen above the baseline for the rumen was used to evaluate the effects. (b) 15 min after the administration of methysergide (10 μg/kg), the ruminal response to 5-HT was nearly halved. (c) 15 min after hexamethonium bromide (0.5 mg/kg), the response to 5-HT persisted.

TABLE II. Increased muscle tone of the rumen expressed as the area under the curve (AUC in cm^2) induced by the intravenous injection of serotonin 15, 75 and 135 min after the administration of 5-HT antagonists (91).

5-HT antagonists	15 min	75 min	135 min
Methysergide (10 μg/kg)	29.4 & 26.5*	27.7 & 21.4	41.2 & 43.4
(20 μg/kg)	17.4 & 4.1	21.4 & 7.0	36.4 & 40.6
R 50970 (50 μg/kg)	8.4 & 12.0	8.2 & 6.1	39.4 & 41.4
(100 μg/kg)	9.3 & 9.7	9.9 & 5.0	29.3 & 40.9

*The control AUC was 46.3 ± 9.7 (means ± SD for n = 14 in the same sheep). The values were obtained in the same sheep at weekly intervals and correspond to two trials.

V.2. Role of the lower oesophageal sphincter (LES) tone.

Oesophageal balloon pressures are accepted as a means of indirectly estimating pleural pressure (92,93). This means that pleural pressure could be one of the mechanisms involved in the regulation of the LES pressure: increase in pleural pressure results in an increase of LES pressure. This reflex mechanism could be involved in the chronic tympania problems, frequently observed in animals with pneumonia. In standing sheep, both end-expiratory pressures and inspiratory pressure swings were similar when pleural pressures were equal. When pleural pressures were made unequal, as during lateral recumbency or unilateral pneumothorax, the oesophageal pressure reflected predominantly the right pleural pressure (94).

In man and dogs, pressure changes inside the antrum also resulted in similar pressure changes in the LES (95).

V.3. Alleviation of free gas bloat

Relaxation of the LES by $5-HT_2$ antagonists is observed during ruminal distension in both sheep and cattle. The insufflation of air or nitrogen in the rumen of cattle slightly increases the cyclical activity of the reticulo-rumen, hence the increased volume of eructated gas (6.2 1/10 min vs. 3.7 1/10 min). After pretreatment with R 55667 (ritanserin 0.1 mg/kg s.c.), the volume of eructated gas is further increased (9.2 1/10 min vs. 4.1 1/10 min) from 10 to 30 min after its injection (Table III).

Table III. Effects of R 55667, a $5-HT_2$ antagonist, on the volume of eructated gas and frequency of secondary ruminal contractions following ruminal distension in cattle during 30 min (87).

Time (min)	10-0 min	0 to 10 min	10 to 20 min	20 to 30 min
Eructations after insufflation during 30 min*				
Volume (liter/10 min)	3.70 ± 0.27	6.28 ± 0.21	6.50 ± 0.43	6.80 ± 0.52
Secondary contractions (per 10 min)	4.1 ± 0.1	6.3 ± 0.4	7.4 ± 0.1	6.7 ± 0.3
Eructation after R 55667 (0.1 mg/kg) pretreatment				
Volume	4.10 ± 0.4	7.61 ± 0.3**	8.41 ± 0.5**	9.12 ± 0.6**
Secondary contractions	4.3 ± 0.1	6.2 ± 0.9	7.1 ± 0.8	8.1 ± 0.6

* Mean ± SD for four experiments
** Significantly different from control without treatment ($p < 0.05$)

As shown in Fig. 16, it is rather the volume of each bolus of gas expelled which is increased than the rate of eructation (87). Similar effects were observed after R 50970, another 5-HT$_2$ antagonist (91) but not with methysergide or cyproheptadine, suggesting that 5-HT$_2$ receptors play a major direct or indirect role in the control of LES pressure. Another possibility of action may be the blockade by ritanserin of substance P, the companion peptide of 5-HT. Substance P has recently been shown to play a role in the tonic motor control of the pylorus in a similar way as 5-HT (96).

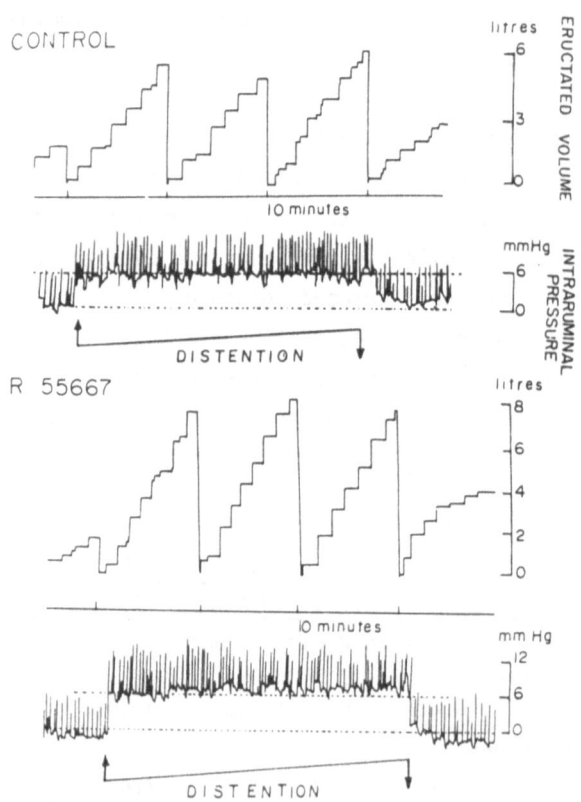

FIGURE 16. The effect of ruminal distension on the eructated volume (1) and on the intraruminal pressure changes in cattle. The resting intra-ruminal pressure was maintained at 6 mm Hg for 30 min.
Figures represent the effect of saline and R 55667 pretreatment.

Also important in the alleviation of gas accumulation is the coordi-

nation of the rumen- and reticular contractions and the muscle tone. The
fetal bovine rumen appears to be highly sensitive to 5-HT since the
effective dose of the drug was relatively small: on strips of ruminal wall
from bovine fetuses, incubated in an organ bath with 5-HT only (1.10-2.56
microg/l), it was shown that the sensitivity to 5-HT increased with age
until 4 months, when the magnitude stabilized. The effect of 5-HT was
antagonized by methyserigde, suggesting that 5-HT acts directly on the
ruminal smooth muscle fiber, because its contractile effect persists after
the addition of hexamathonium and atropine (97). These contractile effects
are very similar to those described in the adult ruminant. : the
effect increased with the increment of the local concentration of 5-HT
(98). In vitro, on the longitudinal smooth muscle from the reticulum and
the rumen of the bovine forestomach, 5-HT potentiated the contraction
evoked by stimulation of the intramural cholinergic nerves, but did not
show any effect on the relaxation produced by the non-adrenergic inhibitory nerve excitation. 5-HT alone caused a contraction and a relaxation of
the ruminal strips while it produced only an excitatory effect on the
reticular strips. These effects were blocked by methysergide, LSD-25 and
phenoxybenzamine. 5-HT seems to have direct effect on the smooth muscles,
but also to induce presynaptic activation of the local cholinergic
nerves (99).

In sheep, serotonin injected i.v. inhibits the rumino-reticular motility
in vivo (100).

V.4. Effects of ritanserin in milk-fed calves

The time intervals between primary and secondary ruminal contractions
were monitored in implanted (electrodes and strain gauges) milk-fed calves
with chronic tympania problems. When tympania developed after the intake
of milk, an increase in this time interval was observed and the number of
antegrade or primary contractions decreased (Fig. 17). If bloat disappeared spontaneously, the time interval and also the number of antegrade
contractions were normalized. If bloating still persisted, either a
stomach tube was used or the animals were injected with R 55667 (0.2 mg/kg
i.v.). Insertion of the stomach tube resulted in immediate debloating,
while after injection of ritanserin, debloating was observed after a lag
period of 10-15 min. Insertion of a stomach tube or injection of R 55667
resulted in a normalization of the time interval between antegrade and

298

retrograde contractions, and also of the number of primary contractions in the same time period (Fig. 17). This suggests that ritanserin is directly acting on the rumen muscle. Indeed, an immediate decrease of muscle tone was observed.

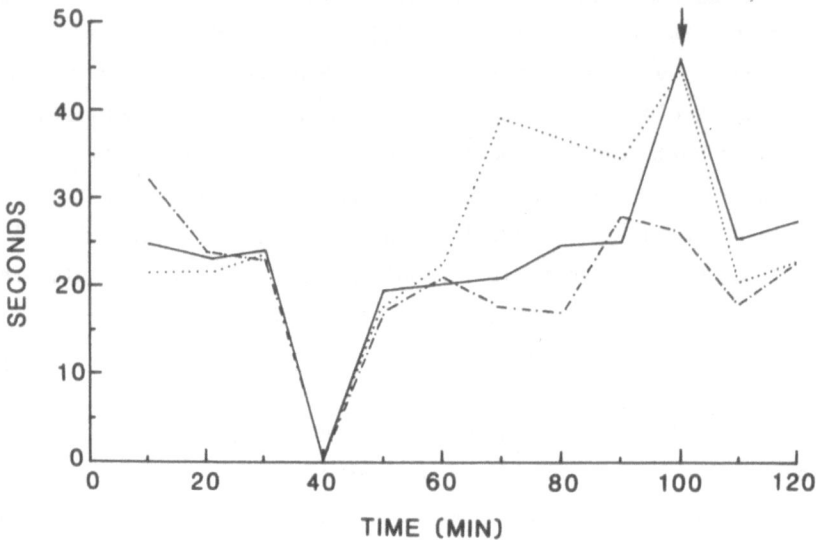

FIGURE 17. Time period (sec) between primary and secondary contractions before and after intake of milk(min 40-43): dotted line (normal); full line and dashed line: bloating after intake of milk. Arrow: treatment with ritanserin (0.2 mg/kg i.v.; full line); insertion of stomach tube (dashed line).

In calves (implanted with electrodes and strain gauges) with a history of bloating after intake of milk, ritanserin added to the milk (0.2 mg/kg), resulted in an increase in the number of reticular-, antegrade- and retrograde contractions (Fig. 18). The number of boli also increased. In these animals, bloating never developed after adding ritanserin in the milk.

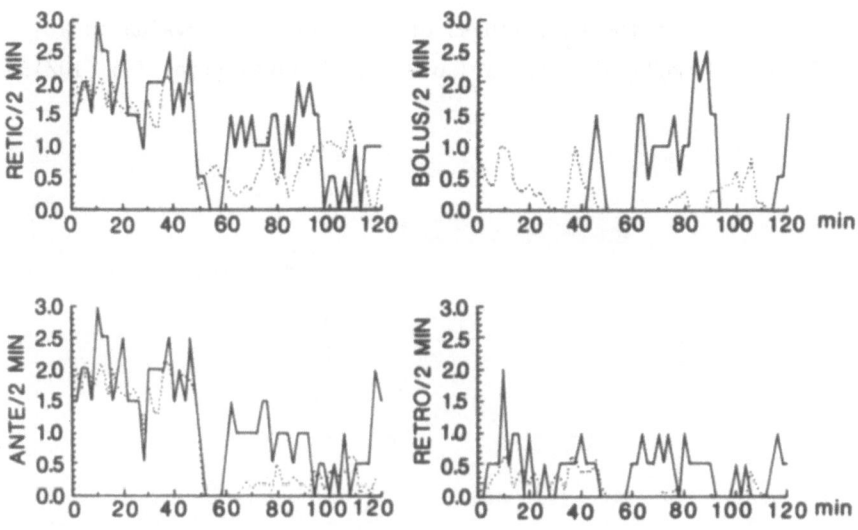

FIGURE 18. Number of reticular contractions (n/2 min), primary- and
secondary ruminal contractions (n/2 min) and boli (n/2 min) in calves
before and after intake of milk with (line) or without (dotted line)
ritanserin added in the milk (0.2 mg/kg).

V.5. Clinical observations

Milk fed calves (± 60 kg body weight; blue-white) as well as 5-12
month-old bulls (red-white) were used in these studies. The milk-fed calves
belonged to a fattening farm, in which bloating was a frequent problem.
An increased frequency of bloating occurred with increasing age (increased
milk-ration). Classical treatment before the experiment consisted of
restriction of the milk volume and relief of free gas bloat with a stomach
tube. At the start of the experiment, only those calves with daily bloating
for at least one weak were included in the study. Treatment consisted of
0.2 mg/kg added to the milk (b.i.d.) for at least 6 consecutive days.
Treatment was very successful: in all treated animals (n = 15) bloating
disappeared.

In a preclinical study, the preventive and curative treatment of gas
bloating with ritanserin was evaluated in cattle (n = 46) with both acute

and chronic gas bloating. At the dose levels used (0.05-0.2 mg/kg i.v. or
i.m.), efficacy of treatment was as follows: treatment of acute bloating:
89.5%; treatment of chronic bloating: 72.5%; prevention of acute bloating
(100%) and of chronic bloating (93%) (101).

In a clinical study the usefullness of ritanserin was evaluated at
dose levels of 0.1 mg/kg i.v. (1 day) or s.c. (5 days) (fig. 19) (102).

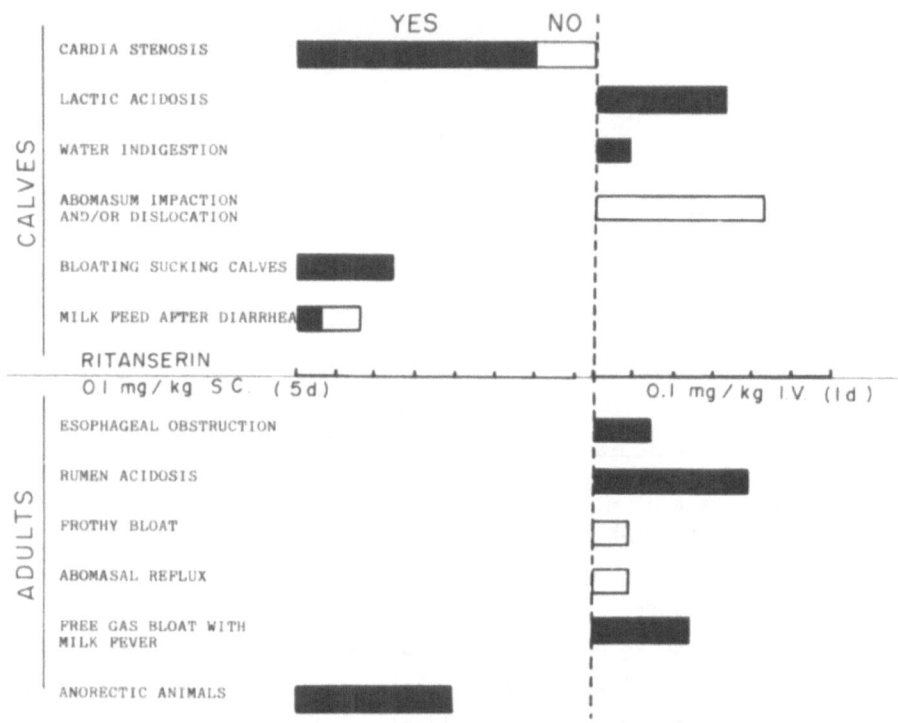

FIGURE 19. Therapeutic use of ritanserin in cattle (102).

VI RUMEN MOTILITY AND RUMEN METABOLISM

Substances used to control rumen metabolism include antibiotics and
especially the ionophores. Antibiotics, used at low dose levels are of
limited use because most of the bacteria develop resistance. Ionophores
(e.g. monensin) are useful substances to improve economy of rumen
metabolism.

In a study on rumen motility in cattle fed hay and concentrates, a significant increase of the number of antegrade and retrograde contractions was observed with R 51619, a substance stimulating the release of acetylcholine (103). In another study, the motor-stimulating properties were evaluated on rumen metabolism. A significant increase of the ruminal contents of propionic- and butyric acid was observed (104,105). Acetic acid content was also increased (not significant). These studies show that forestomach motility is of importance in the control of rumen metabolism and offers opportunities for the future to improve rumen economy.

TABLE IV. Rumen volatile fatty acid content (mM/l) in cattle (mean of 3) fed hay and concentrates (C: control; R: R 51619 0.2 mg/kg or).

	Acetic acid		Propionic acid		Butyric acid	
C	22.93	3.90	6.07	1.04	1.8	0.39
R	26.93	5.41	7.93	1.54*	2.66	0.70*

*: $p \leq 0.05$

VII CONCLUSIONS

To summarize, these data reveal some major new findings in the pharmacological control of the pre-ruminant and ruminant stomach: (i) the tonic-type activity is present in most smooth muscles of the forestomach and may play a major role in controlling phasic activity and transit of digesta; (ii) it is possible to manipulate the oesophageal groove reflex by means of drugs known as gastrokinetic agents like domperidone or cisapride; (iii) studies with a $5-HT_2$ antagonist (ritanserin) were relevant for long-lasting improvement of intrinsic and extrinsic ruminal dysfunction involved in bloating of cattle; (iiii) studies with cisapride were relevant for the involvement of rumen motility in rumen metabolism.

REFERENCES

1. Cooke, R.G. and Nicholson, T.: J. Vet. Pharmacol. Therap. 4, 311-313 (1981)
2. Newhook, J.C. and Titchen, D.A.: J. Physiol. (London) 237, 243-258

(1979)

3. Reid, A.M. and Titchen, D.A.: Can. J. Anim. Sci. 64, 91-92 (1984)
4. Clarke, R.T.J., Ulyatt, M.J. and John, A.: Appl. Environ. Microbiol. 43, 1201-1204 (1982)
5. McManus, W.R.: Austr. J. Agric. Res. 13, 907-923 (1962)
6. Kay, R.N.B.: World Rev. Nutr. Diet 6, 292-325 (1966)
7. Sudweeks, E.M.: J. Anim. Sci. 44, 694-701 (1977)
8. Von Engelhardt, W. and Hales, J.R.S.: Am. J. Physiol. 232, E53-E56 (1977)
9. Little, W., Sansom, B.F., Manston, R. and Allen, W.M.: Res. Vet. Sci. 37, 283-289 (1984)
10. Ruckebusch, Y. and Bardon, T.: C.R. Acad. Sci. 296, 921-926 (1983)
11. Ruckebusch, Y.: In: Physiologie, Pharmacologie, Thérapeutique Animales. Y. Ruckebusch (ed), Maloine, Paris, 418 (1981)
12. Casteels, R. and Droogmans, G.: Fed. Proceedings 41, 2879-2882 (1982)
13. Somlyo, A.V. and Somlyo, A.P.: J. Pharmacol. Exp. Ther. 159, 129-145 (1968)
14. Bolton, T.B.: Physiol. Rev. 59, 606-718 (1979)
15. Edman, A.P. and Schild, H.O.: J. Physiol. (London) 161, 424-441 (1962)
16. Van Breemen, C., Aaronson, P. and Loutzenhiser, R.: Pharmacol. Rev. 30, 167-208 (1979)
17. Wuytack, F., De Schutter, G. and Casteels, R.: Biochem. J. 198, 265-271 (1981)
18. Wuytack, F., De Schutter, G. and Casteels, R.: FEBS Lett. 129, 297-300 (1981)
19. Wuytack, F., De Schutter, G., Verbist, J. and Casteels, R.: FEBS Lett. 154, 191-195 (1983)
20. Brockeroff, H. and Ballou, C.E.: J. Biol. Chem. 236, 1907-1911 (1961)
21. Dawson, R.M.C.: Biochem. 97, 134-138 (1965)
22. Kirk, C.J., Bone, E.A., Palmer, S. and Michell, R.H.: J. Receptor Research 4, 1-6, 489-504 (1984)
23. Streb, H., Irvine, R.F., Berridge, M.J. and Schulz, I.: Nature (Lond.) 306, 67-69 (1983)
24. Takai, Y., Kishimoto, A. and Kawahara, Y.: Adv. Cyclic Nucleotide Res. 14, 301-313 (1981)
25. Nishizuka, Y.: In: International Congress Series. Shizume, K., Imura, H. and Shimizu, N. (eds). Endocrinology 598, 15-24 (1983)

26. Weiss, G.B.: In: New perspectives on calcium antagonists. Weiss, G.B. (ed), Williams and Wilkins, Baltimore, 83-94 (1981)

27. Weiss, G.B.: In: Advances in General and Cellular Pharmacology. II. Narahashi, T. and Bianchi, C.P. (eds), Plenum, New York, 71-154 (1977)

28. Triggle, D.J.: In: New perspectives on calcium antagonists. Weiss, G.B. (ed), Williams and Wilkins, Baltimore, 1-18 (1981)

29. Karaki, H. and Weiss, G.B.: Gastroenterol. 87, 960-970 (1984)

30. Ito, Y., Kuriyama, H. and Sakamato, I.K.: J. Physiol. (London) 211, 445-460 (1970)

31. Osa, T. and Kuriyama, H.: Jap. J. Physiol. 20, 626-639 (1970)

32. Milanov, M.P., Stoyanov, N. and Boev, K.K.: Gen. Pharmacol. 15, 99-105 (1984)

33. Cohen, P.: Nature, Elsevier-Biomedical, Amsterdam 1, 255-268 (1980)

34. Burns, D.L., Hewlett, E.L., Moss, J. and Vaughan, M.: J. Biol. Chem. 257,14035-14040 (1983)

35. Piascik, M.T., Babich, M. and Rush, M.E.: J. Biol. Chem. 258, 10913-10918 (1983)

36. Seamin, K.B. and Daly, J.W.: J. Biol. Chem. 256, 9799-9801 (1981)

37. Schultz, K.D., Schultz, K. and Schultz, G.: Nature 265, 750-751 (1977)

38. Ooms, L.A.A. and Degryse, A.-D.: Unpublished observations.

39. Levitt, D.G., Hakim, A.A. and Lifson, N.: Am. J. Physiol. 217, 777-783 (1969)

40. Hill, F.W.G., Kidder, D.E. and Frew, J.: Vet. Rec. 87, 250-255 (1970)

41. Toullec, R., Thivend, P. and Mathieu, C.M.: Ann. Biol. Anim. Biochem. Biophys. 11, 435-453 (1971)

42. Ruckebusch, Y., Dardillat, C. and Guilloteau, P.: Ann. Rech. Vét. 14, 360-374 (1983)

43. Juhasz, B., Szegedi, B. and Keresztes, M.: Acta Vet. Acad. Sci. Hum. 26, 281-285 (1976)

44. Nicholson, T.: Can. J. Anim. Sci. 64, 187-188 (1984)

45. Pearson, E.G. and Aldwin, B.H.: The Cornell Vet. 71, 288-296 (1981)

46. Orskov, E.R., Benzie, D. and Kay, R.N.B.: Br. J. Nutr. 24, 785-795 (1970)

47. Woodford, S.T., Murphy, M.R., Davis, C.L. and Holmes, K.R.: J. Dairy Sci. 67, 2471-2474 (1984)

48. Sasaki, Y.: Jap. J. Zootech. Sci. 39, 333-340 (1968)

49. Titchen, D.A. and Newhook, J.N.: In: Digestion and Metabolism in the

Ruminant. McDonald, I.W. and Warner, A.C.I. (eds), Armidale, The Univ. New Engl. Publ., 15-29 (1975)

50. Schalk, A.F. and Amadon, R.S.: N. Dak. Agric. Exp. Sta. Bull. 216, 1-64 (1928)

51. Kay, R.N.B. and Ruckebusch, Y.: Br. J. Nutr. 26, 301-309 (1971)

52. Ruckebusch, Y.: J. Vet. Pharmacol. Therap. 6, 245-272 (1983)

53. Ormsbee, H.S.: In: Dopamine Receptor Agonists. Poste, G. and Crooke, S.T. (eds), Plenum Publ. Corp., New York, 333-353 (1984)

54. Wolf, K.U.: Drug Res. 35, 136-137 (1985)

55. Van Nueten, J.M., Vandaele, P.G.H., Reyntjens, A.J., Janssen, P.A.J. and Schuurkes, J.A.J.: In: Proc. 9th Int. Symp. GI Motility, Aix-en-Provence, 513-520 (1983)

56. Blair, E.L., Venables, C.W. and Wilkinson, J.: J. Physiol. (London) 238, 72-73 (1973)

57. Mylrea, P.J.: Res. Vet. Sci. 7, 333-341 (1966)

58. Mathieu, C.M.: Ann. Biol. Anim. Biochem. Biophys. 8, 581-583 (1968)

59. Bell, F.R. and Watson, D.J.: J. Physiol. (London) 259, 445-456 (1976)

60. Bell, F.R., Green, A.B., Wass, J.A.H. and Webber, D.E.: J. Physiol. (London) 321, 603-610 (1981)

61. Winship, D.H., Zboralske, J.F., Weber, W.N. and Soergel, K.H.: Am. J. Physiol. 207, 1189-1194 (1964)

62. Deswysen,A. and Ehrlein, H.J.: Ann. Rech. Vét. 10, 208-221 (1979)

63. Ruckebusch, Y. and Candau, M.: C.R. Soc. Biol. 162, 897-902 (1968)

64. Alborch, E., Torregorosa, G., Terrasa, J.C. and Estrada, C.: Brain Res. 321, 103-110 (1984)

65. Deetz, L.E. and Wangness, P.S.: J. Nutr. 110, 1976-1982 (1980)

66. Bowen, J.M.: Am. J. Vet. Res. 24, 73-76 (1963)

67. Nicholson, T.: Ann. Rech. Vét 10, 231-233 (1979)

68. Gorewit, R.C.: Am. J. Vet. Res. 41, 1769-1772 (1980)

69. Roming, L.G.P.: Dtsch. Tierärztl. Wschr. 91, 154-157 (1984)

70. Guard, C.L. and Schwark, W.S.: The Cornell Vet. 74, 312-321 (1984)

71. Poncet, C., Dimova, E., Leveille, C. and Dardillat, C.: Ann. Biol. Anim. Biochem. Biophys. 17, 515-522 (1977)

72. Spencer, G.S.G., Garssen, G.T. and Hart, I.E.: Livest. Prod. Sci., 10, 25-37 and Ibidem 10, 469-477 (1983)

73. Lagneau, F. and Gallard, P.: Rech. Méd. Vét. 122, 310-313 (1946)

74. Bost, J., Boivin, R. and Ribot, J.: Bull. Soc. Sci. Méd. Comp. 71,

277-282 (1969)

75. Jean-Blain, C., Boivin, R. and Bost, J.: Ann. Nutr. Alim. 25, 121-138 (1971)
76. Leslie, R.A. and Osborne, N.N.: Brail. Bull. Res. 13, 357-362 (1984)
77. Bost, J., McCarthy, L.E., Colby, E.D. and Borison, H.L.: Physiol. & Behav. 3, 877-881 (1968)
78. Ruckebusch, Y. and Laplace, J.P.: Psychopharmacologia 12, 104-114 (1968)
79. Ruckebusch, Y. and Bardon, T.: Can. J. Anim. Sci. 64, 13-15 (1984)
80. Kitzman, J.V., Booth, N.H., Hatch, R.C. and Wallner, B.: Am. J. Vet. Res. 43, 2165-2168 (1982)
81. Weiss, K.E.: Onderstepoort J. Vet. Res. 26, 251-283 (1953)
82. Ruckebusch, Y. and Tomov, T.: J. Physiol. (London) 235, 447-458 (1973)
83. Kolling, K.: Zbl. Vet. Med. A 23, 97-105 (1976)
84. Dziuk, H.E., Sellers, A.F.: Am. J. Vet. Res. 16, 499-504 (1955)
85. Dougherty, R.W.: In: Handbook of Physiology, Section 6. Alimentary Canal. Code, C.F. (ed), American Physiological Society, Washington, D.C., 2695-2698 (1968)
86. Goyal, R.K. and Rattan, S.: Gastroenterology 74, 598-619 (1978)
87. Ruckebusch, Y., Ooms, L.A.A., Degryse, A.-D. and Allal,C.: Am. J. Vet. Res. 46, 434-437 (1985)
88. Bolton, T.B.: Physiol. Rev. 59, 606-718 (1979)
89. Somlyo, A.V. and Somlyo, A.P.: J. Pharmacol. Exp. Ther. 159, 129-145 (1968)
90. Ooms, L.A.A., Degryse, A.-D., Weyns, A. and Ruckebusch, Y.: Unpublished observations.
91. Ruckebusch, Y. and Ooms, L.A.A.: J. Vet. Pharmacol. Therap. 6, 127-132 (1983)
92. Gillespie, D.J., Lay, Y. and Hyat, R.E.: J. Appl. Physiol. 35, 709-713 (1973)
93. Wohl, M.E.B., Turner, J. and Mead, J.: J. Appl. Physiol. 24, 348-354 (1968)
94. Hurewitz, A.N., Sidhy, U., Bergofsky, E.H. and Chanana, A.D.: J. Appl. Physiol.: Respirat. Environ. Exercise Physiol. 56, 1162-1169 (1984)
95. Jennewein, H.M., Hummelt, H., Siewert, R., Weiser, F. and Waldeck, F.: Acta Hepato-Gastroent. 23, 449-454 (1976)
96. Lidberg, P.: Acta Physiol. Scand., Suppl. 538 (1985)

306

97. Arias, J.L., Zurich, L. and Bastias, J.: Pharmacol. Res. Comm. 12, 975-985 (1980)

98. Zurich, L., Brantes, J., Burgos, H. and Lencannelier, S.: Arch. Biol. Med. Exp. 2, 18-21 (1965)

99. Taneike, T.: J. Vet. Pharmacol. Therap. 2, 59-68 (1979)

100. Ruckebusch, Y., Fargeas, J. and Bueno, L.: Annales de Recherches Vétérinaires 3, 131-148 (1969)

101. Ooms, L.A.A., Degryse, A.-D. and Quirijnen, L.: Janssen Research Product Information. Unpublished Report (1985)

102. Bouisset, S. and Ruckebusch, Y.: In: The Ruminant Stomach, Vol. I. Ooms, L.A.A., Degryse, A.-D. and Marsboon, R. (eds), Janssen Research Foundation, 355-361 (1985)

103. Schuurkes, J.A.J., Van Nueten, J.M., Van Daele, P.G.H., Reyntjens, A.J. and Janssen, P.A.J.: J. Pharmacol. Exp. Ther. 234, 775-783 (1985)

104. Ooms, L.A.A., Degryse, A.-D. and Quirijnen, L.: Janssen Research Product Information. Unpublished Report (1986)

105. Ooms, L.A.A., Degryse, A.-D. and Van Roosbroeck, D.: Janssen Research Product Information. Unpublished Report (1986)

INDEX

Lactate 177, 229
  food intake 177
  production 238-239
lactic acidosis
  effects of antibiotics 217
laidlomycin 230, 239
Lama guanacoe 164
lamina propria
  VIP 79
lasalocid 216, 219, 230, 236
          239-240
lasiocarpine 204
Leucaena leucocephale 210, 214
Leu-enkephalin 291
leukotrines 275
leupeptin 230
levamisole 256-258
longitudinal smooth muscle
  abomasum 278-279
  omasum 278-279
  pylorus 278-279
  reticulo-rumen 117, 124-125,
                 277-279
loperamide 127, 292
lupinosis 208

Madoque kirki 160
malathion 208
markers
  digesta flow 146-148, 164-165
  reticular groove reflex 280,
                          282
mastication 13, 133, 161, 163
  digesta flow 140, 163
  food intake 140
  particle size reduction 133,
                          141
meal size and frequency
  see food intake
mechanoreceptors 15
  rapidly adapting 14-16
  slowly adapting 16-18
  VIP 72
meclofenamate 121, 259-261, 263,
              281
Meissner's plexus 116
  Sub P 86
  VIP 75
merthiolate 230
methane 203, 227
  analogues 230-231, 233-235
methanogenesis 228-245
  inhibition 229, 231, 233
  inhibitors 230-240, 242
methicillin 216

methoxyverapamil 92, 275
methylene blue
  reduction test 218
3-methylindole 213
methylnaloxone 39, 127, 292
methysergide 34, 39, 125, 293-294,
                 296-297
mepyramine 124
metoclopramide 27, 283-284
microbial adaptation
  feed additives 219, 300
  rumen function 219
microbial degradation 220
  see also biodegradation
microbial digestion
  see rumen
microbial N-flow 235-240
microbial N-yield
  effect of antibiotics 235-244
mimosine 206, 210, 214-215
miserotoxin 203, 214
monensin 150, 217, 219, 229, 231,
                 233, 235
  loss of appetite 188, 239
moose 161
morantel 268
morphine 94, 125, 127, 290-291
motilin 68
mousedeer 155, 156, 167
mule deer 159
musk-ox 160
mycotoxins
  rumen metabolism 208-209
myenteric plexus 3, 32, 45-46, 52-59,
                 116
  acetylcholinesterase 52-57
  noradrenaline 57-59
  Sub P 85
  VIP 75-76
myoelectric complex 21-22, 31, 34-35,

Naloxone 30, 127, 186, 189, 290-291,
                 292
naltrexone 127
narasin 219, 230, 239
neomycin 216, 267
neostigmine 2, 7, 72
Nesotragus moschatus 160
neuropeptides 39, 47, 128, 182-186,
                 289-291
nicotinic acid 229
nifedipine 92, 275
nipple feeding
  duodenal pH 27, 282